REMEDIES POTIONS & Razzmatazz

REMEDIES POTIONS & Razzmatazz

EDITED BY

DON ROBERTS

Nostalgia Press
P.O. Box 301031
Escondido, CA 92027

This book has been transcribed from the "What To Do and How To Do It" section of the *Peoples Cyclopedia of Universal Knowledge,* published in 1891 by Hunt and Eaton. Material has been organized and edited to facilitate reading. Much of the original spelling and punctuation has been maintained to emphasize the character of the period. All illustrations, notes and quotes have been selected by the editor. Illustrations done in pen and ink by Gary Roberts.

Library of Congress Catalog Card Number: 91-90424

ISBN Number: 0-9628676-0-8

First Printing July, 1991
Nostalgia Press
P.O. Box 301031
Escondido, CA 92027

Printed in the United States of America

PREFACE

I don't remember the month but the year was 1964. I lived on the ground floor of an apartment in West Los Angeles. The day was Saturday and one of my chores was to empty the waste baskets into the trash dumpster in the alley. I completed my duty and just as I was ready to go back to the apartment, I noticed the trash cans across the alley. They were chucked full, and pieces of trash were scattered all over the place. What particularly interested me though, was something which protruded from the top of one of the cans. This appeared to be a large book. Always fascinated with books, I wandered over and took a closer look. I reached in and pulled out the third volume of The People's Cyclopedia of Universal Knowledge. It was somewhat beat, but leather bound and intact.

So feeling somewhat akin to a street person searching for treasures in a trash pile, I began rummaging through the cans in pursuit of other volumes. After a while I managed to come up with the entire set, volumes one through four. I gathered them up, almost hoping that no had seen me as I hustled them into my apartment.

I sat down at the dining-room table with Volume I, wiped off the cover, and began reading. After turning the first few blank pages I came across a two-page color spread of "The World." On the next page, protected by a sheet of vellum, was a reproduction of an etching depicting an outdoor scene of a woman and children. They were busily engaged in reading and learning with such trappings as a divider, an anvil, a paint pallet, a steamship, an oil lamp a world globe and a large mechanical gear. I had to examine the Volume II before learning that the set was published in 1891 by Hunt and Eaton. This encyclopedia set is called a condensed version as opposed to the larger Britannica encyclopedias which were also being published during this time.

As one can imagine, the set is fascinating from cover to cover (as I believe most encyclopedias are), but when I opened Volume IV at about half-way through, I came across a section called *What to Do and How to Do It,* and became mesmerized with what I read. It is printed in 6-point type, double column, with paragraph breaks only for the main subject headings. In some instances I fought through entire pages with no paragraph breaks; squinting my eyes and often losing my place—but I could not stop reading. Here I found scores of 100-year-old remedies and adages. How to cure baldness, how to cure drunkenness, how to dress for the kitchen, how a young lady behaves herself in a hotel lobby. I vowed at this time that eventually I would republish this section.

Guests would come over and we would sit around the table while one individual would scan through the pages, reading that which seemed interesting to him. We would all end up laughing—sometimes so hard our sides would ache. About five years later I copied some of the pages and sent them to various publishers, hoping that *What to Do and How to Do It* could be published again. All of the responses I received were nil. Finally, in 1987 I acquired a personal computer, and decided to publish it myself. I painstakingly prodded through the pages, searching for those items which I believed would interest the general reader. However just as the first disk was about filled, something happened to the word processing program, and I lost everything I had entered—hundreds of hours down the drain.

Since I wasn't about to let one of man's electronic contrivances win out, I started again. This time, however, as I began reading, a sense of confusion came over me; it was becoming difficult to distinguish which of the items might be interesting to a reader. Slowly I began to get the point, and I reasoned, "Who was I to judge the merit of this information?" So with the exception of those sections which were boringly repetitive and obvious typographical errors, I began to enter the entire text into the computer. I made only minor spelling and punctuation changes to make the sentences more readable. I then broke up the sections into paragraphs and used bullets for additional highlighting. It was also very evident that so many out-of-use terms were in the text that much of the original meaning might become lost to the average reader. So I purchased an old dictionary set (the 1884, 5357 page edition of The Encyclopædic Dictionary) and added footnotes wherever I felt the need.

As I continued I began to notice how involved I was becoming with the work. Before long, a period almost unknown to me, the Victorian era in the United States, was becoming vividly real. The life-style in the home, on the farm, how meals were taken and how time was spent for pleasure and for work, how to live a healthful life, and most fascinating, how to properly behave. Then to give the book more of an air of antiquity, I commissioned my son Gary to do pen-and-ink sketches depicting some of the material in the text.

I have found that there are two ways to enjoy this literature. The first is to search the pages, stopping occasionally when something catches your eye, and the second is to curl up with this book, and—starting from the beginning,—page by page, gradually digest the essence of this now-strange near past. I hope you have a chance to do both.

Don Roberts

LIST OF ILLUSTRATIONS

By *Gary Roberts*

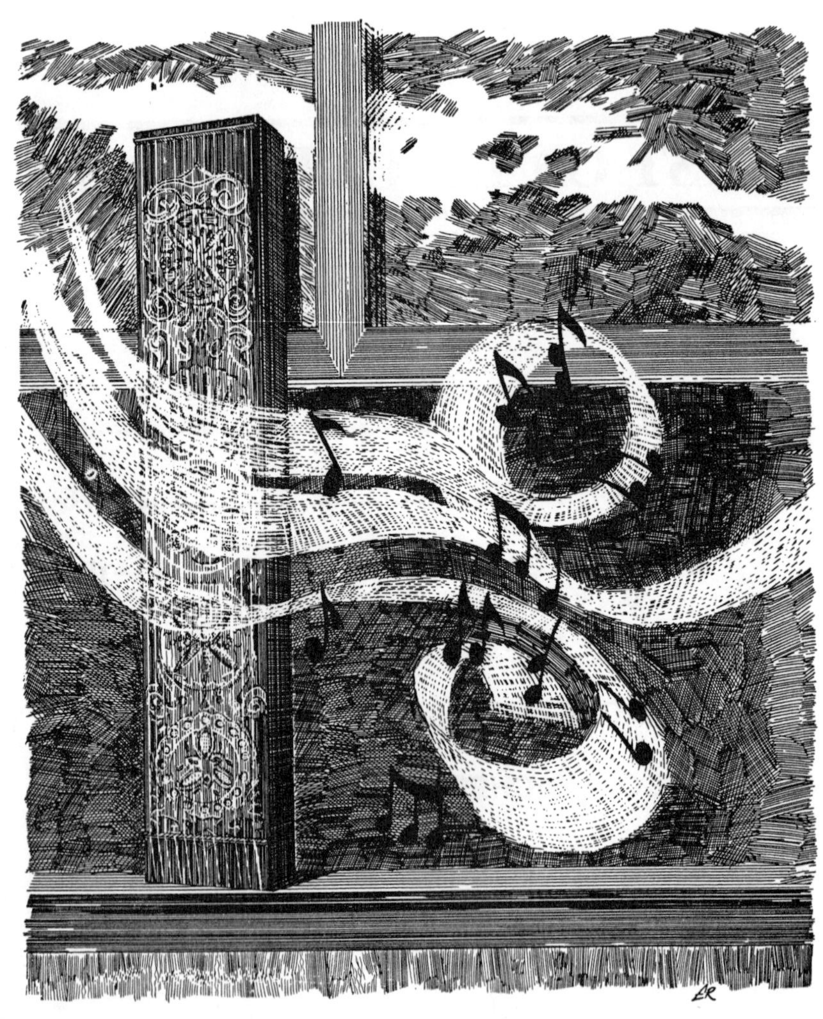

• *Æolian Harp* •

TABLE OF CONTENTS

A

B

C

D

E

F

G

H

I

J-K

L

M

N

O

P

Q

R

S

T

U-V

W-Z

REMEDIES, POTIONS & RAZZMATAZZ

edited by

Don Roberts

A

ABSCESS:

In some particulars an abscess resembles a large boil. There is an inflammatory condition, with heat, pain, and swelling. The result of this inflammation is the discharge of degenerated matter or pus. They may be opened as soon as pulsation is detected, the same as boils, or the operation may be delayed until by using hot water compresses, flax-seed poultice(1), bread and hot milk poultice, they come to a point or head. The matter or pus should be completely discharged by gentle pressure, and the cavity freely washed out by injecting a mixture of 1 part carbolic acid and 20 of warm water, and pressure exerted by a bandage, when healing will rapidly take place.

ACCIDENTS, OR FIRST AID TO THE INJURED:

Always send off for the surgeon immediately an accident occurs, but treat as directed until he arrives.

Burns: If the skin is much injured, spread some linen pretty thickly with ointment, and lay over the part, and give the patient some brandy and water if much exhausted; then send for a medical man. If not much injured and very painful, use ointment or apply carded cotton dipped in lime-water and linseed oil.

Scalds: Treat the same as burns, or cover with scraped raw potato, but chalk ointment is the best. In the absence of all these, cover the parts with molasses, and dust on plenty of flour.

(1) See Poultices and Their Application.

Body in Flames: Lay the person down on the floor of the room, and throw the tablecloth, rag, or other large cloth over him, and roll him on the floor.

Dirt in the Eye: Place your forefinger upon the cheekbone, having the patient before you; then draw up the finger and you will probably be able to remove the dirt; but if this will not enable you to get at it, repeat this operation, while you have a knitting-needle or bodkin(1)placed over the eyelid; this will turn it inside out, and enable you to remove the sand, or eyelash, etc., with the corner of a fine silk handkerchief. As soon as the substance is removed, bathe the eye with cold water and exclude the light for a day.

Lime in the Eye: Syringe it well with warm vinegar and water. (1 ounce to 8 ounces of water); take a purgative(2) and exclude light.

Iron or Steel in the Eye: Drop a solution of sulphate of copper (from 1 to 3 grains of the salt to one ounce of water) into the eye, or keep the eye open with a wine-glassful of the solution. Take a purgative, bathe with cold water, and exclude light to keep down inflammation.

Dislocated Thumb: This is frequently produced by a fall. Make a clove hitch by passing two loops of cord over the thumb, placing a piece of rag under the cord to prevent it cutting the thumb; then pull the same line as the thumb.

Cuts and Wounds: Cut thin strips of sticking-plaster(3) and bring the parts together; or if large and deep cut two broad pieces so as to look like the teeth of a comb, and place one on each side of the wound, which must be cleaned previously. These pieces must be arranged so that they shall interlace one another; then, by laying hold of the pieces on the right-hand side with one hand and those on the other side with the other hand, and pulling them from one another, the edges of wound are brought together, and without any difficulty.

Ordinary Cuts: Ordinary cuts are dressed by thin strips applied by pressing down the plaster on one side of the wound and keeping it there and pulling in the opposite direction, then suddenly depressing hard when edges of wound are brought together.

Contusions: When very severe, lay a cloth over the part, and keep it always wet.

Hemorrhage: Hemorrhage, when caused by an artery being divided or torn, may be known by the blood jumping out of the wound, and being of a bright

(1) A large--eyed dull-pointed threading instrument for leading a cord through a hem.
(2) Having the power of purging; a cathartic or laxative.
(3) Adhesive tape.

scarlet color. If a vein is injured, the blood is darker and flows continuously. To stop the latter, apply pressure by means of a compress and bandage. To arrest arterial bleeding, get a piece of wood—part of a broom-handle will do—and tie a piece of tape to one end of it; then tie a piece of tape loosely over the arm, and pass the other end of the wood under it, twist the stick round and round until the tape compresses the arm sufficiently to arrest the bleeding, and then confine the other end by tying the string round the arm. If the bleeding is very obstinate, and it occurs in the arm, place a cork underneath the string, on the inside of the fleshy part, where the artery may be felt beating by any one; if in the leg, place a cork in the direction of a line drawn from the inner part of the knee a little to the outside of the groin.

It is an excellent thing to accustom yourself to find out the position of these arteries, or indeed any that are superficial, and to explain to every one in your house where they are and how to stop bleeding. If a stick cannot be got, take a handkerchief, make a cord bandage of it, and tie a knot in the middle; the knot acts as a compress, and should be placed over the artery, while the two ends are to be tied around the thumb. Observe always to place the ligature between the wound and the heart. Putting the finger into a bleeding wound and making pressure until a surgeon arrives will generally stop the violent bleeding.

Bleeding from the Nose: From whatever cause, may generally be stopped by putting a plug of lint into the nostrils; if this does not do, apply a cold bandage to the forehead, raise the head, and place both arms over the head, so that it will rest on both hands; dip the lint plug, slightly moistened, into some powdered gum arabic, and plug the nostrils again: or dip the plug into equal parts of powdered gum arabic and alum, and plug the nose.

Violent Shocks: Violent shocks will sometimes stun a person, and he will remain unconscious. Untie strings, collars, etc., loose any thing that is tight and interferes with the breathing; raise the head; see if there is bleeding from any part; apply smelling-salts to the nose and hot bottles to the feet.

Concussion: In concussion, the surface of the body is cold and pale and the pulse weak and small, the breathing slow and gentle, and the pupil of the eye generally contracted or small. You can get an answer by speaking loudly, so as to arouse the patient. Give a little brandy and water, keep the place quiet, apply warmth, and do not raise the head too high.

In Compression of the Brain: From any cause, such as apoplexy(1), or a piece of fractured bone pressing on the brain, there is loss of sensation. The pulse is slow and labored; the breathing slow, labored and snoring; the pupils enlarged. Raise the head, unloose strings or tight things, and send for a

(1) A stroke.

surgeon. If one cannot be got at once, apply mustard poultices to the feet and leeches to the temples.

Choking: When a person has a fish-bone in the throat, insert the forefinger, press upon the root of the tongue, so as to induce vomiting; if this does not do, let him swallow a large piece of potato or soft bread; and if these fail, give a mustard emetic.

Fainting, Hysterics, etc.: Loosen the garments, bathe the temples with water or eau de Cologne; fresh air; avoid bustle, and excessive sympathy.

Drowning: *Attend to the following essential rules:*

(1) Lose no time

(2) Handle the body gently

(3) Carry the body with the head gently raised, and never hold it up by the feet.

(4) *Send for medical assistance immediately, and in the meantime act as follows:*

- Strip the body, rub it dry; then rub it in hot blankets, and place it in a warm bed in warm room.
- Cleanse away the froth and mucus from the nose and mouth.
- Apply warm bricks, bottles, bags of sand, etc., to the armpits, between the thighs, and soles of the feet.
- Rub the surface of the body with hands enclosed in warm, dry worsted socks.
- If possible, put the body into a warm bath.
- To restore breathing, put the pipe of a common bellows into one nostril, carefully closing the other and the mouth, at the same time drawing downward and pushing gently backward the upper part of the windpipe, to allow a more free admission of air; blow the bellows gently, in order to inflate the lungs, till the breast be raised a little; then set the mouth and nostrils free, and press gently on the chest; repeat this until signs of life appear. When the patient revives apply smelling-salts to the nose, give warm wine or brandy and water. *Caution.*—Continue the remedies for 12 hours without being discouraged if no results appear.

Hanging: Loose the cord, or whatever suspended the person, and proceed as with drowning, taking the additional precaution to apply 8 or 10 leeches to the temples.

Apparent Death from Drunkenness: Raise the head, unloosen the clothes, maintain warmth of surface, and give a mustard emetic as soon as the person can swallow.

Apoplexy and Fits Generally: Raise the head, unloosen all tight clothes, string, etc.; apply cold bandages to the head, which should be shaved; apply leeches to the temples, and send for a surgeon.

Suffocation from Noxious Gases: Remove to the fresh air; dash cold vinegar and water on the face, neck, and breast; keep up the warmth of the body; if necessary, apply mustard poultices to the soles of the feet, and try artificial respiration, as in apparent drowning.

ACID STOMACH:

A little magnesia and water will sometimes correct the acidity of a child's stomach, and render unnecessary any stronger medicine. Powder a tea-spoonful of magnesia, and put it in a half glass of water; it will not dissolve, of course, but will mix with the water so that an infant can swallow it. Give a tea-spoonful of this three times a day until indications warrant you in discontinuing it.

ACNE:

This eruptive disease of the skin chiefly attacks the face and forehead, having its origin in the sebaceous follicles which secrete the oily matter that lubricates the surface of the skin. Youths of both sexes are very subject to it, and it sometimes continues later in life. The retained secretions inflame the skin, giving rise to small red pimples, in some of which matter forms. The end of a pimple, when blackened by dust and smoke, resembles the head of a worm. When there are many such pimples it is called spotted acne.

Treatment: Take sulfur, cream of tartar, of each 1 ounce; enough syrup or molasses to make a paste; take a desert-spoonful night and morning before eating, until the bowels are affected and an odor of sulfur is perceived from the skin. A tea-spoonful of Epsom salts every morning, or of Husband's magnesia, with like frequency, may have an equally favorable result. Bathe the face frequently with hot saleratus(1) water, 1 dram of saleratus to the pint of water, and often give it a thorough washing, using only refined soap with hot water. Cultivate as much as possible the general health, and take three times a day a desert-spoonful of the following tonic: Corrosive sublimate, 1 grain; iodine of potassium, 2 drams; water, 3 fluid ounces; mix.

(1) An impure bicarbonate of potash.

ACONITE LINIMENT:

Tincture of aconite root, tincture of arnica(1) flowers, laudanum(2) in equal parts; mix thoroughly. A very useful liniment.

ACONITE(3), POISONING BY:

This root has been sometimes swallowed for horseradish. The symptoms of poisoning by this means, or by an overdose, are tingling and numbness of the tongue, throat, and limbs, pain in the stomach, vomiting, purging, feeble pulse, labored breathing, and great prostration. Give an emetic of sulphate of zinc in water, or 3 or 4 spoonfuls of table-salt and water. Use an alcoholic stimulant, and in the meantime send for the family physician.

ADJECTIVES, GAME OF:

A sheet of paper and a pencil are given to the players, upon which each is requested to write five or six adjectives. In the meantime, one of the company undertakes to improvise a little story, or, which will do quite as well, is provided with some short narrative from a book. The papers are then collected and the story is read aloud, the reader of the same substituting for the original adjectives those supplied by the company on their papers, placing them without any regard to sense in the order in which they have been received. The result will be something of this kind:

"The sweet heron is a bird of hard shape, with a transparent head and an agitated bill set upon a hopeful neck. Its picturesque legs are put far back in its body, the feet and claws are false, and the tail very newfangled. It is a durable, distorted bird, unsophisticated in its movements, with a blind voice, and tender in its habits. In the mysterious days of falconry the places where the heron bred were counted almost shy, the bird was held to be serious game, and slight statutes were enacted for its preservation," and so on.

ÆOLIAN HARP, TO MAKE:

This instrument, when placed in a window in a draft of air, produces the most pleasing music. We here give directions whereby any one may construct one for himself:

Length, 32 in. by 6 in.; depth, 1 3/4 in. The strings are attached to the small hooks at the end, corresponding to the pegs. The strings must be about the thickness of the first string of the violin. These strings answer well, but if too expensive the small gut used by whip manufacturers may be used.

The bottom plank of the harp should be oak, 3/4 in. thick, length 3 ft.,

(1) Arnica Montana, or German Leopard's-bane; for treating paralysis, rheumatism, convulsions, etc.
(2) Tincture of opium.
(3) The blue monkshood, a very poisonous plant, especially the roots.

breadth 10 in. The bridges may be any sonorous wood, (but steel will give the best sound), 1/2 in. in height, cut angular to a blunt point. They must not be flattened down, but must be made to fit very flat to the bottom board, or it will jar and never play well. This is the great defect in all harps made by amateurs.

The ends of the harps should be oak, 1 in. thick, and must be fixed very firmly to the bottom board, but not with metal screws or glue; and in these the pins are fixed for tightening the strings. Use fiddle-pins, half at each end. The top should be 1/2 in. thick, and sycamore wood is the best, and may be polished; it should be very slightly fastened on, for it has to be removed every time to tune.

Common catgut does nearly as well as German. Get as thick a string as you can for one side, and a thin one for the other; then graduate them from the thick to the thin, so as not to have two alike. They are in general tuned to treble C, but it is preferable to tune to low C, and then each string an octave higher. This is easily altered, if desirable. The instruments must be very strong in all respects, for the strings exert almost incredible strength.

The position for placing the harp at the window to be with the upper surface inclined toward the draft of air.

AFTERNOON AT-HOMES:

Afternoon at-homes have come to the rescue of both the great and the little ones of the earth. All feel the relief to their purses that this modest and inexpensive form of entertainment offers. It is an act of discourtesy not to answer an invitation, whether it is to be accepted or declined, for if invitations remain unanswered the usual conclusion is that absence from home is the reason for this. To render an at-home a success, the right people should be invited to meet each other, those who have something in common, for instance, and are well acquainted, or those whose acquaintance it would be pleasant to make.

When a lady has a large acquaintance, and gives a series of at-homes, if she wishes to make them pleasant to all, she issues her invitations with this end in view, bearing in mind the prejudices and partialities of her friends; but when giving an occasional at-home her course is not so clear, and she is fearful of wounding the susceptibilities of some of her acquaintances by leaving them out of her invitations list. On the other hand, if she asks them to meet each other they feel that they have not been asked to the large at-home, and consider the invitation a doubtful compliment; this is a dilemma that many experience, and circumstances and self-interest often influence the decision arrived at for and against.

A difficulty often presents itself when a card is received for a series of "at-homes," as to whether the recipient is expected to go at all. If the "at-homes" are to take place every week, it would be advisable to put in an appearance fortnightly, and to mention the first date of acceptance in answering an invitation of this nature. But a visiting card with an "at-home" day written on it cannot be regarded in the light of an invitation; it is merely an intimation that if the friends of a certain lady call upon her on a given day, mentioned on the card, they will find her at home. But this does not necessitate a call being made, if convenient, or any excuses offered for non-appearance on the "at-home" day.

AGUE CURE:

Cut three lemons into thin slices and pound them with a mallet, then take enough coffee to make a quart; boil it down to a pint and pour it while quite hot over the lemons. Let it stand till cold, then strain through a cloth, and take the whole at one dose, immediately after the chill is over, and before the fever comes on.

AGUE PILL:

Quinine, 20 grains; Dover's powders, 10 grains; subcarbonate of iron, 10 grains; mix with mucilage of gum arabic and form into about 20 pills. Dose, 2 each hour, commencing 5 hours before the chill should set in. Then take 1 night and morning until all are taken.

AIR WE BREATHE, THE:

The Wonder of Breathing: The perfection of the organs of respiration excites our wonder. So delicate are these organs that the slightest pressure would cause exquisite pain, yet tons of air surge back and forth through their intricate passages, and bathe their innermost cells. Every year we perform 7,000,000 acts of breathing, inhaling 100,000 cubic feet of air, and purifying over 3,500 tons of blood. This gigantic process goes on constantly, and never wearies or worries us, and we only wonder at it when science reveals to us its magnitude. In addition, by a wise economy, the process of respiration is made to subserve a second use no less important, and the air we exhale, passing through the organs of voice, is transformed into prayers of faith, songs of thanksgiving and praise, and words of love and social enjoyment.

Fresh air Constantly Needed: None of the wants of the human body are so constant and pressing as that of air. Other demands may be met by occasional supplies, but the air must be furnished every moment, or we sicken and die. Our exhaled breath is the air robbed of its vitality, and containing in its place a gas which is fatal to life as it is to a flame, and effete matter which at the best is disagreeable to the smell, injurious to the health, and may contain the germs of disease. Air containing only 3 or 4 per cent. of carbonic acid gas acts as a narcotic poison, and a much smaller proportion will have an injurious effect. Careful investigations show that air containing more than six tenths of 1 per cent. of carbonic acid(1) in 1,000

(1) Carbon dioxide.

parts of air is really adverse to comfort, and obnoxious to health, the vitiated condition increasing in proportion to the increase of the carbonic acid.

Capacity of the Lungs for Air: There are in an averaged sized and well-developed human body about 600,000,000 of air-cells, into which the air passes in order to purify the blood. According to Hutchinson, a man of medium height will expel at a single full breath about 230 cubic in., or a gallon, and for each inch in height between 5 and 6 ft. there will be an increase of 8 cubic in. which cannot be expelled, thus making their entire contents about 330 cubic in., or 11 pints. The extra amount always on hand in the lungs is of great value, since thereby the action of the air goes on continuously, even during a violent expiration.

Amount of Air we Breathe: A full-sized man takes into his lungs at each breath about a pint of air; while in there all the life-nutriment is extracted from it; and on its being sent out of the body it is so entirely destitute of life-giving power that if re-breathed into the lungs again without the admixture of pure air the individual would suffocate, would die in 60 seconds. As a man breathes about 18 times a minute, and a pint at each breath, he consumes over 2 hogsheads(1) of air every hour, or about 16 hogsheads during the 8 hours' sleep, extract from it every atom of life-nutriment, and would die at the end of 8 hours, even if each breath could be kept to itself, provided no air came into the room from without.

Healthful Respiration: Respiration consists of two acts, inspiration, taking in the air, and expiration, expelling it from the lungs. When we draw in a full breath we straighten the spine, and throw back the head and shoulders so as to give the greatest advantage of the muscles. At the same time the diaphragm descends and presses the walls of the abdomen outward, both of which processes increase the size of the chest. Then the elastic lungs expand to occupy the extra space, while the air rushing in through the wind-pipe pours along the bronchial tubes and crowds into every cell.

When we forcibly expel the air from our lungs, the operation is reversed. This is called expiration. We bend forward, draw in the walls of the abdomen, and press the diaphragm upward, while the ribs are pulled downward, all together diminishing the size of the chest, and forcing the air outward. Ordinary, quiet breathing is performed mainly by the diaphragm, one breath to every four beats of the heart, or 18 per minute.

Evil Effect of Breathing Respired Air: If we take back into our lungs that which has been expelled we soon feel the effect. The muscles after a time become inactive, the blood stagnates, the heart acts slowly, the food is undigested, the brain is clogged. The constant breathing of even the slightly impure air

(1) A measurement of 63 gallons.

of our houses cannot but to undermine the health. The blood is not purified, and is in a condition to receive the seeds of disease at any time.

The system uninspired by the energizing oxygen is sensitive to cold. The pale cheek, the lusterless eye, the languid step, speak too plainly of oxygen starvation. In such a soil catarrh(1), scrofula(2), pneumonia, and consumption(3) run riot. The foul air which passes off from the lungs and the pores of the skin does not fall to the floor, but diffuses itself through the surrounding atmosphere. A single breath will to a trifling extent taint the air of a whole room.

Air in Rooms Vitiated by Fires: It is estimated that a light or a fire will vitiate as much air as a dozen persons. Carbonic oxide gas, a product of combustion more deadly than carbonic acid gas, leaks out from a stove through the pores of the hot iron, and, that which we breathe. Many breaths and lights rapidly unfit the air of a room for use.

Impure air in Small Rooms and Tenement Houses: Small, ill-ventilated sleeping rooms, in which reheated air is ever present, are nurseries of consumption, and an eminent physician says that this disease could as effectually be guarded against by proper attention to ventilation as small-pox by vaccination. To a lack of pure air may be attributed the existence of nearly all the prevalent disease classed under the head of scrofulous diseases. Some physicians attribute the prevalence of intemperance among the lower classes to the effect of bad ventilation in the crowded tenements, which produces a degree of lethargy sufficient to drive them to the rum-shop for stimulants.

How to Ventilate Houses: Every sleeping apartment should have a fireplace with an open chimney, and in cold weather it is well if the grate contains a small fire, enough to create a current and carry the vitiated air out of the room. In such cases, however, it is necessary to see that the air drawn into the room comes in from the outside of the house. Summer or winter, it is well to have a free ingress for pure air. The aim must be to purify the air without causing a great fall of temperature. To accomplish this the windows may be drawn down an inch or two from the top, and a fold of muslin placed over the aperture to prevent draught. Where the body is kept warm and pure air only inhaled, there is no more danger of taking cold in sleeping directly between two windows all the year round than there is of taking cold in riding an open sleigh when thoroughly warmed by the wrappings of furs and robes; and such a thing as taking cold under such conditions never occurs, providing, always, the thorough warming of the feet and back, which are often neglected.

(1) A discharge from various outlets of the body, when from the nose or eyes, a cold in the head.
(2) Inflamation of neck glands.
(3) Tuberculosis of the lungs.

Air in Sick-rooms: Fresh air is one of the most important and difficult things to obtain and retain in a sick-room. The following simple arrangement will remedy the evil of foul gas, generated by burning a kerosene lamp all night in a nursery or sick-room:

Take a raisin box or any other suitably sized box that will contain the lamp when set up on end. Place the lamp in the box, outside the window, with the open side facing the room. When there are blinds, the box can be attached to each by leaving them a little open, and fastening with a cord; or the lamp box can be nailed to the window casing in a permanent manner. The lamp burns quite as well outside, and a decided improvement of the air in the room is experienced.

Bad Air in School-rooms: School-rooms, heated by furnaces or red hot stoves, often have no means of ventilation, or, if provided, these are seldom used. Pupils starved by scanty lung food (and we might add brain food) are stupefied by foul air, and are listless and dull. This process goes on from year to year, and the weakened and poisoned body at last succumbs to disease, and a "mysterious Providence" is charged with sickness and death. The voice of nature, as well as nature's God, cries aloud, "Do thyself no harm." Those who violate the God-given laws of life and health may expect the penalty. Whatsoever we sow we shall inevitably reap. If we sow the seeds of disease, we must reap sickness and death. To breathe the atmosphere of many school-houses, lecture-rooms, and theaters is to breathe the atmosphere of death.

Teachers and Bad Air: With the vile atmosphere of the school-room constantly pouring over the lining membranes of the nasal cavities, surging about the linings of the throat and vocal organs, driving down the bronchial tubes, and deluging the lungs, what wonder the teacher first suffers from vitiated blood, then from clogged membranes, and lastly from catarrh, bronchitis, dyspepsia(1), and perhaps pulmonary consumption! It is next to impossible that the more nervous constitutions should not succumb.

Foul Air in Churches: We sit in our churches, from which the air and light of heaven have been excluded six days out of seven, and, though ventilated as well as heated for the seventh, we bewail our listlessness and want of interest in the life-giving Gospel, and we charge it either to the preacher or to our depravity, when the fact is, no temporary ventilation can take from the carbonic-impregnated crypts and walls the depravity which has there fixed its abode. The foul air left by the congregation on Sunday is often shut up during the week and heated for the next Lord's day, when the people assemble, to be re-breathed as polluted atmosphere.

(1) Indigestion.

How to Remove "Foul Air" from Churches: The best time to change the air in the churches is immediately after the congregation has departed. When the services for the day are concluded, and while the audience room is still warm, if the windows and doors are left open for a short time the cooler air of out-doors will rapidly displace that which has been breathed over and over again by the throng of worshipers. Better arrangement would be to so provide for ventilation in the structure of the church that the foul air shall be constantly passing out and fresh air shall be constantly supplied; but in the absence of such an arrangement the sexton or janitor should, in the way here suggested, thoroughly ventilate the church edifice after each service. If the intervals between the services are long, it may be well, also, to rechange the air a short time before the succeeding service.

Night Air Healthy: Many are afraid of night air. Florence Nightingale replies to this objection by asking, "What can we breathe at night except night air?" Her rule is to keep the air within as pure as that without the house. Don't be afraid to sleep by an open window. It is a common fallacy that cold air is necessarily pure, and that apartments need less ventilation in winter than in summer. Coolness does not always indicate freshness, and disagreeable warmth does not indicate chemical impurity. Draughts are pernicious in their effects, and must be avoided. In sleeping in an unavoidable draught, turn the face to meet it.

Water as Purifier: A pan of water standing in an inhabited room becomes utterly filthy and unfit for drink in a few hours. This depends on the fact that the water has the faculty of condensing, and thereby absorbing, all the gases, which it does without increasing its own bulk. The cooler the water is, the greater its capacity to contain these gases. The "breathed" atmosphere of the room is, therefore, improved by the water, if often changed.

Sea Air: Sea air, as a rule, is beneficial to health. This is shown by the fact that the average life among seamen is larger than among those of most vocations on land. The occupations of the former are such that, were it not for the healthfulness of the sea air, their lives would probably be shorter than those of the latter.

Are Winds Healthful? Stagnation in the air or water is always harmful. The wind expels the stagnant air, and introduces fresh. Railway trains or street cars passing rapidly and frequently by a dwelling stir up the atmosphere, and in this respect render important service. It often occurs that in localities where fevers prevail those persons who reside close to a railway escape the disease.

Damp Air and Health: Dry air as a rule is healthier than damp or humid air.

Hence, if rains continue long, or if fogs prevail for several days, the system suffers by the increased saturation. While oxygen and nitrogen and pure air itself are almost entirely diathermous, the absorptive power of moisture is very great. It seems that a molecule of aqueous vapor has 16,000 times the absorptive power of an atom of oxygen or of nitrogen; and carbonic acid, marsh gas, ammonia, etc., are also extremely absorptive. Now, when the sun shines on an atmosphere that is dry, his rays pass through in all their power, but when the air is damp the rays are much weakened before they reach the earth. On the other hand, when the air is dry, the heat from the earth radiates into space much faster than when it is moist. The importance of these facts from a medical stand-point is very great.

All the agents just mentioned as powerful absorbents of heat are found in greatest abundance near the earth; consequently they absorb a large amount of the heat radiated from the earth, diffused in the atmosphere. Usually over 10 per cent. of the heat from this source is absorbed within 10 ft. of the ground. On the northern Atlantic coast the south and east winds are, as a rule, moist winds; next come the northerly; next the south-west; next the west; next the north; and last the north-west. The sudden veering of a wind from a southerly to a northerly wind is usually attended with a precipitation of moisture; and the same is true of a sudden change of a northerly to an easterly.

Sea and Mountain Air Compared: An able Italian physician, Dr. Alberto, says: "The marine air produces the same benefit as that of a mountain, but each has a different *modus efficiendi*; the former acts more forcibly and energetically on the constitution which retains some robustness and internal resources to profit by it, while the second acts more gently, with slower efficacy, being thereby more suitable to the weaker and less excitable organizations. From this important distinction the conscientious physician who takes the safety of his patient much to heart ought to be able to discriminate whether the alpine or the marine atmosphere is the better suited to the case he has before him."

ALABASTER, TO CLEAN:

For cleaning it there is nothing better than soap and water. Stains may be removed by washing with soap and water, then whitewashing the stained part, letting it stand some hours, then washing off the whitewash, and rubbing the stained part.

ALCOHOL, EFFECT OF, ON LIFE:

A special committee of the British Medical Association investigated the effect of alcohol upon life, and came to the conclusion, so often preached in barrooms, that alcohol is a preservative. The committee found that total abstainers lived an average life-time of 51 yrs. and 22 days; habitually temperate drinkers lived 63 yrs. and 13 days; unsystematic, happy-go-lucky drinkers, who were not drunkards, but simply good fellows, lived 59 yrs. and 67 days; free drinkers lived 57 yrs. and 59 days, and drunkards lived 53 yrs. and 13 days, two years longer than total abstainers. The committee obtained those findings by investigating the lives of 4,234 dead Englishmen. These figures cannot be credited with conclusive importance. The highest testimony points in the other direction and away from alcohol.

Sir Henry Thompson thinks that to every healthy man each drop of alcohol is so much injury. It must be remembered that a similar investigation in America would not be at all likely to produce a similar series of averages. The English climate is widely different from ours. It is continually moist and cloudy, with a small proportion of clear sunlight. It has been noticed by Americans that alcohol has less effect upon the human system there than in our country, where for the greater part of the year the atmosphere itself is stimulating.

It has been argued that artificial stimulus is needed in Great Britain to offset the loss of sunlight and to combat the dampness. Then, again, it must be remembered that the drinking habits of the English are systematized by centuries of experience and usage, so that sensible drinkers over there drink only with their meals and after dinner at night. The drinking is confined almost wholly to spirits, it is true, but every glass of liquor is "drowned," as an American would say, with water. Liquor drowned may not be as harmless as a witch subjected to the same operation used to be considered in New England, but the deviltry of it is lessened in proportion as water is poured into it. "Undoubtedly," said one conspicuous physician, "the less that men drink the better. The least harmful alcoholic beverage is whisky and water—little whisky and much water."

ALCOHOLISM:

This term includes: (1) Intoxication; (2) dipsomania(1), or the acute alcoholism of delirium tremens; and (3) the state of chronic inebriety.

Treatment of: In a case of intoxication, empty the stomach with an emetic of 20 grains of ipecac, or, if that is not at hand, with a large spoonful of mustard. Apply cold water to the head, but keep the feet and body warm; mustard plasters to the feet and pit of the stomach are useful. As soon as the patient can drink, give strong hot coffee, without milk or sugar, in table-spoonful doses, every 5 minutes. Give iced milk for nourishment, and, as tonic, three times a day, tincture nux vomica(2), 10 drops, mixed with a dram each of compound tincture of gentian(3) and compound tincture of colombo(4).

In delirium tremens the first thing is to secure quiet and sleep, and

(1) The brain fever of drunkards.
(2) A medicine made from the poisonous seed of the strychnos nux vomica.
(3) The sweet smelling yet bitter testing root of the genus Gentiana plant family.
(4) The alcoholic extract of the colombo root (Jateorhiza Calumba).

no drug has been more efficient for this object than chloral hydrate, in $^1/_2$ dram doses; repeated, if necessary, two or three times. The bromide of potassium has also succeeded in some cases, 20 grains every hour, until the nerves are quieted and the patient rests. The strength must now be supported by nutritious diet of eggs, soups, and milk, and by mild stimulants, as 10 drops tincture of capsicum(1)or aromatic ammonia in one half ounce of water every hour. These means, with good nursing, will generally succeed; where they fail, a very rare and moderate allowance of opium and brandy is sometimes permitted.

In chronic inebrioty, most physicians now insist on entire cessation from the use of liquor at the beginning of the treatment; then give 1 fluid dram tincture of ginger or tincture capsicum every 3 hours, combined with $^1/_2$ dram of bromide of ammonia, or 15 grains of chloral hydrate, as nervines. Sustain also as much as possible with generous diet.

Homeopathic: If the patient lies in a state of stupor, eyes open, stertorous breathing, pupils contracted, give opium; if of a full habit, with flushed face, red eyes, dilated pupils, give belladonna(2); if there is trembling of the limbs and spasmodic twitching of muscles, give nux vomica. The best remedies for the inclination to drink and the evil effects of habitual drunkenness are arsenic, nux vomica, and sulphur.

Administration: Of a solution of 3 drops or 12 globules in 10 tea-spoonfuls of water, give 2 tea-spoonfuls every two or three hours in urgent cases; but in milder forms of the disease a dose two or three times a day will be sufficient.

AMMONIA, USES OF:

For washing paint, put a table-spoonful of spirits of ammonia in a quart of moderately hot water, dip in a flannel cloth, and with this simply wipe off the wood-work; no scrubbing will be necessary. For taking grease-spots from any fabric, use the ammonia nearly pure, then lay white blotting-paper over the spot and iron it lightly. In washing laces, put about 12 drops in a pint of warm suds. To clean silver, mix 2 tea-spoonfuls of ammonia in a quart of hot soap-suds, put in your silverware and wash it, using an old nail-brush for the purpose. For cleaning hair-brushes, etc., simply shake the brushes up and down in a mixture of 1 tea-spoonful of ammonia to 1 pint of hot water; when they are cleansed, rinse them in cold water, and stand them in the wind or in a hot place to dry. For washing finger-marks from looking-glasses or windows, put a few drops of ammonia on a moist rag, and make quick work of it. If you wish your house plants to flourish, put a few drops of the spirits in every pint of water used in watering. A tea-spoonful in a basin of cold water adds much to the refreshing effects of

(1) The dried ripe fruit of Capsicum fastigiatum from Zanzibar, used as a stimulant and gargle.
(2) A medicine made from the leaves of the deadly nightshade plant with black poisonous berries.

bath. In every case rinse off ammonia with clear water. Liquid ammonia is the most powerful and useful agent for cleaning silk stuffs and hats, and for neutralizing the effects of acids. In this later case it is often enough to expose the spots to the vapors of ammonia, which makes them disappear entirely.

ANTI-FAT DIET:

For those people whose embonpoint(1) is a matter of solicitude, whether because it is uncomfortable or unfashionable, the following diet is proposed by a doctor:

Lean mutton and beef, veal and lamb, soups not thickened, beef-tea and broth; poultry, game, fish and eggs; bread in moderation; greens, cresses, lettuce, etc.; green peas, cabbage, cauliflower, onions; fresh fruit without sugar.

ANTISEPTICS:

Boracic acid is said to be one of the best antiseptics; 1 part of a 10 per cent. solution added to 8 of milk is said to keep it fresh a week. Dr. Zollner states that carbon disulfide in a state of vapor is capable of acting as a powerful antiseptic. Two drops allowed to evaporate spontaneously in a closed vessel of the ordinary temperature were found to keep meat, fruit, vegetables, and bread in a perfectly fresh condition for several weeks. The articles submitted to the process acquire neither smell nor taste, the carbon disulphide evaporating entirely when they are exposed to the air at the ordinary temperature. The vapor of carbon disulphide being very inflammable, all experiments should be performed during daylight.

ANTS, TO DESTROY:

(1) Drop some quicklime on the mouth of their nest and wash it in with boiling water, or dissolve some camphor in spirits of wine, then mix with water and pour into their haunts; or tobacco water, which has been found effectual. They are averse to strong scents. Camphor will prevent their infesting a cupboard, or a sponge saturated with creasote. To prevent their climbing trees, place a ring of tar about the trunk or a circle of rag moistened occasionally with creasote.

(2) Grease a plate with lard and set it where the ants are troublesome; place a few sticks around the plate for the ants to climb upon; occasionally turn the plate over a fire where there is no smoke, and the ants will drop off into it: reset the plate, and in a few repetitions all the ants will be caught; they trouble nothing else while lard is accessible.

(3) Sprigs of wintergreen or ground ivy will drive them away.

(1) Plumpness.

(4) They may be kept away from any thing by surrounding it by a chalk mark.

ANUS, FISSURE OF:

A common and very painful affection, especially of middle life, more frequently in females. Neglected constipation and piles are the most frequent causes. The symptoms are, at first, slight smarting or soreness, which later becomes severe, with intense pain, burning, aching, and throbbing, lasting sometimes for hours.

Treatment: Bathe the part frequently with cold water, or weak lead water; wash thoroughly after every evacuation; anoint with equal parts of benzoated oxide of zinc ointment and belladonna ointment; if the pain is very severe use a suppository of opium and extract of belladonna, $^1/_2$ grain of each to 20 grains of cocoa butter. In obstinate cases it may be necessary to touch the fissure occasionally with nitrate of silver. The bowels should be kept soluble by fruit or mild laxatives, or the daily use of an injection of water or weak soap-suds.

APARTMENTS, TO PERFUME:

The best and most simple method to diffuse the odor of any perfume throughout an apartment is to make use of a spirit lamp. Into this lamp put the essence or scent, which should not contain water. Provide the lamp with a thick wick, and place slightly above a small ball of spongy platinum; then light the wick, and when the platinum is red-hot, which will be the case in a few seconds, blow out the flame. The platinum ball will continue in a state of ignition as long as any spirit remains in the bottle, throwing off the perfume and vapor as it rises by means of the wick, and diffusing it generally throughout the whole apartment. In the absence of a spirit lamp a narrow-necked bottle may be made use of; but care must be taken that it does not crack when the wick is alight. The lamp is safe.

APERIENTS(1):

In the spring time of the year the judicious use of aperient medicines is often to be commended.

Spring Aperients: *For children, nothing is better than:*

(1) Brimstone and molasses; to each tea-cupful of this, when mixed, add a tea-spoonful of cream of tartar. As this sometimes produces sickness, the following may be used:

(2) Take of tartrate of soda $1^1/_2$ drams; powered jalap and powdered rhubarb, each 15 grains; ginger, 2 grains; mix. Dose for a child above 5 yrs., 1 small tea-spoonful; above 10 yrs., a large tea-spoon-

(1) Laxatives.

ful; above 15, half the whole, or 2 tea-spoonfuls; and for a person above 20, 3 tea-spoonfuls or the whole, as may be required by the habit of the person. This medicine may be dissolved in warm water, common or mint tea. This powder can be kept for use in wide-mouthed bottle, and be in readiness for any emergency. The druggist may be directed to treble or quadruple the quantities, as convenient.

Aperient Pills: *To some adults all liquid medicines produce such nausea that pills are the only form in which laxative medicine can be exhibited. The following is a useful formu*la:

(3) Take of compound rhubarb pills 1 dram and 1 scruple; or powdered ipecacuanha(1), 6 grains, and of extract of hyoscyamus(2), 1 scruple. Mix and beat into a mass, and divide into 24 pills. Take one or two, or, if of a very costive habit, three, at bed-time.

(4) For persons requiring a more powerful purge, the same formula, with 10 grains of compound extract of colocynth(3), will form a good purgative pill. The mass received this addition must be divided into 30, instead of 24 pills.

Black Draught: *The common aperient medicine known as black draught is made in the following manner:*

Take of senna leaves, 6 drams; bruised ginger, 1/2 dram; sliced liquorice root, 4 drams; boiling water, 1/2 imperial pint. Keep this standing near the fire for 3 hours, then strain, and after allowing it to grow cool, add of sal volatile 1 1/2 drams; of tincture of senna and of tincture of cardamoms, each 1/2 ounce. (This mixture will keep a long time in a cool place). Dose, wine-glassful for an adult; 2 table-spoonfuls for young persons above 15 yrs. of age. It is not a suitable medicine for children.

APPLE CHERMES, TO EXTIRPATE:

The eggs are laid in September, on different places of the twigs of the apple-tree, usually in the furrows of the knots. To secure the blossoms and fruit of trees in pots, or dwarf trees, brush away the young chermes with a fine brush when they appear, or, at latest, when the first changing of skin takes place in April. It is also necessary to examine the small trees in spring, when the blossoms begin to appear, to ascertain if any insects are upon them, and if so to destroy them.

APPLE-ROOT PLANT-LOUSE, TO EXTIRPATE:

This forms wart-like excrescences upon the roots of apple-trees, which contain in their crevices the insects which suck their juices; is said to

(1) An emetic and expectorant from the dried root of the Cephaelis Ipecacuanha plant found in Brazil.
(2) From the fresh dried leafs of the hyoscyamus niger plant used to prevent the griping of purgatives.
(3) A drastic purgative from the dried fruit, freed from seeds, of the Citrullus Colocynthis (cumuis).

be destroyed by an application of boiling hot water. Mulching round infested trees has been found to have the effect of bringing the lice to the surface of the ground, where they can be more easily reached by the hot water.

APPLES, TO DRY:

Pare and cut the apples in slices; then spread them on cloths, tables, or boards, and dry them out-doors. In clear, dry weather, this is the most expeditious way. It is a good plan to use frames. These combine the most advantages with the least inconvenience of any way, and can be used either in drying in the house or out in the sun. In pleasant weather the frames can be set out-doors against the side of the building or any other support, and nights or cloudy and stormy days can be brought into the house and set against the side of the room near the stove or fire-place.

Frames may be made in the following manner:

Two strips of board, 7 ft. long, 2 or 2½ in. wide; 2 strips, 3 ft. long, 1½ in. wide; the whole ¾ in. thick. Nail the short strips across the ends of the long ones, and it makes frame 7 by 3 ft., which is a convenient size for all purposes. On one of the long strips nails are driven 3 in. apart, extending from the top to the bottom.

After the apples are pared, quarter and core, and with a needle and twine or stout thread string them into lengths long enough to reach twice across the frame; the ends of the twine are then tied together, and the strings hung on the nails across the frame. The apples will soon dry, so that the strings can be doubled on the nails and fresh ones put on, or the whole of them removed and others put in their place. As fast as the apples become sufficiently dry they can be taken from the strings, and the same strings used to dry more on.

Dried apples are bleached by exposure to the fumes of burning sulphur. This may be done by making a tight box with shelves to slide in or out at the front. The shelves should have wire gauze bottoms on which the dried fruit is to be placed. The box is set up on legs 1 ft. high. Under the box is a sheet-iron close receptacle, from which a pipe passes into the bottom of the box. A quantity of ignited charcoal is put into the iron vessel and covered with sulphur, the fumes of which pass into the box and through the fruit, making them very white and clear. Any other convenient arrangement which will answer the same purpose may be adopted, but the fumes must be confined in a close receptacle, and the fruit should be arranged so that they pass through it.

To Pack:

(1) Assort them so as to run uniform in size and quality. Pack in new, sound barrels of the standard size, flat hops preferred; only one variety in a barrel; turn the upper end of the barrel down; take out the lower head, and commence packing by placing a tier of apples

snugly with stem ends upon the head; then fill up the barrel without bruising the fruit; shake down gently, but thoroughly, and press, flattening the last tier of apples; then, fastening the head, turn the barrel over, and mark plainly with a stencil plate, or red chalk, or ink, the variety contained.

(2) Wrap each one in manilla tissue paper; then pack as solidly as possible, putting a layer of soft chaff at the bottom of the barrel, and sifting more over every layer; when the barrel is full, place plenty of packing on top, and press the head firmly down. In this condition apples will travel months without injury.

APPLES WITHOUT SUGAR:

Sugar added to apples only robs them of their specific and delicate aroma, reduces their quality, and renders them insipid and commonplace. The finest apples for cooking are, without doubt, the Ribston and Newtown pippins at their best, and both are not only greatly deteriorated, but half spoiled in flavor by any additions of foreign sugar. The best eating apples are also the best cooking ones.

Convenience, the possession of kitchen varieties, and the perversity of cooks in heavily dredging all apples with sugar frequently overthrow one's convictions, and go far to ruin the best apple pies and puddings. As a fact, the popular custom of adding paste and sugar to most cooked apples is largely responsible for the loss of most of their richest and most delicate aroma, as well as the source of their unwholesomeness to so many consumers. Butter, batter, and sugars of the rankest, roughest character, but little superior to molasses, why should these be allowed to destroy all the most delicate and delicious flavors of our choicest apples?

If we wish to enjoy the latter in perfection let us either roast them in their skins, or skin and core and place in a pipkin, as you did the Newtown pippins, and enjoy a feast of apples pure and simple, and free from the suspicion of paste, molasses, and fat. Heads of families are advised against providing sweets to be added to this kind of fruits, precaution which would have the double benefit of "opening the eyes" of the people to the enormous consumption of sugar in reducing all apples to a sort of dead level of mediocrity, and the most wholesale deterioration and destruction of flavor; and in the end promote the growth of only the best varieties, regardless of the present absurd market preference for bright color of skin.

APPLE-TREE LOUSE, TO EXTIRPATE:

Feeds on leaves and twigs of apple trees. The wingless female is pale green, with yellowish head and dark green stripes on the back. The winged ones of both sexes have black heads, green abdomens, and a row of blacks dots on each side. A mixture of tobacco-juice and lime will kill them.

AQUARIA, HOW TO MANAGE:

For fresh water, the simplest and least expensive aquarium is the bell glass. It is preferable to the globe, exposing a larger surface to the atmosphere. It is also free from any contaminating influences. Where space is no object, an oblong tank may be selected. The frame-work may be of wood, zinc, iron or glass pillars, with glass sides; but the best are slate, with glass front, or slate ends, with a glass front and back. If not made from slate, the bottom should be lined with glass or slate, embedded in a layer of Portland cement. Wood frames are least durable, and soon leak.

Sand or pebbles may be used for the bottom, but sand is to be preferred. Wash the sand till the water runs from it clear, and then lay it in the bottom of the tank to the thickness of 2 in., to hold the plants and allow them to root. Or, the plants may be fastened in one of the terra-cotta ornaments sold for that purpose, with enough sand or broken rock to cover the bottom.

The plants will root readily if the aquarium has light. A few large pebbles improve the appearance, and afford sheltering nooks to which the fish may retire. Shells and corals are out of place. Floating islands may be made of pieces of cork, on which may be grown small ferns. For rock-work or caverns, pile up small blocks of granite, fastening them with Portland cement, (other cements are apt to injure the fish); this cement must remain in water for a week, in order that it may part with any soluble matter it may contain.

Having laid your sand and gravel, and built your rockery, let the cement get firm, then add water, and empty and refill till the water is clear, when it will be fit to receive plants. These must be put in the aquarium several days before the fish, to enable the plants to commence growing vigorously. Do not put in the fish till this is the case, and then put in only a moderate number. The most important consideration is light. A certain amount of sunlight is necessary.

Frequent removal of sediment is required. For this purpose use the lifting tube, which is a simple glass tube, 1/2 in. in diameter, and 2 or 3 in. longer than the depth of the water, and drawn in a little at one end, so that the finger may cover it more are easily. Hold it in the right hand, with the finger over the smaller end, insert it into the water, placing the open end over the object to be removed. Then remove the finger, when the air will escape, allowing the water to rush into the tube, carrying the dirt with it. By placing the finger again over the opening at the top, the tube may be lifted out with its contents and emptied into a vessel held in the other hand, by again removing the finger from the opening.

Never take fish in your hand. If the aquarium needs cleansing, make a net of mosquito netting, and take the fish out in it. Keep the aquarium clean and the water clear. Watch the fish, and you will find out when they are all right. Feed them with worms, meat, fish wafer or fish spawn. Dace, roach, and other cyprinidonts are vegetable feeders, and may be kept in good condition on the wafer food, sold by dealers. The addition of shreds of lean meat and oysters, or small worms, will be enjoyed. Sun-fish may be kept healthy on meat, oysters or worms; the oysters should first be washed. Where a brook is accessible, small net, dipped among the plants, dead leaves, or sedimentary deposits, will furnish crustaceous larvae, on which all classes of fish feed. The sticklebacks(1) require this, and will not thrive on dead food. All food which is not eaten within 2 or 3 hours should be removed with the lifting tube.

ARTICLES OF DRESS, TO RENOVATE:

Oils and fats are the substances which form the greater part of simple stains. They give a deep shade to the ground of the cloth; they continue to spread for several days; they attract the dust and retain it so strongly that it is not removable by the brush; and they eventually render the stain lighter-colored upon dark ground, and of a disagreeable gray tint upon a pale or light ground. The general principle of cleansing all spots consists in applying to them a substance which shall have a stronger affinity for the matter composing them that this has for the cloth, and which shall render them soluble in some liquid menstruum, such as water, spirits, oil of turpentine, etc. Alkalies would seem to be proper in this point of view, as they are the most powerful solvents of grease; but they act too strongly upon silk and wool, as well as change too powerfully the colors of dyed stuffs, to be safely applicable in removing stains.

The best substances for this purpose are:

(1) Soap

(2) Chalk, fuller's earth, soap-stone. These should be merely diffused through a little water into a thin paste, spread upon the stain, and allowed to dry. The spot requires now to be merely brushed.

(3) Ox-gall(2) and yoke of eggs have the property of dissolving fatty bodies without effecting perceptibly the texture of colors of cloth, and may therefore be employed with advantage. The ox-gall should be purified, to prevent its greenish tint from degrading the brilliancy of dyed stuffs, or the purity of whites.

(4) The volatile oil of turpentine will only take out recent stains, for which purpose it ought to be previously purified by distillation over quicklime. Wax, resin, turpentine, pitch and all resinous bodies in general form stains of greater or less adhesion, which may be dissolved out by pure alcohol.

(1) A popular name for any of the species of gasterosteus, a very active carnivorous fish.
(2) Fresh bile of the ox, purified and used when there is insufficient bile; used for dyspepsia also.

ARTIFICIAL SKIN, FOR BURNS, BRUISES, ETC.:

Take gun-cotton and Venice turpentine, equal parts of each, and dissolve them in 20 times as much sulphuric ether, dissolving the cotton first, then adding the turpentine; keep it corked tightly. Water does not effect it, hence its value for cracked nipples, chapped hands, surface bruises, etc.

ASPARAGUS BEETLES, TO EXTIRPATE:

These are troublesome pests found on asparagus. There are two kinds:

(1) Blackish-green, the thorax red, with two black dots, yellow wing-cases, the suture and three spots united to it on both sides being black.

(2) Twelve-spotted Leaf-beetle, red, the wing-cases lighter, each having six black dots; the horns, eyes, breast, edge of the abdomen, tips of the thighs and palpi, black. The larva is spindle-shaped, flat beneath, arched, fleshy, wrinkled, covered with single hairs, bordered at the sides, of an olive color; the head and legs black.

The only remedy is to pick off and kill both beetles and larvæ.

ATTAR OF ROSES, TO MAKE:

Fill a large earthen jar or other vessel with the leaves of rose-flowers picked over and freed from all dust and dirt. Pour upon them as much pure spring water as will cover them, and from sunrise to sunset, for six or seven days in succession, set the vessel where it will receive the sun's rays. At the end of the third or fourth day a number or particles of fine yellow oily matter will float on the surface, which, after a day or two, will gather into a scum. This is the attar of roses. It must be taken up as often as it appears, with a piece of cotton tied to a stick and squeezed from this into a small vial, which must be kept corked and tied over.

AUTUMN LEAVES:

(1) Gather the leaves from the trees before frosts, getting all the shades and tints possible, singly and in sprays suitable for pressing, and at once placed between the leaves not too near together, of books or newspapers, and several pounds' weight laid upon them. Keep while pressing in a cool place, and as often as every other day change into new books; this is important because the paper absorbs the dampness from the leaves.

They should be kept in press between two and three weeks. They are then ready for a coating of oil or varnish. Mixture of 3 ounces of spirits of turpentine, 2 ounces of boiled linseed oil, and 1/3 ounce of white varnish is preferable to either alone. Get a perfectly smooth board, large enough to lay a spray upon, with no reaching of the leaves beyond the outer edges; take a piece of soft cloth to apply the dressing; after the application the leaves must be laid carefully on boards or papers, not overlapping each other, until dry. Then disposed of as taste suggests, avoiding as much as possible a stiff, unnatural arrangement; the stem can be broken off and a fine wire attached in its place, which makes them a little more yielding to handle.

(2) Spread the fresh leaves and press them in a suitable dish, with alternate layers of fine sand, which is thoroughly dry and smoothed under a hot iron, dipped for a moment in clear French spirit varnish, and allowed to dry in the air. By many, melted white wax or paraffine is preferred to the varnish. These latter must not be too hot.

AWNINGS, TO MAKE WATERPROOF:

Plunge first into a solution containing 20 per cent. soap and afterward in another solution the same percentage of copper. Wash afterwards.

AXLE-GREASE, TO MAKE:

Take one part good plumbago (black-lead) sifted through a coarse muslin so as to be perfectly free from grit, and stir it into five quarts of lard, warmed so as to be stirred easily without melting. Stir vigorously until it is smooth and uniform. Then raise the heat until the mixture melts. Stir constantly, remove from the fire, and keep stirring until cold. Apply cold to the axle or any other bearing with a brush. If intended for use where the axle or bearing is in a warm apartment, as the interior of mills, etc., 2 ounces of hard tallow or one ounce of beeswax may be used to every 10 pounds of the mixture. This grease is cheaper in use than oil, tallow or tar, or any compound of them.

B

BABY, HOW TO TRAIN THE:

Judicious "letting alone:" is a great gift. Happy the babies whose mothers possess it. Unfortunately there are comparatively few who do, and still fewer nurses. Babies, especially first babies, are great sufferers from too much attention. They are very often, too, the victims of experiment, or even worse, of prejudice. Grandmothers and old nurses have very rigid ideas concerning their training and discipline, while young mammas have, on their side, a good many theories. Between these different influences, the little nursery despot is often called upon to suffer many things.

The child should from the first be accustomed to absolute regularity in regard to its meals; but, although this is essential, it is a very great mistake to apply the same rule to other matters—dressing, for instance. An infant's sleep should never be broken in upon. Even when the nursing hour arrives, it is exceedingly injudicious to arouse the baby for the sake of punctuality; but so easily are habits formed that if the child is nursed at regular intervals from the beginning it will naturally stir about the right time, and can be gently lifted up and nursed without arousing it entirely. It is really better to let the infant remain unwashed than to waken it because the time for the bath has come.

Little children beginning to notice and to babble out their monosyllable utterances are so engaging that the temptation all the time is to wake up their faculties; they are always on exhibition, always being roused up to show their pretty ways, tossed and dangled and played with, when they had far better be left lying in the crib. A very great deal in the direction of training can be accomplished by accustoming the baby to lie still in the cradle when awake.

It is not a welcome fact, but it is a very pregnant one, that the less babies are talked to and noticed the first year the better. All success in training them indeed, depends upon this calm letting them alone. The children of the working poor are in this respect far better off than those of the well-to-do; if later they miss much of the culture of good habits, they are, as babies, let so much alone that, take them all in all, they are peaceable and quiet. One rarely hears the washwoman or seamstress talk of walking up and down all night with a fretful, excitable baby.

BABY, TO KEEP CLEAN:

A baby that is not kept perfectly sweet and fresh loses half its charm, and is defrauded of its just rights. It should be bathed in warm water every morning, and as it grows older the temperature gradually lowered, until, at five months old, the chill is just taken off the water. Most babies love their baths, and are more apt to scream at being taken out of it than when put into it.

If there is a shrinking from the plunge, a small blanket can be spread on the tub, the child laid on it, and gently lowered into the tub. At night it should be held on the lap, and quickly sponged with a sponge, wrung out of warm water. Its mouth should be washed with a soft piece of linen dipped in cool water. All creases where the flesh touches should be powdered with pulverized starch, or any good toilet-powder. This is most important, and must never be omitted, as the delicate skin easily chafes. Where there is redness, or any symptom of chafing, lycopodium powder should be used; it is most healing, and can be applied even if the skin is broken. When there are frequent discharges, the parts should be washed in thin, boiled starch, instead of water. It is criminal neglect to allow a baby to suffer from chafing.

BABY BASKET:

This can be made as elaborate or as plain as you wish. Most mothers prefer the double basket with stand, instead of the old-fashioned one without stand, which used to be placed on top of the chest of drawers. Line the basket with pink or blue soft-finished cambric, and then cover with dotted muslin. Make three small pockets on the inside of basket, and line one of them with oilsilk. Have a deep ruffle of the muslin around the outside of the basket with plaited ribbon. Place bows of wide ribbon on two sides of basket.

Contents: Small comb and brush, (soft and very fine); powder box, filled with sifted starch; powder puff; metal or ivory soap-box, with cake of white castile or Skin Success soap; small soft sponge; three linen wash-clothes; three small-sized linen face towels, (these come especially for infants); pair of sharp scissors; roll of linen bobbin or narrow tape; pincushion sewed to inside of basket, filled with large and small-sized safety-pins.

BACON, HOW TO SELECT:

Bacon should have a thin rind, and the fat should be firm and tinged red by the curing. The flesh should be of a clear red, without intermixture of yellow, and it should firmly adhere to the bone. To judge the state of a ham, plunge a knife into it to the bone; on drawing it back, if particles of meat adhere to it, or if the smell is disagreeable, the curing has not been effectual, and the ham is not good. It should, in such a state, be immediately cooked. In buying a ham, a short, thick one is to be preferred to the long and thin.

BAD BREATH, TO RELIEVE:

Bad breath, from catarrh(1), foul stomach, or bad teeth, may be temporarily relieved by diluting a little bromochloralum with 8 or 10 parts of water and using it as a gargle, and swallowing a few drops.

BALDNESS:

It is not uncommon for the hair to fall out during or after severe sickness; but very often between 30 and 40 years of age, without any assignable cause, it commences falling out, and if not arrested, more or less complete, and often permanent, baldness results.

Treatment:

(1) As soon as the hair commences to come out cut it short and bathe the entire scalp regularly in fresh or salt water, or water having in it a small quantity of spirits of ammonia; after rubbing vigorously with the fingers for a few moments, brush well with a moderately stiff brush. If the hair is dry and harsh, rub into it after each bathing a few drops of glycerine, or a mixture of 8 to 10 parts glycerine with 1 part of tincture of cantharides and a little oil of rosemary, which will be stimulating to the scalp.

(2) Muriate of pilocarpia(2) in subcutaneous injections, to be administered only by a physician.

(3) *The decoction of boxwood, successful in cases of baldness, is thus made:*

Take of the common box, which grows in garden borders, stems and leaves 4 large handfuls; boil in 3 pints of water, in a closely covered vessel, for a quarter of an hour, and let it stand in a covered earthenware jar for 10 hours or more; strain, and add an ounce and a half of eau de Cologne, or lavender water, to make it keep. The head should be well washed with this solution every morning.

(4) *Erasmus Wilson's lotion against baldness:* Eau de Cologne, 2 ounces; tincture of cantharides, 2 drams; oil of lavender or rosemary, of each 10 drops. These applications must be used once or twice a day for a considerable time; but if the scalp becomes sore they must be discontinued for a time, or used at longer intervals.

BALLS AND PARTIES, ETIQUETTE OF:

A hundred guests constitute a ball; over that, a large ball; under that, a "dance." One of the first requisites of a ball-room is thorough ventilation. Have a beautifully arranged room; the floor well waxed, and even: and draw

(1) A running discharge from various bodily outlets, commonly called a head cold when from the eyes or nose.
(2) A salt solution of Pilocarpus from the leaves of the jaborandi plant used to stimulate sweating.

a cord across two thirds of it, not admitting more than can dance inside the space. The dressing-room should be provided with servants; small cards, with the names of invited guests, should be in readiness to pin to the wraps of each: or checks used. All the requisites of the toilet should be on hand.

If a gentleman acts as escort to a lady, he must call at the hour she appoints, with a carriage, and in the course of the afternoon send a bouquet. Upon reaching the house of the hostess he must escort his charge to the dressing-room, leave her at the door, make his own toilet, and return to meet her there again; escort her to the ball-room, and to the hostess. She is obliged to dance the first dance with him, but after that she may select other partners.

He must be her escort to supper, and ready to escort her home. If a gentleman is unaccompanied by a lady he must solicit one of the ladies of the house for the first dance, and yield gracefully if she declines, and consent smillingly if she requests him to lead out the homeliest of her wall-flowers. Do not strive to obtain a particular position in the quadrille(1). If a stranger, apply to the managers for a partner, and you will be presented to a lady with whom you may dance. This does not entitle you to claim her acquaintance afterward. Never solicit a strange lady to dance until you have been presented to her for that purpose. If you should see a lady in the ball-room to whom you have been introduced at some previous time, and she recognizes you, it is no breach of etiquette to ask her to dance; but it is better to secure the services of the manager.

Gentlemen cannot be too careful not to injure the dresses of the ladies. White or light tinted gloves are indispensable. Lead the lady through the quadrille; do not drag her or clasp her hand too tight. Never dance unless acquainted with the figures and with some of the steps. Dance quietly. Let your motion be from the hips down. Do not pride yourself on the neatness or your steps. When waltzing with a lady do not press her waist, but touch it lightly with the open palm of your hand. If a lady should civilly decline to dance with you, making an excuse, and you see her dancing afterward, do not notice it, nor be offended.

The music must be first a march, then a quadrille, a polka, a waltz, a galop, and so on, with 2 or 3 round dances to each quadrille, until 14 dances are completed, when another march announces supper; 7 to 10 dances may follow. Each guest must be provided with a printed programme of the dances, and space for engagements upon it, and with a pencil attached. After a dance conduct the lady to a seat, if she does not decline.

The supper-room must be thrown open at midnight, and remain so until the ball closes. It shows bad taste for gentlemen to cluster round the table in groups and remain there. The hostess should see that no young lady loses her supper for want of escort. If there are no young gentlemen in the family, she must request one of her guests to act. No gentleman should

(1) A dance consisting of five movements, executed by four sets of couples, each forming the sides of a square.

wait until the music has commenced before selecting his partner. A lady who declines dancing on pretext of fatigue must dance no more, unless she wished to rest for that dance alone. If a gentleman offers to dance with a lady she should not refuse, unless for some particular reason, in which case she can accept the next offer. It is a breach of manners to offer a partner in dancing an ungloved hand. When a lady is standing in a quadrille a gentleman not acquainted with her partner should not converse with her. No lady should converse with a gentleman while engaged with a partner, unless certain that her gentleman acquaintance is on familiar terms with her partner.

Unless a man has a graceful figure, and can use it with elegance, it is better for him to walk through the quadrilles. Do not withdraw from a quadrille when your assistance is needed to complete the pleasure of others.

The master of the house should see that all the ladies dance. He should take notice of those who seem to serve as drapery to the walls, and should see that they are invited. Ladies who dance much should not boast of the number of dances for which they are engaged. They should also recommend less fortunate ladies to gentlemen of their acquaintance. For any members of the family at whose house the ball is given to dance frequently denotes ill breeding. The ladies should not occupy places in a quadrille which others may wish to fill, and they should be at leisure to attend to the rest of the company; and gentlemen should entertain married ladies and those who do not dance. Confidential conversation is in bad taste. A misunderstanding of any kind at a public ball should be refereed to the master of ceremonies, and his decision accepted. A lady should not enter or cross the ball-room unattended. While a dance is in progress it is in bad taste to make arrangements for another.

In tendering a lady an invitation to dance she should be allowed to designate the set, and the gentleman should fulfill the engagement. It is impolite for a gentleman to enter the ladies' dressing-room. To remain too late is not well-bred, and implies that you are unaccustomed to such pleasures. In extending an invitation to a lady to dance, various forms may be used, such as "May I have the honor of dancing this set with you?" "May I have the pleasure?" etc. Or if the lady be engaged for the first dance following the introduction, the gentleman may request the favor of putting his name upon her card for another. No gentleman should take the vacant seat next to a lady unless acquainted, and not then without permission.

A gentleman must offer his arm to lead a lady to and from the dance. A lady must be careful not to engage herself to two gentlemen for the same dance, unless, for a round dance, she states, "I am engaged for the first half of the waltz, but will dance the second part with you; then she must tell her first partner. A young lady should not dance more than twice with the same gentleman. Every gentleman must invite the ladies of the house to dance; and he will devote himself or a portion of the evening to those ladies for whom the May of life has passed away. Decline the invitation of a lady you may accompany home to enter the house; but you may request permission to call. It is a breach of etiquette for a lady or gentleman to forget an engagement. Excepting for the first dance, it is not etiquette for married people to dance together. Do not cross a room in an anxious manner, and force your way up to a lady to receive a bow. Should you desire to withdraw before the party breaks up, go quietly out without saluting even the mistress of the house, unless you can do so without attracting attention.

BALM OF GILEAD:

Opodeldoc(1), spirits of wine, sal ammoniac, equal parts of each; shake; bottle and label. Relieves neuralgia, pains, aches, etc. Apply as a lotion.

BALSAM, INDIAN:

Clear, pale resin, 3 pounds, and melt it, adding spirits of turpentine, 1 quart: balsam of tolu, 1 ounce; balsam of fir, 4 ounces: oil of hemlock, origanum, with Venice turpentine, of each 1 ounce; strained honey, 4 ounces; mix well and bottle. Dose, 6 to 12 drops; for a child of 6, 3 to 5 drops, on a little sugar. The dose can be varied according to the ability of the stomach to bear it and the necessity of the case. It is a valuable preparation for coughs, internal pains, or strains, and works benignly upon the kidneys.

BANDAGES:

Bandages can be made by tearing a sheet into narrow strips, rolling each one tightly and fastening the end with a pin. Old linen does not mean worn-out shirt-fronts, but soft pieces of table-clothes, napkins, or cambric handkerchiefs.

BANNERS, TO PAINT:

Stretch the fabric upon a frame and finish your design and lettering. Use a size made of bleached shellac dissolved in alcohol, thinned to the proper consistence, go over such parts as are to be gilded or painted, overrunning the outlines slightly, to prevent the color from spreading. For inside work the white of an egg makes a good size; lay the gold while the size is still wet; when dry, dust off the surplus gold, and proceed with the shading, painting, etc. A little honey, combined with thick glue, is another good size.

BARBER'S ITCH, OR SYCOSIS:

Little pimples on the hairy parts of the face and nape of the neck, with matter at the top, and with the shaft of a hair passing through them; are of a pale yellowish color, and in a few days burst; the matter forms into

(1) A camphorated liniment made of camphor and essential oils.

hard, brownish crusts, which fall off in one or two weeks, leaving purplish, sluggish pimples behind, which disappear very slowly.

Treatment: Shaving had better be discontinued and the beard merely cropped off with scissors; all intemperance in eating and drinking, and exposure of the face to heat, must be avoided; a light, cool diet will do much toward curing the disease. The nitrate of mercury ointment, or the iodide of lead ointment, or carbolized oil, (1 part carbolic acid to 10 of olive or linseed oil), with frequent sponging with carbolic acid soapsuds, are useful applications.

BARK-LICE:

Judicious pruning of the branches, draining the land where the trees stand, manuring the soil and keeping it free from grass and weeds—all have the effect to promote vigorous growth, and are, therefore, useful in preventing the depredations. For killing the lice, the best things are strong lye made of wood ashes, a solution of caustic soda of potash, diluted soft soap, or a mixture of lime whitewash and kerosene oil. If the latter is employed, the proportions of the mixture should be 1 pint of kerosene to 1 gallon of whitewash.

BARNS, LOCATION OF:

It is not well to build barns too near the road, observes a recent writer, and we indorse his further criticism on the subject. It looks bad to see the road used for the barn-yard, with a lot of old drays, wagons, and plows standing by the fence, and hay and straw scattered in front. This is not the worst objection, for when threshing barns are near the road it is often the case that horse-power or engine is placed in the road and travel obstructed for two or three days. Barns should be from six to a dozen rods from the highway.

BAROMETER, TO MAKE:

(1) Take a long, narrow bottle, and put into it $2\frac{1}{2}$ drams of camphor; spirits of wine, 11 drams. When the camphor is dissolved add to it the following mixture: Water, 9 drams; saltpeter, 38 grains; sal ammoniac, 38 grains. Dissolve these salts in the water prior to mixing with the camphorated spirit; then shake all well together, cork the bottle well, wax the top, but afterward make a very small aperture in the cork with a red-hot needle. By observing the different appearances which the materials assume as the weather changes, it becomes an excellent prognosticator of a coming storm or a sunny sky.

(2) *One that answers the purpose of indicating the approach of fair or foul weather can be made as follows:*

Take an 8-ounce bottle, the glass being clear and white, and put into it 6 ounces of the highest-colored whiskey to be obtained, and put into it all the gum camphor it will dissolve and a little more. Set in some convenient place. On the approach of rain or bad weather the camphor will settle toward the bottom of the bottle; the heavier the rain or the more sultry the weather is indicated by the feather-like appearance of the camphor, which rises and floats in the liquid. If alcohol is used it must be diluted so that it will not be stronger than the whisky, for if it is, so much of the camphor will be held in solution that the atmosphere will have no perceptible effect upon it.

(3) Take an 8-ounce phial and put in it 3 gills of water, and place in it a healthy leech, changing the water in summer once a week and in winter once a fortnight, and it will most accurately prognosticate the weather. If the weather is to be fine, the leech lies motionless at the bottom of the glass and coiled together in a spiral form; if rain may be expected, it will creep up to the top of its lodgings and remain there till the weather is settled; if we are to have wind, it will move through its habitation with amazing swiftness, and seldom goes to rest till it begins to blow hard; if a remarkable storm of thunder and rain is to succeed, it will lodge for some days before almost continually out of the water, and discover great uneasiness in violent throes and convulsive-like motions; in frost, as in clear, summer-like weather, it lies constantly at the bottom; and in snow, as in rainy weather, pitches its dwelling in the very mouth of the phial. The top should be covered with a piece of muslin.

BASKETS:

The life of a splint or willow basket can be indefinitely prolonged if, when it begins to give way, strips of cotton are woven into it and wound round the frame-work. This treatment will not only lengthen the life of the basket, but will keep it from catching and tearing every garment that comes in contact with its broken splints. Where wood is used as a fuel, a basket for carrying into the house is a very great saving of litter. Fasten into the basket a lining of strong bagging, and this will prevent strain on the basket, and also keep the bits of bark and sawdust from rattling through it. A bushel basket with two strong handles is best for this use.

BATH-BAG:

Make a small square bag of flannel, leaving one end partly open. In this put all the remnants of soap as the pieces become too small to handle easily. When the bag is filled, baste up the opening, and it makes a good bath-tub arrangement.

BATHERS, HINTS TO:

(1) Open-air bathing suggests itself as a timely subject for discussion. It is a

luxury which in hot weather all long to indulge in, and yet many deny themselves the gratification, fearing that harm may possibly follow. They rightly recognize that cold bathing is salutary under certain conditions of the system, while in others it is capable of doing much harm. As no rule can be fixed for the guidance of all, in order to assist the doubtful reader we must consider certain facts regarding the application of cold to the skin; when these are understood he will be much better able to judge whether open-air bathing is likely to be beneficial or injurious to him.

(2) A bath is considered cold when the water is below 70 degrees Fahr. The first or direct effect of it is sedative, or, properly speaking, depressing to the system. If one remains long in cold bath this is the only influence it has. But if it is left quickly, in a place tolerably warm, a reaction occurs, and the temperature of the surface of the body rises about 1 degree above what it was before the water was entered. If a person on leaving the cold bath experiences a sense of unusual heat in the skin, is refreshed, stronger, lighter, then he may feel certain that the nerves, blood vessels, and all the organs of the body are excited to a more healthy and energetic action.

(3) Of course, as before stated, if one, no matter how healthy, remains too long in a cold bath the depressing symptoms are sure to follow, and therefore the duration must be considered in estimating whether its effect is beneficial or injurious.

(4) It is safe to say that for those persons who are strong and robust cold bathing is salutary(1).

(5) There is a large class of persons who, while not having any actual disease, are yet weakened by excesses, such as dissipation, confinement within doors, deep study, and other close mental application; for them cold bathing is indicated and proves bracing and salutary. It is also beneficial in sleeplessness, nervous disquietude, and debility, constipation, chronic catarrhal troubles, corpulency, dyspepsia, where the circulation is sluggish, and in a very great variety of other affections. In fact, cold bathing is one of the most efficient tonic measures, and physicians depend upon it in the treatment of no inconsiderable proportion of their patients.

(6) Sea-bathing in the North can be considered cold bathing, for the surf temperature is rarely 70 degrees. It differs considerably from the fresh-water bathing. Salt-water is more stimulating, and some of its constituents are to a certain extent absorbed by the skin. Again, the surroundings of sea-bathers are more cheerful. During their

(1) Promoting or preserving health.

sojourn at coast resorts they are, as a rule, free from care, and hence in a condition mentally favorable for improvement.

(7) During the summer those who are vigorous can bathe in salt or fresh water every day if they care to; the less strong should not do so oftener than on alternate days. All bathers should enter the water quickly. The immersion should be sudden, and a bold dive is the best. The effect is then uniform. If one wades into the water hesitatingly the blood is driven from the lower extremities to the upper parts, and temporary congestion therein is induced.

(8) The ancient theory that after exercise and while perspiring freely the body should be allowed to cool before bathing is no longer accepted. It is well to exercise first, for thereby general circulation is stimulated, the temperature of the body elevated, and prompt reaction is insured.

(9) An hour before noon and before going to bed are the best times to bathe. The average duration of the bath should be from 5 to 10 minutes for children, 15 minutes for women, and but little longer for men. To delay much beyond these periods is a pernicious practice, inviting debility and injury. As has been said, how often one sees, in a stroll along a popular sea-beach, groups of drenched, miserable objects, with blue lips, chattering teeth, and wrinkled, clammy skin, who have been spending half a morning in alternately plunging into the waves and walking about, dripping in the cool air. All trace of reaction has disappeared in these too enthusiastic bathers, and they return from what should have been an invigorating dip in a condition approaching collapse, and often requiring the use of alcoholic stimulates to restore the system to full vitality. Such abuse of sea-bathing is, unfortunately, too common, even among those who have sought the sea-side for the improvement of impaired health.

(10) On leaving the water one should rub down with a coarse towel, until the skin is heated and reddened, and, after dressing rapidly, a brisk walk for a short distance should be taken to quicken circulation. Those who feel weak and depressed after a bath will do well to take a cup of hot tea or coffee; rarely will the use of more powerful stimulants be indicated. They should also, if possible, determine the cause of the depression; it may be due to some systematic disturbance which must be overcome before cold bathing will be admissible.

BATHING AND HEALTH:

Bathing in Ancient Times: In the early ages among all the leading nations of the East bathing was one of the most flourishing institutions. The baths were celebrated for their magnificence. They often formed parts of buildings of vast extent and grandeur, termed Gymnasia, and were large enough to accommodate several thousand persons at the same time. In these baths were centered all that was elaborate in workmanship, elegant in design, and beautiful in art. Nothing was thought too grand or magnificent for their decoration. Precious gems and metals, and the finest works of the painter and sculptor, were to be found within their walls. The great hall of the bath was generally ornamented with the statues of Hercules, the god of strength, Hygeia, the goddess of health, and Æsculapius, the god of medicine.

The Object of the Ancient Bath: The chief and ever-guiding purpose of the bath was to give health and strength to the physical system, and thus make accomplished warriors. The bath was not merely for luxury or pleasure. It bore an important part of the imperatively enjoined system of thorough training for the future. In modern times the people, during their leisure hours, patronize places of amusement; in the ancient times those hours were largely devoted to the baths and the gymnasia. These were very properly fostered by the national authorities, as the "tribute money" of the people was wisely made to cover their support.

Fresh and Salt Water Bathing: Salt-water is a stimulant to the skin, and in many cases is to be preferred for the bath. It is, however, more exhaustive to the system, and special care should be taken in its use by invalids that it should not be prolonged or severe. The sea-water is found by experience to be milder than salt-water artificially prepared, and to possess tonic properties superior to the latter.

Caution in Sea-side Bathing: "We love this air of the sea," writes a correspondent, "and taken aright, which one soon learns, is a tonic to drink in with exquisite delight. That does not mean than an invalid should face an ocean storm, or that he should ever allow himself to get chilly; for, though cold is often healthful, real chilliness never is. To be borne at all, it must be very temporary. If you do not know how to breathe, and forget that the nose is the chimney, and rush to the sea with the mouth wide open and a yell, you may get as hoarse as the waves, and be the shorn lamb to which the wind will not be tempered. But, if only very briefly, you will adjust yourself to the changed air, avoid at first the dampness of morning or evening, and have changes of clothing ready to adjust and to get full vigor of the ocean life."

Season for Sea-Bathing: In the Middle Atlantic States the bathing season extends from the middle of June to the middle of September. Farther north the season is shorter, and farther south longer. In the Middle States, if there are no indications of unhealthfulness of the place, the season may be safely extended from four to six weeks later.

Duration of the Sea-Bath: *On this head much ignorance prevails, and much damage to health and needless delays in the cure of disease are caused by such ignorance. Very many persons, especially of the younger class, stay in the water until they are tired, and are often surprised that they should pay the tax for their rashness in subsequent suffering from some one or more of the following disorders:* viz., Defective reaction, as shown by paleness of the skin, blueness of the lips, sleeplessness, loss of appetite, rheumatic pains, headache, bronchitis in those with a delicate chest, earache, fullness of the head, giddiness, and various spasmodic affections. From the same care arises disturbed digestion, manifested by pains of the stomach, nausea, and diarrhea.

Surf-Bathing: This kind of sea-bathing is a luxury to those who are strong and vigorous. An eminent physician, however, expresses the opinion that the high surf, which many seek, is more harmful than helpful to a majority of those who indulge in it. A low or gentle surf is to be preferred. We strongly recommend the erection of strong inclosures in the surf in such manner as to permit the free ebb and flow of the tide, and yet break the force of the surf wave. Such inclosures in time of the heavy surf would be exceedingly serviceable to a large proportion of sea-side bathers.

Best Hour for Bathing: A rule of the most general, if not universal, application is, that the bath should be taken before a meal, and never on a full stomach, or during the first stages of digestion. By general consent, a morning hour is preferred for sea-bathing. Comparatively few, however, choose the time before breakfast for the purpose. Invalids with a cold skin and languid circulation will require a slight refreshment, a cup of good chocolate, a plate of plain soup, or a soft boiled egg with a roll, before bathing. If an early or noon-day dinner be taken, an evening bath may be used with advantage, and in some cases it is found to agree better with invalids than in the morning.

Bathing Indoors: This should be frequent and thorough. The bath-room should be an essential part of every dwelling. Every person should use it for "health's sake" once a week, at least. In many cases twice a week would be still better, and in some cases a daily bath would be useful. When taken frequently, it should be used only for a few minutes.

The "Towel Bath:" A thorough rubbing daily, first with a coarse and then with a soft towel, immediately after the morning wash, is always healthful, providing it can be done without chilliness or exhaustion of the strength. Continue the towel exercise until the body is thoroughly dry, and until the glow of the skin becomes assured.

Temperature of Baths: The cold bath is a tonic, and must be used with caution. The tepid and warm bath is slightly tonic and sedative, and induces sleep. It should generally be taken immediately before retiring. Hot baths are debilitating when used for any length of time. It is very rarely beneficial to take hot baths unless they are followed at once by a cold shower-bath to tone down the system.

Best Baths for Children: We have no hesitation in recommending a warm bath early in the day, followed by simple douche of cold water, as far preferable to the cold bath; or a warm bath at night for the sake of cleanliness, and none at all in the morning. It may be taken as a rule that, in the case of children, sudden changes of temperature are dangerous, and that 58 degrees to 60 degrees may be taken as the safe average temperature in which they should be constantly kept.

Turkish and Russian Baths: The only difference between Turkish and Russian baths is that in the former the bather is first submitted to hot air, and in the latter to hot vapor. The processes of shampooing, showering, plunging, rubbing, and kneading, are the same in both. In both baths the bather reclines for some time, until he is thrown by the hot air or vapor into a profuse perspiration. He is then rubbed by an attendant, and afterward receives a shower or douche of cold water. The duration of the bath depends upon the constitution and habits of the bather, and may be 2 minutes or 2 hours. These baths are of excellent service in rheumatism, neuralgia, and various nervous conditions, aside from their general cleansing and invigorating qualities.

Medicated Baths: The alkaline bath is especially efficient in curing itching and other diseases of the skin, and is made by putting 8 ounces of impure carbonate of potash into 30 gallons of tepid water. The nitro-muriatic bath is for diseases of the liver, and is composed of 2 ounces of nitric acid, 3 ounces of muriatic acid, and 10 1/2 gallons of water.

Convenient Vapor Baths: Simple and convenient vapor baths may be made by placing a large pan or pail containing boiling water under a cane-bottomed chair. The patient seats himself upon it, enveloped from head to foot in a blanket, which covers the bath as well. Sulfur, spirit, herbal and other baths may be obtained in the same manner.

Electric Baths: (1) In these baths electricity is diffused through the water of the bath-tub. Special advantages arise from the improved method of applying electricity in the treatment of disease over the more ordinary methods. The friends of this system argue that water, at blood temperature, is a better

(1) Experimenting with electric baths could be fatal!

conductor of electricity than the human body; hence the diffusion of the electric current through the water and to the whole periphery of the body intensifies and insures more certain results. Moreover, they claim its influence thus conditioned, in promoting the absorption of the medicines dissolved in the water, and its power to "through chemical affinity, to facilitate the elimination from the body of certain metallic substances, and to further the absorption of morbid deposits." A number of cases are related in support of the theories advanced, and a category of diseases given deemed to be especially amenable to this kind of treatment.

Hot Sand Baths: One of the most attractive therapeutical novelties for some time past in London, recently introduced from the Continent, consists in the erection of establishments for administering hot sand baths as a remedy for rheumatism, recent cases of nervous disorders, affections of the kidneys, and all cases where heat is needed as the chief remedial agent. The advantages claimed on behalf of this method of treatment are, that it does not suppress respiration like the hot water bath, but rather increases it, and does not interfere with the respiration, after the manner of the steam bath or Turkish bath. It is found that the body can endure the influence of this kind of bath for a much longer time, and a much higher temperature can be applied.

Bathing Dresses: There is no doubt that the less cumbersome the clothing the more beneficial the bath, and ladies who are fortunate in having private bathing places will find a flannel dress, made with a loose blouse waist and short closed drawers, very nearly perfection; but for the ordinary bather, who has to take her chances with many others, there is no better design than the one which serves also as a gymnastic suit, and consists of a sailor blouse, skirt, and trousers. Twilled flannel, dark blue or Russian gray, is the most serviceable material for bathing dresses, as it does not chill or hold the water. White, black, or red braids are the usual trimmings, put on broad and clusters, or simply as bindings, according to taste.

BATHING AND PERSONAL BEAUTY:

Tepid water is preferable for every season of the year. Milk baths have been in favor from time immemorial with ladies, and nothing is better than a daily hot bath of milk. Mme. Tallien was among the historical women who bathed in milk, to which she added crushed strawberries to give it an agreeable perfume.

For a full length bath a bag of bran will soften the water and make the skin deliciously smooth and fair; but no bath is perfect in its results without the long and brisk friction of hands or a coarse towel afterward. Friction not only stimulates circulation, but it makes the flesh firm and polished like Parian marble. It is sometimes astonishing to see the change made in an ugly skin by friction, and any lady who wishes to possess a healthful body, firm to the touch and fair to the eye, with the elasticity of youth well prolonged into age, must give willingly of her strength to the daily task of rubbing the body thoroughly.

For healthy persons of good physique warm baths are admirable at times for cleansing purposes. Very stout persons find hot baths useful for reducing corpulence, but that is a medicinal and not a sanitary measure. Every one who prizes good health and intends to maintain it should indulge in a dry rub upon going to bed. A fresh brush is good for the purpose, but a good rough towel is better. The object is to keep the pores open and in healthy activity. Turkish and Russian baths are luxuries and sometimes remedies and so they should always be regarded. If a man wishes to indulge, better take the Turkish.

BATTLEDOOR AND SHUTTLECOCK(1), THE GAME OF:

This is a game indulged in by adults as well as by the youngsters, but although a capital game, in that it affords good exercise and amusement, it is not so popular as it once was. Ordinarily, battledoors are either made entirely of wood, or else with wooden handles and "drum" heads of parchment. A more expensive kind of battledoor is made of box-wood for handle, with a strained net, like the bat used in lawn tennis. Either of the first two may be purchased for a small sum at any toy-shop, and they will be found much better than home-made battledoors.

The shuttlecock also is better bought than made; it consists mainly of a bit of cork, in which goose feathers of equal size have been stuck obliquely. The object of the game when played by one player is, after having thrown the shuttlecock in the air, to keep it bounding and rebounding, by repeated strokes of the bat end of the battledoor, as long as possible. It will be found that the shuttlecock ascends and descends with the feathers downward and upward respectively. When more than one player indulges in the game, the players should be stationed at equal distances round the ground, each armed with a battledoor, and by the aid of the battledoors a shuttlecock, or more than one if it is desired, should be kept passing round and round.

BAY RUM, TO MAKE:

Saturate $^{1}/_{4}$ pound of carbonate of magnesia with oil of bay; pulverize the magnesia, place it in a filter, and pour water through it until the desired quantity of obtained, then add alcohol. The quantity of water and alcohol employed depends on the desired strength and quantity of the bay rum.

(1) Badminton.

Another: Oil of bay, 10 fluid drams; oil of pimento, 1 fluid dram; acetic ether, 2 fluid drams; alcohol, 3 gallons; water 2 $^1/_2$ gallons. Mix, and after two weeks' repose, filter.

BED-BUGS:

(1) Take the furniture in which they harbor to pieces and wash all the joints with soap and boiling water, carefully exploring all the cracks and openings with a stiff piece of wire; when the wood is dry, saturate the joints with kerosene oil, using a small paint-brush; fill up the cracks with a mixture of plaster and linseed oil; if the rooms are papered, saturate the places where the paper joins the baseboard with benzine, using a brush or a sponge, and carefully avoid the presence of a light; do the same with the linings of trunks; if the floor cracks are infested fill these with plaster and linseed oil.

(2) Two ounces of red arsenic, $^1/_4$ pound of white soap, $^1/_2$ ounce of camphor dissolved in a tea-spoonful of spirits rectified, made into a paste of the consistency of cream; place this mixture in the openings and cracks of the bedstead.

(3) Touch all you can with a feather duster dipped in carbolic acid; remove all clothing, and then fumigate the room and bedding with brimstone; close the room tightly, and in 24 hours all bugs will have vanished.

BED DRESSING, A PRETTY:

A pretty way to dress a bed is to make a set, cover and long sham of cheesecloth of pale pink or blue, or any color that harmonizes with the general tone of the room. The sham is to be long enough to cover the two pillows or a bolster. Cut a center-piece of the desired size and turn over the hem 2 in. in width, feather-stitch this down with wash embroidery silk or some of the new flax floss in white or any tint liked. Around this sew a 2-in. insertion of torchon or crochet lace, then another hem 2 in. wide of the cheesecloth. A spray of flowers may be embroidered in the center if desired, and the edge may be finished with lace. When lace is put on the spread it is only run along the sides, which are not tucked in, but allowed to fall over the wood-work.

A very pretty set is make of cream-colored cheesecloth, with sprays of woodbine(1) painted in rich autumn tints, the feather stitching being done in the pale blue. Line the spread and sham with cambric, and if cream-colored cheesecloth is used, some tint may be placed underneath to show slightly through.

(1) European climbing honeysuckle.

BED-MAKING:

The first item of bed-making is demanded from the occupant of the couch. Her duty it is, immediately upon rising, to throw back the covers over the foot of the bed on to a couple of chairs placed there for that purpose. They should never be tossed in a heap on the floor to gather dust from the carpet or matting. The mattress should then be half turned, that the air may get at both sides of it, and the windows opened at top and bottom, admitting a sluice of fresh outer atmosphere. Even in the coldest weather this should be done for a few minutes, while in summer the bed should stand uncovered for at least an hour before making.

The habit of leaving one's room in perfect order when one goes to breakfast is not commendable as far as the bed is concerned. The other arrangement necessary may be done then, but the couch should be left stripped until the unpleasant vapors generated by the body during the night have been dispersed and the bed thoroughly sweetened.

BEDROOMS, SOME HINTS ABOUT:

The care of a bedroom is sometimes neglected because of the apparent simplicity of the work. The style in which it is usually accomplished is known to every one. The bed is not all that needs close care in the sleeping-room. The dusting is far more important than many people suspect. Accumulations of fluff and dust form a favorite nesting-place for disease germs and unsavory smells. On this account many ornaments are not to be commended in a bed-chamber. The bits of drapery, the brackets, the gay Japanese fans, the photographs and the pieces of bric-a-brac that are admirable in other parts of the house are out of place here. Whatever furniture there is should be carefully wiped off each day with a soft cloth and this shaken out of the window afterward.

The room should receive a thorough sweeping at least once a week, and at this time every article in it should be moved and no nook nor corner left unbrushed. If there are curtains at the windows they should be well shaken, that no dust may linger in their folds. The receptacles for waste water should be washed out every day and scalded three times a week. In hot weather the scalding would take place every day, and the utensils be sunned, if possible.

Wash-cloths should be wrung out in boiling water every other day. Without this they soon become offensive. Shoes and other articles of apparel should not be left lying about the room to gather dust and look untidy. Soiled clothes should never be left in a sleeping-room. They contaminate the atmosphere. When all these precautions are closely followed there will be no trouble with the close, unpleasant odor that one finds often in even handsome and apparently well-kept bedrooms. Such malodors are not only disagreeable, but positively unwholesome, especially for delicate persons and children.

BEDS, DAMPNESS IN:

After the bed is warmed put a glass globe in between the sheets, and if the bed be damp a few drops of wet will appear on the inside of the glass.

BEDS, TO WARM:

(1) Take a long stone quart bottle, let it be filled with boiling hot water, with a good cork; wrap it up in 2 or 3 folds of flannel or woolen cloth; this done about $^1/_2$ hour before bedtime, introduce it between the sheets at the foot of the bed; the water thus bottled will be found to retain its heat till the next morning.

(2) Providing one has neither warming-pan(1) nor soapstone(2), bricks make a very good substitute; heat them well, wrap in thick brown paper so as not to scorch, and move about between the sheets.

(3) To heat a bed at a moment's notice, throw a little salt into a warming-pan and suffer it to burn for a minute previous to use.

To Ascertain when a Bed is Aired: Introduce a glass goblet between the sheets for a minute or two, just when the warming-pan is taken out; if the bed be dry, there will only be a slight cloudy appearance on the glass; but if not, the damp on the bed will assume the more formidable appearance of drops, the warning of danger.

BEDS AND BED-CLOTHES:

A bed, whatever it be made of, should be so flexible that all parts of the body may rest upon it equally. It ought to adapt itself to the outline of the body in whatever position the body may be placed. The very hard mattress which yields nothing, and which makes the body rest on two or three points of corporeal surface, should be excluded from use. On the other hand, the bed that is so soft that the body is enveloped in it, though it may be luxurious, is too oppressive, hot, and enfeebling; it keeps up a regular fever, which cannot fail to exhaust both physical and mental energies.

The best bed is one of two kinds: A fairly soft feather bed laid upon a soft horse-hair mattress; or a thin mattress laid upon one of the elastic steel-spring beds. Heavy bed-clothes are a mistake; weight in no true sense means warmth. The light down quilts or coverlets are best to use. One of these quilts takes well the place of two blankets, and they cause much less fatigue from weight than layer upon layer of blanket covering. It should be the rule to learn so to adapt the clothing that the body is never cold and never hot while under the clothes.

(1) A long handled covered pan for holding hot coals used in airing and warming beds.
(2) Saponite: essentially hydrated silicate of magnesia and alumina, sometimes resembling soap.

BED-SORES, TO PREVENT:

The patient being often obliged to lie in one position, bed-sores occur, being due to long-continued pressure on parts whose general vitality is weakened. They usually form at the lower end of the backbone. Much may be done to prevent them by keeping the under sheet perfectly smooth, clean, and dry. Pressure on any one point may be avoided by changing position frequently. The parts of the body resting most heavily on the bed, when the skin is not broken, should be sponged three or four times daily with alcohol or whisky and water. Air-cushions, so made as to remove all pressure from the lower end of the backbone, are useful.

BEEF, GOOD, TO CHOOSE:

The grain of ox beef, when good, is loose, the meat red, and the fat inclining to yellow. Cow beef, on the contrary, has a closer grain, a whiter fat, but meat scarcely as red as that of ox beef. Inferior beef, which is meat obtained from ill-fed animals, or from those which had become too old for food, may be known by a hard, skinny fat, a dark red lean, and, in old animals, a line of horny texture running through the meat of the ribs. When meat pressed by the finger rises quickly, it may be considered as that of an animal which was in its prime; when the dent made by pressure fills slowly, or remains visible, the animal had probably passed its prime, and the meat consequently must be of inferior quality.

BEEFSTEAK, HOW TO HAVE GOOD:

The finest beef is required for really good steak. Steaks cut from three different parts of the beef are in request for private tables and restaurants, know as tenderloin, porter-house and round steak. The last is most commonly seen, because, having no fat, suits the many who have Jacks Sprat's taste; yet it is far inferior in juice and tenderness to the two other cuts named. Tenderloin steak cut from prime beef cannot be excelled. Porter-house cut from it is next choice. Beefsteak should be cut in slices 1/2 in. thick.

If the beef is of the right quality, by no means beat it, as in this way much of the sweetness escapes. Have a clear bed of coals over which to place a griddle with slender bars, well warmed and greased. Lay the steak on the bars and cook it just to the degree that pleases the palate of those for whom you are providing. Some persons who like it rare insist that five minutes is ample time to allow for having it done perfectly, while others have a disgust for any save a well done, thoroughly cooked meat, and would prefer their steak to remain over the fire for 15 minutes.

A cook should accommodate herself strictly to the instructions of her employer, and learn how to please parties who widely differ. Cooking beefsteak upon an ordinary stove is to fill a kitchen with a smell of burnt fat, which may be avoided by having a charcoal brazier for this purpose put in some airy place, the charcoal supplying good heat without smoke. No gravy is so good as the pure juice from the meat, joined with a little butter added to the meat as soon as it is lifted from the gridiron. Pepper the steak when first put upon the griddle, but let salt be added to taste at table. Mustard should always be at hand, ready mixed for those who like it as a condiment for their beefsteak.

BEE-HIVE COVERS, TO PREVENT LEAKING:

To prevent bee-hive covers from leaking, tack on flour-sacks and give them two good coats of paint, and they will stand outdoors for years and not leak a drop.

BEER, GINGER:

(1) To a pail half filled with boiling water add one pint of molasses and two spoonfuls of ginger; when well stirred, fill the pail with cold water, leaving room for one pint of yeast, which must not be put in until the preparation becomes lukewarm. Place it on a warm hearth for the night and bottle in the morning.

(2) White sugar, 20 pounds; lemon juice, 18 ounces; honey, 1 pound; bruised ginger, 17 ounces; water, 18 gallons; boil the ginger in 3 gallons of the water for half an hour; then add the sugar, the juice, and the honey, with the remainder of the water, and strain through a cloth; when cold, add the white of an egg and 1/2 ounce of the essence of lemon; after standing 4 days, bottle. This beverage will keep for many months.

BEER, ROOT:

Mix together a small amount of sweet fern, sarsaparilla, winter green, sassafras, princesspine(1), and spicewood. Boil them with 2 or 3 ounces of hops and 2 or 3 raw potatoes, pared and sliced, in 3 or 4 gallons of water. After boiling 5 or 6 hours, strain off the liquor, and add to it common molasses in the proportion of 1 quart to 3 gallons of the beer. If it is too thick, dilute it with water. A half pound of browned bread added to the liquor will increase its richness.

BEES, HOW TO MANAGE:

The great secret, or charm, as many people suppose it to be, can all be summed up in one word—"smoke". One can handle them just as well as another, if they have the nerve and determined will to do so, and this knowledge and the bee-smoker are the first requisites. The bee-smoker is a small bellows with a tin fire-box attached for burning rotten wood or cotton rags, or, in fact, any thing that will burn and make a good smoke. There are now a half-dozen or more kinds in the market that sell from 75 cents to $2,

(1) Probably prince's pine or pipsissewa, a plant of the heath family.

so that no one who keeps even a single hive of bees need have any excuse for being without one. Never go to a hive of bees to do any thing with them without your smoker trimmed and burning.

The first thing before disturbing the hive in any way, puff a few whiffs of smoke in at the entrance; this will generally drive in the sentinels, and also prevent any from coming out. If they are Italians, this will almost always be sufficient; but if they are crosser kinds, it had better be repeated a few times. This will frighten and excite them, and they will at once fill themselves with honey, which makes them very docile, unless they are accidentally pinched.

After waiting a few minutes, the lid or cover to the hive may be raised, but do it gently; in fact, always do every thing gently about them, as all quick motions or jars of the hive tend to exasperate them. As soon as you raise the lid a little, send in more smoke, and enough, if necessary, to drive them down and out of the way; then proceed to put on or take off boxes, or do all the work necessary. If they begin to come up or to dispute your right, use more smoke to convince them you are master of the situation. But from the very start just make up your mind that you can and will, and that is half the battle. With Italians, after the first few puffs of smoke, they can often be handled for an hour or two without any more smoke, but with blacks or hybrids it may be necessary to repeat the dose every few minutes. Smoke does not injure them at all.

BEE STINGS, CURE FOR:

Take a pinch in the finger of common salt, put on the place stung and dissolve with water, rub with the finger. If not relieved in one minute, wet the place with aqua ammonia. Care should be taken not to get the ammonia into the eye.

BEESWAX, TO RENDER:

To render beeswax, put the wax into a thin muslin bag, and add some pebbles to make it sink into a wash-boiler containing water. Let it boil, then press out the wax with a pair of squeezers, (i.e.,two narrow boards fastened together at the end with a cord). Then skim and pour into a bucket partly filled with warm water and set away to cool.

BELLADONNA(1) MIXTURE:

To be taken as a preventive when fevers or any infectious complaints are prevalent. Extract belladonna, 5 ounces; aqua cinnamomi, 2 ounces. Take 15 drops of the above in a table-spoonful of water every morning for 10 or 12 days. Children to have as many drops as they are years old.

(1) The leaves of the deadly nightshade plant, used for treating fevers, palsy, pertussis, epilepsy, etc.

BENZINE, USES OF:

Benzine dissolves fats and oils, resins, varnishes, paint, etc., so readily that it is largely used for the purpose of cleaning clothing and other fabrics. It is within the recollection of many that benzine was once rather costly, and could only be purchased in small bottles at a high price. Now it is cheap; the makers of kerosene produce so much more benzine than there is a demand for that, at wholesale at least, it bears but a nominal price. Benzine, in careless hands, is a very dangerous article, and no one should use it without understanding its properties, that accidents may be guarded against. It boils at 140 degrees Fahr., and at all ordinary temperature rapidly evaporates. When this vapor is mingled with the air, the two form a mixture which, in contact with a flame, will explode violently. The vapor of the benzine, when not mixed with air to form an explosive mixture, will readily take fire and burn rapidly. A bottle partly filled, in a warm room, will give off the vapor so freely that it will take fire even when at a distance of several inches from a lamp.

In working with benzine, always use it by daylight and in a room without a fire, or so far from a fire that there can be no danger. These facts cannot be too thoroughly impressed upon all who have occasion to use this liquid for any purpose. In using benzine and other solvents for removing grease or other spots from fabrics, a mere wetting often is given, and after the benzine has evaporated the place looks worse than before.

By applying a little benzine, the grease or other substance is dissolved, and this solution spreads to the surrounding portions of the cloth, and the evil is increased. We must use the liquid in such a manner as to dissolve the grease and then to carry away the solution; we must, in fact, wash out the spot with benzine. To do this, it is not necessary to immerse the article or a large portion of it. In removing a spot, first fold some old woolen cloths, or even porous newspapers, to form a thick pad. Place this pad under the article, and wet the spot with benzine. Use a sponge or a roll of woolen cloth and rub the spot, adding more benzine as it is taken up by the pad below. In this manner the benzine holding the grease, etc., in solution, is absorbed by the pad, and the solution is washed out of the cloth by successive quantities of benzine, to be also carried down into the pad.

Success depends upon using sufficient benzine; it is cheap ,and one need not be sparing of it. Gloves are cleaned by immersing them in benzine in a wide-mouthed, glass-stoppered bottle. The gloves are shaken up with the liquid for a few minutes, taken out, squeezed, and hung under a chimney to dry. If any spots are left, these are rubbed with a rag wet with benzine. If the gloves retain any odor, they are placed on a plate, covered by another, and the whole set upon a kettle of boiling water. The heat will soon drive off the odor.

BEVERAGES, SUMMER:

Lemonade and Lemons: Lemonade is a simple and grateful beverage. To make it best, roll the lemons on something hard till they become soft; cut or grate off the rinds, cut the lemons in slices and squeeze them in a pitcher, (a new clothes-pin will answer for a squeezer in lieu of something better). Pour on the required quantity of water, and sweeten according to taste. After mixing thoroughly, set the pitcher aside for half an hour, then strain the liquor through a jelly-strainer and put in the ice. Do not drink lemonade if your physician tells you there is an excess of acid in your system.

Lemons for Excessive Thirst: When persons are feverish and thirsty beyond what is natural, indicated in some cases by metallic taste in the mouth, especially after drinking water, or by a whitish appearance of the greater part of the surface of the tongue, one of the best coolers, internal or external, is to take a lemon, cut off the top, sprinkle over it some loaf sugar, working it downward into the lemon with the spoon, and then suck it slowly, squeezing the lemon, and adding more sugar as the acidity increases from being brought up from a lower point.

Lemons at Tea-time: A lemon or two thus taken at tea-time, as an entire substitute for the ordinary supper of summer, would give many a man a comfortable night's sleep and an awakening of rest and invigoration, with an appetite for breakfast, to which they are strangers who will have their cup of tea or supper of relish or cake and berries or peaches and cream.

Various Drinks: If any thing is added to the summer drink it should contain some nutriment, so as to strengthen the body as well as to dilute the blood, for the purpose of a more easy flow through the system; as any one knows that the thinner a fluid is the more easily does it flow.

Some of the nutritious and safe drinks are given below, especially for those who work in the sun of summer; all to be taken at the natural temperature of the shadiest spot of the locality; to any of them ice may be added, but it is a luxurious, not a beneficial, ingredient, nor a safe one.

(1) Buttermilk; (2) a pint of molasses to a gallon of water; (3) a lemon to half a gallon of water and a teacupful of molasses, or as much sugar; (4) vinegar, sugar, and water are substitutes, but the vinegar is not a natural acid, contains free alcohol, hence it is not as safe or healthful; (5) a thin gruel made of corn or oats, drank warm, is strengthening; (6) a pint of grapes, currants, or garden berries to half a gallon of water is agreeable.

Orangeade: *It is thus composed:* Take of dilute sulphuric acid, concentrated infusion of orange peel, each 12 drams; syrup of orange peel, 5 fluid ounces. This quantity is added to 2 imperial gallons of water. A large wine-glassful is taken for a draught, mixed with more or less water, according to taste.

BILIOUSNESS(1), SYMPTOMS AND CURE:

Bad blood, too much blood, giving headache, bad taste in the mouth mornings, variable appetite, sickness at stomach, chilliness, cold feet, and great susceptibility to taking cold. No one person may have all these symptoms when bilious, but one or more is always present. Sometimes a bilious person has a yellow tinge in the face and eyes, called bilious because the bile, which is yellow, is not withdrawn from the blood; it is the business of the liver to do that, but when it does not do it, it is said to be lazy, does not work, and the physician begins at once to use remedies which are said to promote the action of the liver.

It has been discovered within a few years that acids act on the liver, such as nitric acid, elixir vitriol, vinegar; but these are artificial acids, and do not have the uniform good effect of natural acids—those found in fruits and berries.

Almost all persons become bilious as the warm weather comes on; nine times out of ten nature calls for her own cure, as witness the almost universal avidity for greens, for spinach in the early spring, these being eaten with vinegar; and soon after by the benign arrangement of Providence the delicious strawberry comes, the raspberry, the blackberry, the whortleberry; then the cherries and peaches and apples, carrying us clear into the fall of the year, when the atmosphere is so pure and bracing that there is general good health everywhere. The most beneficial method of using fruits and berries as health promoters is to take them at dessert, after breakfast and dinner; to take them in their natural, raw, ripe, fresh state, without cream or sugar, or any thing else besides the fruit themselves. Half a lemon eaten every morning on rising, and on retiring, is often efficacious in removing a bilious condition of the system, giving a good appetite and greater general health.

First, on getting up and going to bed, drink plenty of cold water. Eat for breakfast, until the bilious attack passes, a little stale bread, say one slice, and a piece as large as your hand of boiled lean beef or mutton. If the weather is warm, take instead a little cracked wheat or oatmeal porridge. For dinner take about the same thing. Go without your supper.

Exercise freely in the open air, producing perspiration, once or twice a day. In a few days your biliousness is all gone. This result will come even though the biliousness is one of the spring sort, and one with which you have from year to year been much afflicted. Herb drinks, bitter drinks, lager beer, ale, whisky, and a dozen other spring medicines are simply barbarous.

(1) An ailment of the bile or liver.

BILLS OF FARE, TWELVE:(1)

(1) **Dinner for Six Persons:** (January.) *First course*: Palestine soup; fried smelts; stewed eels. *Entrées:* Ragout of lobster; broiled mushrooms; vol-au-vent of chicken. *Second course*: sirloin of beef; boiled fowls and celery sauce; tongue, garnished with Brussels sprouts. *Third course:* Wild ducks; Charlotte aux pommes; cheesecakes; transparent jelly, inlaid with brandy cherries; blanc-mange; Nesselrode pudding.

(2) **Dinner for Eight Persons:** (February.) *First course*: Mock-turtle soup; filets of turbot à créme; fried filleted soles and anchovy sauce. *Entrées:* Curried mutton; macaroni à la Milanaise. *Second course*: Stewed rump of beef la jardinière; roast fowls; boiled ham. *Third course:* Roast pigeons; rhubarb tartlets; meringues; clear jelly; cream; iced pudding; soufflé. Dessert and ices.

(3) **Dinner for Five Persons:** (March.) *First course:* Bonne femme soup; boiled turbot and lobster sauce; salmon cutlets. *Entrées:* Compôte of pigeons, fillet of mutton and tomato sauce. *Second course:* Roast lamb; boiled half calf's head, tongue, and brains; boiled bacon-cheek, garnished with spoonfuls of spinach; vegetables. *Third course:* Ducklings; plum-pudding; ginger cream; trifle; rhubarb tart; cheese-cakes; fondues, in cases. Dessert and ices.

(4) **Dinner for Six Persons:** (April.) *First course:* Tapioca soup; boiled salmon and lobster sauce. *Entrées:* Calf's head en tortue; oyster patties. *Second course:* Saddle of mutton; boiled capon and white sauce; tongue; vegetables. *Third course:* Soufflé of rice; lemon cream; Charlotte à la Parisienne; rhubarb tart. Dessert.

(5) **Dinner for Twelve Persons:** (May.) *First course:* White soup; asparagus soup; salmon cutlets; boiled turbot and lobster sauce. *Entrées:* Chicken vol-au-vent; lamb cutlets and cucumbers; fricandeau of veal; stewed mushrooms. *Second course:* Roast lamb; haunch of mutton; boiled and roast fowls; vegetables. *Third course:* ducklings; goslings; Charlotte rum; vanilla cream; gooseberry tart; custards; cheese-cakes; cabinet pudding and iced pudding. To conclude with dessert and ices.

(6) **Dinner for Eight Persons:** (June.) *First course:* Vermicelli soup; trout à la Genévé; salmon cutlets. *Entrées:* Cotelettes d'agneau purée de pois; Madras dry curry. *Second course:* Roast beef; tongue; boiled ham; vegetables. *Third course:* Roast ducks; compote of gooseberries; strawberry jelly; pastry; iced pudding; cauliflower with cream sauce. Dessert.

(1) See "French Terms Used in Cooking".

(7) Dinner for Ten Persons: (July.) *First course:* Soup à la Paysanne; crimped salmon and parsley batter; trout aux frais herbes. *Entrées:* Salmi of duck; macaroni with tomatoes. *Second course:* Loin of veal with béchamel sauce; salad; braised ham; vegetables. *Third course:* Turkey poult; lobster salad; cherry tart; lemon cream; marrow pudding. Dessert and ices.

(8) Dinner for Eight Persons: (August.) Soup Julienne; fillets of turbot and Dutch sauce; red mullet. This forms the first course. *For entrées:* Riz de veau aux tomatoes; fillets of ducks and peas. *Second course:* Haunch of venison; boiled capon and oysters; ham garnished and vegetables. *Third course:* Leveret; fruit jelly; compote of greengages; plum tart; custards; omelette soufflé. Dessert and ices to follow.

(9) Dinner for Eight Persons: (September.) *First course:* Palestine soup; red mullet and Italian sauce. *Entrées:* Minced fowl and macaroni; lamb cutlets, with purée de pois. *Second course:* Loan of veal, with bechamel sauce; roast haunch of venison; braised hare; grouse pie; vegetables. *Third cours*e: Roast hare; plum tart; whipped cream; peach jelly. Dessert.

(10) Dinner for Twelve Persons: (October.) *First course:* Carrot soup à la Créci; soup à la Reine; baked cod; stewed eels. *Entrées:* Riz de veau and tomato sauce; vol-au-vent of chicken; pork cutlets and sauce Robert; grilled mushrooms. *Second Course:* Rump of beef à la jardinière; roast goose; boiled fowls and celery sauce; tongue, garnished; vegetables. *Third course:* Grouse; pheasants; quince jelly; lemon cream; apple tart; compote of peaches; Nesselrode pudding; cabinet pudding; scalloped oysters. Dessert and ices.

(11) Dinner for Six Persons: (November.) *First course:* Game soup; slices of codfish and Dutch sauce; fried eels. *Entrées:* Kidneys à la maitre d'hôtel; oyster patties. *Second course:* Saddle of mutton; boiled capon and rice; small ham; lark pudding. *Third course:* Roast hare; apple tart; pineapple cream; clear jelly; cheese-cakes; marrow pudding; Nesselrode pudding. Dessert.

(12) Dinner for Twelve Persons: (December.) Game soup; carrot soup à la Créci; codfish au gratin; fillets of whitings à la maitre d'hôtel. *Entrées:* Fillet de boeuf and sauce piquante; fricasseed chicken; oyster patties; curried rabbit. *Second course:* Roast turkey and sausages; stewed beef la jardinière; boiled leg of pork; vegetables. *Third course:* Partridges; Charlotte aux pommes; mince-pies; orange jelly: lemon cream; apple tart. Dessert and ices.

BILLS OF FARE FOR THE FAMILY:

There should be no fixed routine of the different kinds of food. Fish on Friday should be the only landmark of the week. Nor should the housekeeper, in her desire to preserve the health of her husband and children, make too great a run upon dietetics.

Graham bread, rice-pudding, and oatmeal are very well in their way, but there is such a thing possible as having too much of them. Good food—even rich food if taken in moderation—is not necessarily unwholesome for grown people of undyspeptic constitutions.

Fried articles are not dangerous if the frying is properly done, and consists of a quick browning in boiling fat, instead of a slow soaking in lukewarm grease.

Pastry should never be a daily occurrence. When it is rich it is both good and indigestible; when it is cheap it is bad and still more indigestible.

Many hints may be gleaned by the housekeeper who endeavors to study variety in her menus if she will read the market reports. A suggestion now and then is of infinite value to the woman who has to evolve from her inner consciousness something over 1,000 bills of fare per annum. One woman, who resembled Mrs. Bagnet in so far that she longed to get troublesome matters off her mind, used regularly to write out every Saturday night a bill of fare for each meal of the following week. The plan is worthy of imitation. Where there are wide variances of taste and digestion, individual peculiarities have to be consulted by the caterer, but a general outline can almost always be put down in black and white to serve as a guide.

BIRD-CATCHER, THE GAME OF:

One of the party is chosen to be the bird-catcher. The rest fix upon some particular bird whose voice they can imitate when called upon, the owl being the only bird forbidden to be chosen. Then sitting in order round the room with their hands on their knees, they listen to the story their master has to tell them.

The bird-catcher begins by relating some incident in which the feathered tribe take a very prominent position, but particularly those birds represented by the company. Each one, as the name of the bird he has chosen is mentioned, utters the cry peculiar to it, never for a moment moving his hands from his knees. Should the owl be referred to, however, every one is expected to place his hands behind him, and to keep them there until the name of another bird has been mentioned, when he must, as before, place them on his knees.

During the moving of the hands, if the bird-catcher can succeed in securing a hand, the owner of it must pay a forfeit, and also change places with the bird-catcher.

When the leader, or bird-catcher, as he is called, refers in his narrative to "all the birds of the air," all the players are to utter at the same time the cries of the different birds they represent.

BIRD LIME:

Take any quantity of the middle bark of the holly. Boil it in water for several hours, until it becomes quite soft. Drain off the water and place the holly bark in a hole in the earth, surrounded with stones; here let it remain to ferment, and water it, if necessary, until it passes into a mucilaginous state. Then pound it well and wash it in several waters. Drain it and leave it for 4 or 5 days to ferment and purify.

BIRDS, TO PRESERVE:

Small birds may be preserved as follows: Take out the entrails, open a passage to the brain which should be scooped out through the mouth; introduce into the cavities of the skull and the whole body some of the mixture of salt, alum, and pepper, putting some through the gullet and whole length of the neck; then hang the bird in a cool, airy place, first by the feet that the body may be impregnated by the salts, and afterward by a thread through the under mandible of the bill, till it appears to be sweet; then hang it in the sun, or near a fire; after it is well-dried, clean out what remains loose of the mixture, and fill the cavity of the body with wool, oakum, or any soft substance, and pack it smooth in paper.

BIRDS AND BIRD-FOOD:

Places for Cages: Place the cages so that no draught of air will strike them. Avoid placing them near the stove, fire-place, or register. About half-way between the floor and ceiling is best, as the temperature there is preferable. The room should never be heated above 70 degrees.

Size of Cage Perches: Very many mean to give their birds all things needed to make them bright and happy, and at the same time are guilty of great cruelty in regard to perches. The perches in a cage should be each one of different size and the smallest as large as a pipe-stem. If perches are of the right sort no trouble is ever had about the bird's claws growing too long; and of all things keep the perches clean.

Food for Canary-birds: Give nothing to healthy birds but rape and canary seed, water, cuttle-fish bone, and gravel-paper or sand on the floor of the cage, no hemp-seed, and a bath 3 times a week. When moulting (shedding feathers) keep warm; avoid all draughts of air. Give plenty of German rape-seed; a little hard-boiled egg, mixed with crackers grated fine, is excellent. Feed at a certain hour in the morning. By observing these simple rules birds may be kept in fine condition for years. For birds that are sick or have lost their song procure bird-tonic at a bird-store.

Care of Young Canaries: Feed young canaries with white and yelk of hard eggs, mixed together with a little bread steeped in water. This should be pressed and placed in one vessel, while in another should be put some boiled rape-seed, washed in fresh water. Change the food every day. When they are a month old put them in separate cages.

Parasites: The red mite, a minute insect, almost invisible to the naked eye, but easily seen through the microscope, is found in large numbers in nearly all cages containing canaries, particularly those which are kept in dark rooms away from the light. These tiny creatures shun the light, and generally leave the birds during the day, concealing themselves in the cracks and crevices of the cage until darkness arrives, when they sally forth to attack the canaries. By continually irritating them, they cause a loss of sleep which occasions many diseases and very often is the cause of their death.

How to Destroy Parasites: The presence of these insects is indicated by the uneasy manner the birds exhibit, becoming dispirited and sitting in a drooping position on the perches or on the ground. It is difficult to get rid of them. A plan simple and effectual is to place in the cage a hollow reed with 3 or 4 gimlet-holes along it, as a substitute for the ordinary perch. The mites hide in the reed with the return of light, and can be readily shaken from it. In a short time the insects can all be destroyed by this easy process.

Food for Mocking-birds:

(1) One medium-sized boiled potato (without salt) and the yelk of one hard-boiled egg, chopped together very thin when warm. In cold weather this may last 2 days, but in summer should be made fresh daily.

(2) Ground or bruised hemp-seed, 16 ounces; ground or bruised rice, 4 ounces; dust of butter-crackers, 8 ounces; flax-seed meal, 2 ounces; mix and put in a pan with 2 ounces of lard, and cook until it has a brown color stirring with a spoon to keep it from sticking or getting into lumps; 1 or 2 table-spoonfuls a day, with grated carrot, is sufficient.

Thrushes—Food: The male bird may be distinguished from a hen by a darker back and the more glossy appearance of the feathers. The breast also is white. Their natural food is insects, worms, and snails. In a domesticated state they will eat raw meat, but snails and worms should be procured for them. Young birds are hatched about the middle of April, and should be kept very warm. They should be fed with raw meat, cut small, or bread mixed in milk with hemp-seed well bruised; when they can feed themselves give them lean meat cut small, and mixed with bread or German paste(1), plenty of clean water, and keep them in warm, dry, and sunny situation.

Bullfinches: Old birds should be fed with German paste, and occasionally rape-seed. The Germans occasionally give them a little poppy-seed, and a grain or two of rice, steeped in Canary wine, when teaching them to pipe, as a reward for the progress they make. Bird-organs, or flageolets, are used to teach them to sing. Bullfinches breed 2 or 4 times a year. The young require to be kept very warm, and to be fed every 2 hours with rape-seed, soaked for several hours in cold water, afterward scalded and strained, bruised, mixed with bread, and moistened with milk. One, two, or three mouthfuls at a time.

Linnets and their Food: Male birds are browner on the back than the hens, and have some of the large feathers of the wings white up to the quills. Canary and hemp-seed, with occasionally a little groundsel, watercress, chickweed, etc., constitute their food.

Blackbirds and their Food: The cock-bird is of a deep black, with a yellow bill. The female is a dark brown. It is difficult to distinguish male from female birds when young, but the darkest generally are males. Their food consists of German paste, bread, meat, and bits of apple. The same treatment as given for the thrush applies to the blackbird.

Skylarks: The cage should be of the following proportions: Length, 1 ft. 5 in.; width, 9 in.; height, 1 ft. 3 in. There should be a circular projection in front to admit of a fresh turf being placed every 2 or 3 days, and the bottom of the cage should be plentifully and constantly sprinkled with river sand. All vessels containing food should be placed outside, and the top of the cage should be arched and padded, so that the bird may not injure itself by jumping about.

Their food in a natural state consists of seeds, insects, and also buds, green herbage, as clover, endive, lettuce, etc., and occasionally berries. When confined they are usually fed with a paste made in the following manner: Take a portion of bread, well-baked and stale, put it into fresh water, and leave it until quite soaked through, then squeeze out the water and pour boiled milk over it, adding two thirds of the same quantity of barley-meal well sifted, or, what is better, wheat-meal. This should be made fresh every 2 days. Occasionally the yelk of a hard-boiled egg should be crumbled small and given to the birds, as well as a little hemp-seed, meal-worms, and elderberries. Great cleanliness should be observed in the cages of these birds.

(1) A paste composed of hard-boiled eggs, pea-meal, sweet almonds, lard, sugar, and hay saffron.

BISCUITS, HOW TO SECURE GOOD:

At present this favorite bread is generally made with baking or yeast powders, but a few general hints concerning their preparation may be useful to inexperienced housekeepers. The cook should be instructed to roll her dough till only half as thick as you wish your biscuits to be when done, if any of the above powders are used, as it will rise a great deal, in spite of being stuck with a fork—a part of the biscuit-making process never to be neglected. Nothing can be more inelegant than a large, thick biscuit.

Let the oven be well heated before the cook begins to make up her dough even, for the quicker the process the more likely it is to be successful. Biscuits should be baked in about 10 minutes, brown and crisp, but not hard. Occasionally a person is found who likes soft, white biscuit; if so, special directions may be given to that effect, for this may be considered an idiosyncrasy of taste. A biscuit should be cut not more than 3 in. in diameter, and not more than one-third in. in thickness. For variety, biscuits may be made out of hand instead of being cut with a cutter. Strange as it seems, so small a matter makes a decided change in the look and the taste of the article, and it is well worth a housekeeper's while to study all these little ways of gratifying that love of novelty so inherent with us all, but with the young especially.

A popular bread for the tea-table is supplied by merely taking as much biscuit-dough as would suffice for one biscuit, dividing it into two parts, and rolling each part out round until the circumference is 5 in. instead of 3. Stick with a fork here and there over the surface. The cakes will be very thin, of course, and can be cooked in 5 minutes, the oven being moderately and steadily heated. Let them brown, but not the least burnt. Prepare as many as your family require. A pint of flour will furnish a nice plateful.

BITES AND STINGS, CURE FOR:

Apply instantly with a soft rag, most freely, spirits of hartshorn(1). The venom of stings being an acid, the alkali nullifies them. Fresh wood ashes, moistened with water and made into a poultice, frequently renewed, is an excellent substitute, or soda, or saleratus, all being alkalies.

BITES OF SNAKES AND DOGS, TREATMENT:

(1) Apply immediately strong hartshorn and take it internally; also give sweet oil and stimulants freely; apply ligature right above part bitten, and then apply a cupping-glass.

(2) In case of a bite of a venomous serpent, the old historic method of sucking the wound with the lips is one of the first things to be resorted to. If the poison is in the circulation, the use of strong brandy or

(1) From the dry distillation of the horn of male deer, consisting mainly of ammonia and volatile bases.

whisky in quantities powerful enough to produce intoxication must be resorted to. The bite of a mad dog should be cauterized at once by a pencil of lunar caustic, or by application of irons heated white. The peculiarity of hydrophobic poison is that it remains in the spot where the bite occurs for several days or weeks, and not until the poison ferments does it become dangerous.

Dr. Hewett, a surgeon of London, allowed himself to be bitten no less than eighty times by rabid dogs, each time successfully cauterized the wound. He fell a victim to his temerity, however, for one day he was found dead with a pistol-shot from his own hand. A statement was left in his papers that he had neglected the cauterization too long, and feeling the first symptoms of hydrophobia, he preferred to die without the long agony.

BLACK, TO COLOR:

Allow 4 pounds of woolen material to 1/2 pound of copperas(1). Wring the goods very dry out of warm water, and put into the copperas that has been boiling in water an hour. Set aside until cool enough to wring, then wash thoroughly in clear cold water. Boil 2 pounds of logwood tied in a bag 1 hour. Allow the articles to remain in this till cool enough to wring, then put them in water that dry clover has been steeped in for about 1/2 hour to prevent smutting. Dry thoroughly and wash.

BLACK ANTS:

Place fresh bones where they congregate; they will gather upon them and may be scalded.

BLACKBERRY BRANDY:

Take 10 gallons of brandy and use 5 quarts nice rich blackberries, mashed; macerate the berries in the liquor for 10 days, then strain off and add 1 ounce sugar to each gallon. If strawberries are used, work the same proportions with half the quantity of sugar.

BLACKBERRY WINE:

The usual process for other fruit juices may be followed. To a gallon of the berries, well braised, add a quart of boiling water. Allow these to stand for 24 hours, stirring occasionally. Then strain and press out the juice, and add 2 pounds of sugar to each gallon. Place the liquid in a jug to ferment. The jug must be kept full by adding from time to time some of the juice kept for the purpose.

When fermentation ceases, cork the jug and keep in a cool place 3 or 4 months, after which the wine may be bottled, carefully pouring it off

(1) Sulphates made up of iron, copper, and zinc, called respectively blue, white, and yellow copperas.

from the sediment. Of course, larger quantities may be made with the same proportions in a cask.

BLACKBIRDS, FOOD OF:

The natural food of the blackbird is berries, worms, insects, shelled snails, cherries, and other similar fruit; and its artificial food lean fresh meat, cut very small, and mixed with bread or German paste.

BLACK CLOTHES, TO RESTORE:

Boil 3 ounces of logwood in a quart of vinegar, and when the color is extracted drop in a piece of carbonate of iron the size of a large chestnut. Let it boil 5 minutes. Have the article to be dyed sponged with soap and hot water, laying it on the table and sponge it all over with it, taking care to keep it smooth and brush downward. When completely wet with the dye, dissolve a tea-spoonful of saleratus in a tea-cup of warm water, and sponge over with this, which sets the color so nothing rubs off. They must not be wrung or wrinkled, but carefully hung up to drain. The brownest cloth may be made a perfect black in this simple manner. So many people have faded garments that this recipe may be of service in restoring them to a lively color.

BLACKING:

For harness: Melt 4 ounces of mutton suet with 12 ounces of beeswax, add 12 ounces of sugar candy, 4 ounces of soft soap dissolved in water, and 2 ounces of indigo finely powdered. When melted and well mixed, add $^{1}/_{2}$ pint of turpentine. Lay it on the harness with a sponge and polish off with a brush.

For Boots and Shoes:

(1) Ivory black, 2 pounds; molasses, 2 pounds; sweet oil, 1 pound; rub together till well mixed, then add oil vitriol, three-fourths pound; add coarse sugar, $^{1}/_{2}$ pound, and dilute with beer bottoms. This cannot be excelled.

(2) Ivory black, $1^{1}/_{2}$ ounces; sperm oil, 3 drams; strong oil of vitriol(1), 3 drams; common vinegar, 1/2 pint. Mix the ivory black, molasses, and vinegar together, then mix the sperm oil and oil of vitriol, and add them to the other mixture.

For Leather: Fill a bottle half full of nails or rusty bits of iron, then fill with sharp vinegar; shake every few days for a while; in a few weeks it will be fit for use. It improves with age. When used down, fill up again with vinegar. When boots become red, wet in the blacking and oil them. They will look

(1) A name for the sulfates of iron, lead, and nickel.

as good as new. The oil sets the color, and it will neither rub nor wash off. It is good for all kinds of leather, and will not injure it in the least.

BLACK TONGUE IN CATTLE:

The symptoms are inflammation of the mouth, swelling of the head and face, discharge of bloody saliva, and high fever marks the first stage. Ulcers soon appear under and on the sides of the tongue. Then the throat and neck swell, and if the disease is not checked gangrene ensues and the animal dies. The disease is said to yield readily to early and proper treatment.

The following has proved very successful:

The animal should be bled from the neck vein. Give him castor oil, 1 pint, to be repeated in 10 hours if it should not operate. Then use the following: Powdered burnt alum, 4 ounces; chloride of lime, 2 ounces; corn meal, 2 quarts. Mix, and with this powder swab the mouth frequently.

BLACK WALNUT, TO POLISH:

To give black walnut a fine polish, so as to resemble rich old wood, apply a coat of shellac varnish, and then rub it with a smooth piece of pumice-stone until dry. Another coat may be given and the rubbing repeated. After this, a coat of polish, made of linseed oil, beeswax, and turpentine, may be well rubbed in with a dauber made of a piece of sponge tightly wrapped in a piece of fine flannel several times folded and moistened with the polish. If this work is not fine enough, it may be smoothed with the finest sand-paper, and the rubbing repeated. In the course of time the walnut becomes very dark and rich in color, and in every way superior to that which has been varnished.

BLANKET, ROMAN, TO KNIT:

Five stripes, 3 of black and 2 of Roman colors. Stripes are 50 stitches wide, and 275 ribs long. Take off the first and seam the last stitch in each row. Crochet strips together with 4 stitches black, 4 white, and 4 yellow.

Material: Germantown wool sixfold, one and five-eights pounds of black, 1/4 pound of cherry, 1/4 pound of blue, 1/4 pound pearl white, and 2 ounces of yellow, shade bordering on orange. For fringe, 1 thread of yellow with 3 of black for black stripes, Roman colors for Roman stripes.

Arrangement of colors: One row of white, 1 row of blue, 1 row of cherry, 1 row of blue, 1 row of yellow, 1 row of cherry, 1 row of white, 12 row of blue, 1 row of white, 1 row of cherry, 1 row of blue, 1 row of yellow, 1 row of white, 1 row of cherry, 1 row of blue, 10 rows of white, 1 row of white, 1 row of cherry, 1 row of blue, 1 row of yellow, 1 row of cherry, 1 row of white, 16 rows of cherry.

BLANKETS, TO STORE:

Spread a large coarse sheet on the floor; fold up the blankets and place them on it, having sprinkled between every fold either shreds of tobacco or bits of camphor; having piled the blankets smoothly, put the remainder of the sheet around them and over them, and pin up tightly in various places; then lay the whole in a large chest or dark closet; let them remain unopened during the summer.

BLANKETS, TO WASH:

Put 2 large table-spoonfuls of borax and 1 pint bowl of soft-soap into a tub of cold water; when dissolved put in a pair of blankets and let them remain there over night; next rub them out and rinse thoroughly in two waters, and hang them to dry; do not wring them. This recipe will also apply to the washing of all kinds of flannels and woolen goods.

BLEACHING COTTON:

(1) Cotton is more easily bleached and appears to suffer less from the process than most other textile substances. In the chemical system of bleaching the goods are "washed" and "bucked" as on the old plan, then submitted to the action of a weak solution of chloride of lime, and afterward passed through water soured with hydrochloric or sulphuric acid, when they have only to be thoroughly washed, and to be dried and finished, for the entire completion of the process.

(2) Into 8 quarts of warm water put 1 lb. of chloride of lime; stir with a stick a few minutes; then strain through a bag of coarse muslin, working it with the hand to dissolve thoroughly; add to this 5 bucketfuls of warm water, stir it well and put in the muslin; let it remain in 1 hour, turning it over occasionally that every part may be thoroughly bleached; when taken out wash well in two waters to remove the lime, rinse and dry. This quantity will bleach 25 yds. of yard wide muslin. The muslin will bleach more evenly and quickly if it has been thoroughly wet and dried before bleaching.

BLEACHING COTTON CLOTHES:

(1) A bleaching preparation may be made by dissolving 2 lbs. of sal soda in 1 gallon of hot water, and add 1 lb. of good lime; stir the mixture a few minutes, allow it to stand for 1/2 hour, and then carefully pour off and bottle the clear liquid; 1/2 pint of this may added to each tub of water.

(2) 1 table-spoon of turpentine boiled with white clothes will aid the whitening process.

BLEACHING LINEN CLOTHES:

(1) Work them well in water, to which some strained solution of chloride of lime has been added, observing to well rinse them to clean water, both before and after the immersion in the bleaching liquor. The attempt to bleach unwashed linen should be avoided, as also using the liquor too strong, as in that case the linen will be rendered rotten.

(2) Linen garments which have become yellow from time may be whitened by being bathed in a lather made of milk and pure white soap, 1 lb. of the latter to 1 gallon of the former. After the boiling process the linen should be twice rinsed, a little blue being added to the last water used.

BLEACHING SILK:

Silk is usually bleached by first steeping it and then boiling it in solutions of white soap in water, after which it is subjected to repeated rinsings, a little indigo blue or archil being added to the last water to give it a pearly appearance. When required to be very white the goods are cautiously submitted, for 2 or 3 hours, to the action of the fumes of burning sulphur, and then finished by rinsing, as before. Boiling or sulphuring is not required for the white silk of China.

BLISTER, TO DRESS:

Spread a little blister compound on a piece of common adhesive plaster with the right thumb. It should be put on just thickly enough to conceal the appearance of the plaster beneath. The part from which a blister has been taken should be covered over till it heals with soft linen rages smeared with lard.

BLISTERED HAND OR FEET:

When the hands are blistered from rowing, or the feet from walking, or other causes, be careful not to allow the blisters to break, if possible. Some persons are in the habit, by means of a needle and piece of worsted, of placing a seton(1) into blisters to draw off the water; but, in our opinion, this is a great mistake and retards the healing. Bathe the blisters frequently in warm water, or, if they are very severe, make a salve of tallow dropped from a lighted candle into a little gin and worked up to a proper consis-

(1) A few horsehairs or small threads passing under the skin to promote drainage.

tence, and on going to bed cover the blisters with this salve and place a piece of clean soft rag over them.

BLOOD, ITS RELATION TO LIFE AND HEALTH:

Change and Waste: A great change is constantly taking place in every part of the human system. The old particles of the body are incessantly passing off in the respiration, perspiration, and excretion. Careful and intelligent observation leads to the belief that the entire body is changed once in 7 yrs. Many parts change much oftener—those which are constantly active many times in a single year. The same body, in its form, appearance, and functions, may remain, but every particle of flesh, bones, skin, etc., is removed and the place occupied by a new particle. So that in all its material element the body is renewed in 7 yrs.

Supply from the Blood: The chief supply in repairing this great waste is furnished by the blood. The blood is "liquid flesh." It is a repository of the ingredients of nutrition. Its materials are so varied and so refined that they penetrate the minutest parts of the physical system, and become assimilated to muscle, bone, skin, hair, cartilage, and nerve.

Quantity of the Blood: The entire quantity of blood in the vessels is but one eighth part, by weight, of the whole body, so that in a man weighing 140 lbs. the quantity of blood is nearly 18 lbs. The quantity of blood, however, as well as its composition varies somewhat at different times. Soon after digestion it is considerably increased, for it has absorbed all the nutritious materials taken with the food, and these materials must necessarily pass through the blood in order to reach the tissues. After long abstinence it is diminished in quantity to a corresponding degree. For the same reason, its composition varies to a certain extent, since its different ingredients will diminish or increase according as they have been discharged or absorbed in greater or less abundance. The blood, therefore, does not coagulate while the circulation is going on, because its fibrine is being incessantly altered and converted into new substances.

It has been found that in certain of the internal organs, especially in the liver and kidneys, the fibrine(1) disappears, and that little or none of it is contained in the blood returning from them. When we come to learn with what rapidity the circulation is carried on, we shall easily understand how coagulation may thus be prevented. But if the blood be withdrawn from the circulation altogether, or confined in any part of a ligature, then its fibrine can no longer go through with the natural changes of its decomposition and it accordingly coagulates, as we have above described.

(1) A protein substance which causes blood to clot & is obtained by stirring blood with a bundle of twigs.

BLOOD BLISTER, TO TREAT:

When a finger is bruised so as to cause a blood blister under the nail it should immediately be drilled with a knife or other sharp-pointed instrument and the blood allowed to escape. This affords instant relief to an injury which may otherwise become exceedingly painful.

BLOOD PURIFIER:

Mix $^1/_2$ ounce sulphate of magnesia with 1 pint water. Dose, a wineglassful 3 times a day. This can be used in the place of iron tonic or in connection with it.

BLOOD-STAINS, TO REMOVE:

(1) These may be obliterated from almost any substance by laying a thick coating of common starch over the place; the starch is to be mixed as if for the laundry, and laid on quite wet.

(2) Steep the article in a solution of iodide of potassium in four times its weight of water. This would probably not injure silk of moderately fast color.

(3) For removing blood-spots from woolen goods of tender colors rub them with the inner side of a crust of bread.

BLOTCHED FACE, WASH FOR A:

Rose water, 3 ounces; sulphate of zinc, 1 dram; mix. Wet the face with it, gently dry it, and then touch it over with cold cream, which also dry gently off.

BLOWING OUT THE CANDLE, GAME OF:

No end of merriment has frequently been created by this simple, innocent game. It is equally interesting to old people and to little children, for in many cases those who have prided themselves on the accuracy of their calculating powers and the clearness of their mental vision have found themselves utterly defeated in it. A lighted candle must be placed on a small table at one end of the room, with plenty of walking space left clear in front of it. One of the company is invited to blow out the flame blindfolded. Should any one volunteer, he is placed exactly in front of the candle, while the bandage is being fastened on his eyes, and told to take 3 steps back, turn round 3 steps, then take 3 steps forward and blow out the light. No directions could sound more simple.

The opinion that there is nothing in it has often been expressed by those who have never seen the thing done. Not many people, however, are able to manage it—the reason why you young people will soon find out if you decide to give the game a fair trial.

BLUING, TO MAKE:

(1) If raw indigo is used to make the bluing water—and in careful hands it is as good as any—a few lumps should be tied gently in a little bag and allowed to soak a short time in the water, which should be cold.

(2) Take best Prussian blue, pulverized, 1 ounce; oxalic acid, also pulverized, 1/2 ounce; soft water, 1 quart; mix; 1 or 2 table-spoonfuls of it is sufficient for a tub of water, according to size of tub.

(3) Dry soluble blue, dissolved in water, makes a good bluing; it can be bought at any drug-store.

(4) 20 lbs. white potato starch, 20 lbs. wheat starch, 20 lbs. Prussian blue, 2 lbs. indigo carmine, 2 lbs. finely ground gum arabic are mixed in a trough, with the gradual addition of sufficient water to form a half-fluid homogeneous mass, which is poured out on a board with strips tacked to the edges. It is then allowed to dry in a heated room until it does not run together again when cut. It is next, cut, with a suitable cutter, into little cubes, and allowed to dry perfectly.

(5) Put a little neutral sulphate of indigo into the water.

BLUING, USE AND ABUSE OF:

An artifice sometimes resorted to by the lazy laundress is an extravagance in bluing. By means of this the dirt is disguised and labor saved. In all these matters the housekeeper must be constantly on the alert. The quality of soap and starch has its share in making the clothes look well. In buying soap it is well to purchase a large quantity and spread it out in a dry place—on the attic floor or upper shelf of a closet; exposure to the air dries and improves it. Old soap lasts much longer than new. A good quality of starch stiffens better than a cheap one. The best brands in both these wares can be ascertained by experiment, taking care always to deal with a reliable firm.

"BOB"-VEAL(1) AS FOOD:

The inquiry is sometimes made why bob-veal is treated with so little consideration by our health officers. It is perfectly true that bob-veal is neither poisonous nor innutritious. The only objections are that it is a watery and rather indigestible substance, standing somewhat in the relation to good veal or beef that skimmed milk does to the pure article. Veal, as would be expected, has almost identically the same amounts of fat, nitrogenous matter, and salts as beef. The tissues, however, have less osmazome, or flavoring matter, are more insipid, and hard to digest. It is a question, however, whether even the bobbest of bob-veal is not better food

(1) Meat from an unborn calf.

than the "lights" which are sold to and eaten by the poor. Bob-veal ought not to be sold for good veal; but under its own name, and at a low price, it might be admitted as an article of food.

BOILS, CURES FOR:

(1) *An experienced and well-known New York physician prescribes the following cure for boils:*

Procure 1 ounce horse-radish root, 1 ounce yellow-dock root, and 1 quart of cider. Boil 10 minutes. Drink a wine-glassful 3 times a day. The physician referred to hinted, sub rosa, that the cider need not be continued after the boils are cured.

(2) As soon as the characteristic culminating point of a boil makes its appearance put in a saucer a thimbleful of camphorated alcohol, and, dipping the ends of the middle fingers into the liquid, rub the inflamed surface, especially the middle portion, repeating the operation 8 or 10 times, continuing the rubbing at each time for about a half minute. Then allow the surface to dry, placing a slight coating of camphorated olive-oil over the affected surface.

One such application in almost all such cases causes boils to dry up and disappear. The application should be made at morning, noon, and in the evening. The same treatment will cure whitlows(1) and all injuries of tips of fingers. As soon as pain and redness appear the fingers should be soaked for 10 minutes in camphorated sweet-oil. The relief is said to be immediate, and three applications are generally enough to affect a cure.

BOOT AND SHOE PRESERVATIVE:

It is said 2 parts tallow and 1 of resin, melted together and applied to the soles of new boots or shoes, as much as the leather will absorb, will double their wear.

BOOTS, RUBBER, TO MEND:

Procure some pure gum, which can be bought at any wholesale rubber house, or you can have your druggist order it for you at a cost of about 5 cents per ounce. At the same time order patching, and it is well to have two thicknesses for mending different goods. Put an ounce or two of gum into 3 or 4 times its bulk of benzine, cork tightly, and allow it to stand 4 or 5 days, when it will be dissolved. Wet the boots with benzine for an inch or more around the hole and scrape with a knife.

Repeat this wetting with benzine and scraping several times until thoroughly cleaned and a new surface is exposed. Wet the cloth side of the patching with benzine and give one light scraping, then apply with a knife a good coating of the dissolved rubber, both to the boot and patch, and allow

(1) Inflammation in the phalanges of the fingers or toes. It may arise spontaneously from a prick of a needle or thorn.

it to dry until it will not stick to your fingers; then apply the two surfaces and press or lightly hammer it into as perfect compact as possible, and set away for a day or two, if possible, before using.

BOOTS, WET, TREATMENT OF:

When boots are wet through do not dry them by the fire. As soon as they are taken off fill them quite full with dry oats. This grain will rapidly absorb every vestige of damp from the wet leather. As it takes up the moisture it swells and fills the boot like a tightly fitted last, keeping its form good and drying the leather without hardening it. In the morning shake out the oats and hang them in a bag near the fire to dry ready for use on another occasion.

BORAX, USES OF:

It may be interesting to some to know that a weak solution of borax-water snuffed up in the nostrils, causing it to pass through the nasal passage to the throat, then ejecting it from the mouth, will greatly relieve catarrh, and in cases not too obstinate or long standing will, if persevered, effect a permanent cure. It is also of great value in case of inflamed or weak eyes. Make a solution, (not too strong), and bathe the eye by opening and shutting it two or three times in the water. This can be done by means of an eye-cup, or equally well by holding a handful of the water to the eye.

Another difficulty with which many persons are afflicted is an irritation or inflammation of the membrane lining the cavities of the nose, which becomes aggravated by the slightest cold, often causing great pain. This can be greatly relieved, if not entirely cured, by sniffing borax-water up the nostrils two or three times a day. The most difficult cases of sore throat may be cured by using it simply as a gargle. As a wash for the head it not only leaves the scalp very white and clean, but renders the hair soft and glossy.

It has been found by many to be of invaluable service in case of nervous headache. If applied in the same manner as in washing the hair the result is wonderful. It may be used quite strong, after which rinse the hair carefully with clear water; let the person thus suffering remain in a quiet, well-ventilated room until the hair is nearly or quite dry, and, if possible, indulge in a short sleep and there will hardly remain a trace of the headache. If clergymen, teachers, and others who have an undue amount of brain work for the kind and quality of physical exercise usually taken would shampoo the head in this manner about once a week, and then undertake no more brain work until the following morning, they would be surprised to find how clear and strong the faculties had become, and there is reason to hope there would be much less premature decay of the mental faculties.

As a toilet requisite it is quite indispensable. If used to rinse the mouth each time after cleaning the teeth it will prevent the gums from becoming diseased or uncleanly. In short, in all cases of allaying inflammation there is probably nothing better in materia medica. The average strength of the solution should be small tea-spoonful to a toilet-glass of water.

BORERS, TO PROTECT TREES FROM:

An Ohio farmer washes his apple-trees every spring and fall with a strong lye that will float an egg, and finds it to be sure death to the borers. He claims that he has not lost a tree since beginning this practice, although he had lost several previously.

BOTANICAL SPECIMENS, TO PRESERVE:

The plants you wish to preserve should be gathered when the weather is dry, and after placing the ends in water let them remain in a cool place till the next day. When about to be submitted to the process of drying place each plant between several sheets of blotting-paper, and iron it with a large smooth heater, pretty strongly warmed, till all the moisture is dissipated. Colors may thus be fixed which otherwise become pale or nearly white. Some plants require more moderate heat than others, and therein consists the nicety of the experiment; but I have generally found that if the iron be not too hot and is passed rapidly, yet carefully, over the surface of the blotting-paper, it answers the purpose equally well with plants of almost every variety of hue and thickness.

In compound flowers, with those also of a stubborn and solid form, as the centaurea, some little art is required in cutting away the under part, by which means the profile and forms of the flowers will be more distinctly exhibited. This is especially necessary when the method employed by Maj. Velley is adopted, viz.: to fix the flowers and fructification down with gum upon the paper previous to ironing, by which means they become almost incorporated with the surface. When this very delicate process is attempted, blotting-paper should be laid under every part excepting the blossoms, in order to prevent staining the white paper. Great care must be taken to keep preserved specimens in a dry place.

BOWELS, BLEEDING FROM THE:

Treatment: Should serious hemorrhage occur, rest and quiet, and cold water poured slowly over the lower portion of the belly, or clothes wet with cold water, or, better, with ice-water, applied over the belly and thighs, and to the lower end of bowels, will ordinarily arrest it. In some cases it may be necessary to use injections of cold water, or even to put small pieces of ice in the rectum.

BOWELS, FALLING OF THE:

A protrusion of a portion of bowel, more commonly in children. It sometimes results from violent purgative medicines, or from the straining at stool in diarrhea or dysentery. In children it sometimes results from allowing or encouraging the child to sit long on the chair.

Treatment: When the bowel is down it should be washed, oiled, and gently returned, then bathed freely with cold water. In children a pad and bandage may be necessary to retain it. The bowels should be carefully regulated, and a seat used so high that the feet cannot touch the floor; the hole should be so narrow as not to draw the buttocks apart. Then the bowel cannot be forced down, and a cure will result. In prolapsus, in the adult, a surgeon should be consulted.

BOW-LEGS:

If the child is healthy, and has good, nourishing food and pure air, it will probably outgrow the bow-legs as its strength increases. Rubbing the legs with the hand in the morning may help to strengthen and straighten them, holding them straight at the same time. If a case is pretty bad, the two legs may be bound together with comfortable bandages during sleep, rubbing them well before and after binding them. If the child is still quite young, it may be kept from standing on its feet for a few months, giving time for the crookedness to straighten while the limbs are growing stronger.

A healthy child, with wholesome food and pure air to breathe, if kept from standing and walking while too young and weak, will not have bow-legs. Scrofulous(1) children are more likely to suffer in this way, and those that are very fleshy.

BOWLS AND SLABS:

Marble bowls and slabs must receive a hebdomadal(2) scrubbing, in addition to the wiping off that should be a daily occurrence. Pumice-stone, sapolio(3) or scourene serves here as upon faucets. On the marble it may be applied with a cloth or a small stiff brush, but for the faucets, stoppers, chains and other plated finishings the brush is preferable, as it carries the soap better into the chinks and interstices. One such scouring as this in a week will keep these platings bright, if it is supplemented by a wiping off with hot water and a rub with a flannel or chamois-skin each morning. The inside of the bath-tub and set foot-tub should also be scrubbed regularly. In the well-regulated house the sinks, washbowls, and faucets should receive attention at least once a week.

When practicable, all drain-pipes should be flushed daily with hot water, if possible, but when that is out of the question, with an abundance of cold. The human body parts with a great deal of greasy matter in the course of its ablutions, and this is apt to form a deposit on the lining of the

(1) An anemic, feeble condition leading to tubercules and ulcerative states of the skin.
(2) Weekly.
(3) Refers to soapstone, hydrated silicate of magnesia and alumina, resembling soap.

waste-pipes that will in time clog them seriously if it is allowed to remain. An excellent compound of potash is sold by druggists and grocers for the special purpose of cleansing waste-pipes. The same work may be accomplished nearly as successfully by a strong solution of washing-soda.

BOX, THE MAGIC:

A quaint story of olden times, recently retold in Golden Days, conveys a pleasing lesson to young people as well as their elders. The story goes that somewhere, many years ago, there lived a housekeeper whose affairs for a long time had been in a very bad way and she knew not what to do. So she went to a wise old hermit who lived in a neighboring cave and told him her trouble. "Things go badly," said she. "Nothing prospers indoors or out. Pray, sir, can you not devise some remedy for my misfortunes?" The hermit reflected, begged her to wait, and retiring to an inner chamber of his cave, after a short time brought out a very curious-looking box, carefully sealed up. "Take this," said he, "and keep it for 1 yr. But you must three times a day and three times a night carry it into the kitchen, the cellar, and the stable, and set it down in each corner. I answer for it that shortly you will find things improve. At the end of the year bring back the box. Now, farewell."

The good woman received the box with many thanks and bore it carefully home. The next day, as she was carrying it into the cellar, she met a servant who had been secretly drawing a pitcher of beer. As she went, a little later, into the kitchen, there she found a maid making herself a very large omelet. In the stable she found the groom selling some hay to a stranger. At the end of the year, faithful to her promise, she carried the box back to the hermit and besought him to allow her to keep it, as it had a most wonderful effect. "Only let me keep it one year longer," she pleaded, "and I am sure all will be remedied." The hermit smiled and replied, "I cannot allow you to keep the box, but the secret that is hidden within you shall have." He opened the box, and lo! it contained nothing but a slip of paper, on which was written this couplet:

"Would you thrive most prosperously
Yourself must every corner see."

BOX MEASURES:

Farmers and market gardeners will find a series of box measures very useful, and they can be readily made by any one who understands the 2-foot rule and can handle the saw and the hammer:

- A box 16 by 16.8 in. square and 8 in. deep will contain a bushel, or 2,150.4 cubic in., each inch in depth holding 1 gallon.

- A box 24 by 11.2 in. square and 8 in. deep will also contain a bushel., or 2,150.4 cubic in., each inch in depth holding 1 gallon.
- A box 12 by 11.2 in. square and 8 in. deep will contain $^1/_2$ bushel or 1,075.2 cubic in., each inch in depth holding $^1/_2$ gallon.
- A box 8 by $8^1/_4$ in. square and 8 in. deep will contain $^1/_2$ peck, or 298.8 cubic in.—the gallon dry measure.
- A box 4 by 4 in. square and 4.2 in. deep will contain 1 quart, or 67.2 cubic in.

BRAIN, HEALTH OF:

Do not overtax the brain. No man should do more work of muscle or of brain in a day that he can perfectly recover from the fatigue of in a good night's rest. Up to that point exercise is good; beyond are waste of life, exhaustion, and decay. In apoplexy a blood-vessel of the brain gives way, and the blood accumulates near its base, and pressing on the cranial nerves, on which the action of the vital organs depends, cuts off the flow of nervous force to the latter.

A slighter effusion may cause only paralysis, from which the patient may recover, the sound healing and the blood being taken gradually up and carried off by the absorbents. Sometimes the serous portion of the blood escapes through the pores of the vessels sufficiently to occasion a similar result. Free livers are especially liable to apoplexy. They keep the vessels too full and the current too strong. Distaste for work, except in one constitutionally lazy, is a sign of cerebral fatigue. Brain-workers should take just enough exercise to keep up a good circulation. For food they require what can be digested easily.

BRASS OR COPPER, TO CLEAN AND POLISH:

(1) First remove all the stains, by rubbing the brass with a flannel dipped in vinegar; then polish with a leather and dry rotten-stone(1).

(2) Rub the surface of the metal with rotten-stone and sweet-oil, then rub off with a piece of cotton flannel and polish with a piece of soft leather. A solution of oxalic acid rubbed over brass soon removes the tarnish, rendering the metal bright. The acid must be washed off with water and the brass rubbed with whiting and soft leather. A mixture of muriatic acid and alum dissolved in water imparts a golden color to brass articles that are steeped in it for a few seconds.

(3) Brass ornaments should be first washed with a strong lye made of rock

(1) Siliceous limestone decomposed for polishing, originally from Tripoli (Tripoli powder).

alum, in the proportion of an ounce of alum to a pint of water. When dry, rub with leather and a fine tripoli. This will give to brass the brilliancy of gold.

(4) Copper utensils or brass articles may be as thoroughly cleaned and look as bright by washing them with a solution of salt and vinegar as by using oxalic acid, and the advantage of running no risk of poisoning either children or careless persons. Use as much salt as the vinegar will dissolve, and apply with a woolen rag, rubbing vigorously, then polish with pulverized chalk, and the article will look like new with little labor, as the acid of the vinegar is very efficient in removing all stains from either copper or brass.

(5) Wash with warm water to remove grease, then rub with a mixture of rotten-stone, soft-soap, and oil or turpentine, mixed to the consistency of stiff putty. The stone should be powdered very fine and sifted, and a quantity of the mixture may be made sufficient to last for a long time. A little of the above mixture should be mixed with water, rubbed over the metal, then rubbed briskly with a clean dry rag or leather, and a beautiful polish will be obtained.

BRASS OR SILVER, TO CLEAN:

To clean brass and silver and polish the same, use aqua ammonia and rotten-stone, followed by rouge, applied with soft leather.

BREAD, STALE TO FRESHEN:

Put a stale loaf into a closely covered tin vessel; expose it for 1/2 hour or longer to a heat not greater than that of boiling water; allow it to cool, when its freshness will be found restored.

BREAD, TO KEEP MOIST:

Keep a large earthen jar—a cover of the same material is better than a wooden one—and have it well aired and fresh; let the bread be well cooled after it is taken from the oven; then place it in the jar and cover closely.

BREAD CRUMBS, TO UTILIZE:

The waste of bits of bread in some families is unpardonable. Every fragment of clean bread, if no bigger than a pea, should be saved and used. If attention be given to this the quantity of crumbs that would otherwise be wasted will astonish one who tries it. Do not allow the crumbs to mold; place them on a plate in the stove-oven with the door open until they are quite dry. Then roll the crumbs until then are as fine as meal, and keep in a carefully closed vessel; a fruit can be excellent. Crumbs prepared in this way are useful to bread chops or cutlets, oysters for broiling, egg-plant for frying; they make the most perfect of bread puddings, and are unequaled for stuffings.

BREAKFAST HINTS:

The housekeeper should study variety in the breakfasts she offers her family, not only from day to day, but changing them as much as possible with the seasons. The things which are the most suggestive of comfort on a cold winter's morning are by no means tempting in July, when we need not only lighter clothing, but lighter food. Too often the meal loses all character in a continual round of steak or chops the year through, and dainty dishes which are really less expensive are ignored. Cold meats and chicken can easily be made into croquettes, or minced and well seasoned and served on slices of water toast. Eggs can be cooked in such a variety of ways that one need never tire of them, and the same may be said of potatoes. In their season, tomatoes sliced and served with Mayonnaise dressing, or a simple dressing of oil and vinegar, are very nice for breakfast.

There is no more wholesome or tempting addition to the morning meal than fruit served as a first course. Oat meal porridge, too, is so healthful an article of food that it should be used universally. If it is necessary in order to economize time in the morning to set the breakfast-table the night before, it should be covered with an old linen table-cloth, or something of the kind kept for the purpose.

The tea or coffee service should be placed in a line at one end of the table before the hostess; it is no longer customary to stand them on a tray. Mats, which are prettiest if they are pure and white, are put at the opposite end of the table for one or more substantial dishes, and at the sides for vegetables. A table set in this way looks much better than when the host and hostess sit opposite each other at the sides of the table, as in that case all the larger dishes are crowded in the center. A fork should be placed at the left of each plate and a knife and spoon at the right. The table-spoons and pepper and salt stands are arranged at the corners of the table.

If fruit which requires handling is to form the first course, as oranges or peaches, a plate upon which is a doily, finger-bowl, fork, and fruit-knife, may be set at each plate. After the fruit has been removed the more substantial part of the breakfast is brought on.

The pot in which the coffee is made should be of a kind which is presentable at table, as the coffee is not so good if it is poured off the grounds into an urn. If it is not possible to have cream for it, boiled milk, with a spoonful of condensed milk in each cup, to make it richer, is the best substitute.

Cakes to be eaten with syrup should be served at the last of the meal, and the plates and knives and forks changed for them. It is well to have all plates which will be needed ready for use on the buffet, except in winter, when they may be consigned to the plate-warmer.

BRITANNIA METAL[1], TO CLEAN:

(1) Rub the article with a piece of flannel moistened with sweet-oil; then apply a little pounded rotten-stone or polishing paste with the finger till the polish is produced; then wash the article with soap and hot water, and when dry rub with soft wash leather and a little fine whiting.

(2) To clean britannia metal use finely powdered whiting, 2 table-spoons of sweet-oil, and a little yellow soap. Mix with spirits of wine to a cream. Rub on with a sponge, wipe off with soft cloth, and polish with a chamois skin.

BROADCLOTH, TO REMOVE STAINS FROM:

Take 1 ounce of pipe-clay that has been ground fine and mix it with 12 drops of alcohol and the same quantity of spirits of turpentine. Moisten a little of this mixture with alcohol and rub it on the spots. Let it remain till dry, then rub it off with a woolen cloth, and the spots will disappear.

BRONCHITIS:

An inflammation of the mucous lining of the bronchia, or smaller ramifications of the windpipe. In the mild form it is called a cold on the chest. The symptoms are hoarseness, dry cough, and fever, followed by expectoration of mucus, at first thin and afterward thick; in the severe forms there is oppression at the chest, with more or less wheezing and rattling, and in the outset a sensation of rawness in the upper chest and windpipe; toward night, generally, the symptoms increase, sometimes giving rise to great distress.

Treatment: A hot mustard foot-bath, with 10 grains of Dover's powder, or a hot lemonade at bed-time, will very often, during the first 24 hours, cut short the attack; a wet towel folded upon the chest and covered with a dry flannel or piece of oiled silk, to prevent evaporation and keep the clothing dry, will generally assist much in breaking up the cold; should these means fail or have been neglected, a brisk saline cathartic (a table-spoonful of Epsom salts or citrate of magnesia) should be given, with a few doses of spirits of niter, 20 to 30 drops, with 3 drops of tincture aconite in each, if there is much fever, a flax-seed tea or other demulcents[2], with frequent doses of some simple cough mixture to ease and loosen the cough; in many cases $^1/4$ to $^1/2$ grain of morphia to each ounce; should the pain in the chest be very severe, a mustard-plaster or friction with turpentine and sweet oil, with or without a little spirits of hartshorn, will be useful; with children especially the chest may be covered with a hot poultice.

(1) Any alloy of brass, tin, antimony and bismuth; used to make cheap spoons and teapots.
(2) Any medicine which protects sensitive parts of the body from the irritating action of other substances.

BRONCOCELE, TO CURE:

Iodide of potassium, (often called hydriodate of potash), 2 drams; iodide, 1 dram; water, 2$^1/_2$ ounces; mix and shake a few minutes, and pour a little into a phial for internal use. Dose, 5 to 10 drops before each meal, to be taken in a little water.

External application: With a feather wet the enlarged neck from the other bottle night and morning until well. It will cause the scarf skin to peal off several times before the cure is perfect, leaving it tender, but do not omit the application more than one day at most, and you may rest assured of a cure, if a cure can be performed by any means whatever.

BRONZE FOR BRASS:

Take 1 ounce of muriate of ammonia, $^1/_2$ ounce of alum, and $^1/_4$ ounce of arsenic, dissolved in a pint of strong vinegar. This will make a good bronze for brass-work.

BROOMS, CARE OF:

Keep a separate broom for the parlor, the dining-room, sleeping room, and kitchen; when the latter is too much worn for use in the house, send it to the barn, take the second best for the kitchen, the broom from up-stairs for the dining-room, the parlor and hall. Leaning heavily on a broom when stooping to pick up articles while sweeping results in bent and broken splinters and a worthless broom; when a new broom is purchased provide a way for hanging it up; always hang or stand it with the brush up; if the broom becomes one-sided, scald it and bend it back; if brooms are wet in boiling suds once a week they will become very tough, will not cut a carpet, will last much longer, and will always sweep like a new broom.

BUFF WITH THE WAND, THE GAME OF:

Blind man's buff is so time-honored and popular with young and old that one would think it impossible to devise a better game of the kind. The newer game of buff with the wand, however, is thought by many to be superior to the long-established favorite. The blind person, with a stick in his hand, is placed in the middle of the room. The remainder of the party form a ring by joining hands, and to the music of a merry tune, which should be played on the piano, they all skip round him. Occasionally the music should be made to stop suddenly, when the blind man takes the opportunity of lowering his wand upon one of the circle. The person thus made the victim is then required to take hold of the stick until his fate is decided. The blind man then makes any absurd noise he likes, either the cry of animals or street cries, which the captive person must imitate, trying as much as possible to disguise his own natural voice.

Should the blind man detect who holds the stick, and guess rightly, he is released from his post, the person who has been caught taking his place. If not, he must still keep the bandage on his eyes, and hope for better success next time.

BUGS, TO DRIVE FROM VINES:

Ashes moistened with kerosene are recommended for keeping striped bugs from cucumber, melon, and squash vines.

BULBS, MANURE FOR:

An ounce of nitrate of soda dissolved in 4 gallons of water is quick and good stimulate for bulbs, to be applied twice a week after the pots are filled with roots and the flower spikes are fairly visible. A large handful of soot, or about a pint, tied up in a piece of old canvas, and immersed in the same quantity of water for a day or two will furnish a safe and excellent stimulant. Also good and safe is 1/4 pound of cow manure mixed in a large garden pot of water, and used as required. Any of these stimulants will do good, or the whole of them, applied alternately, will benefit bulbs that need more sustenance than the soil affords.

BULBS, TO HASTEN THE BLOOMING OF:

Dissolve 12 ounces of nitrate of potash, 4 ounces of common salt, 3 ounces of pearl ash, 5 ounces of moist sugar in 1 quart of rain-water, and put a dessert-spoonful of this liquid into the flower-glass, which should be filled with soft water so as not quite to touch the bulb. Change the water and add some more of the liquid every 9 days. In changing the water do not remove the bulb, but merely tilt the glass on one side.

BUNION REMEDY:

(1) Bunions may be checked in their early development by binding the joint with adhesive plaster and keeping it on as long as any uneasiness is felt. The bandaging should be perfect, and it might be well to extend it round the foot. An inflamed bunion should be poulticed and larger shoes be worn. Iodine 12 grains, lard or spermaceti(1) ointment 1/2 ounce, makes a capital ointment for bunions. It should be rubbed on gently twice or three times a day.

(2) Bunions may be cured by applying iodine freely twice a day with a feather. For cure of corns or chilblains(2) the same is recommended.

BURDOCK, HOW TO EXTIRPATE:

A coarse, rank, bitter weed, with very large burs. Cut the leaves off near the ground and pour a small quantity of coal-oil into the crown of the plant. In some cases it will take years to completely exterminate it.

(1) White waxlike substance taken from the oil in the heads of whales or dolphins.
(2) A painful swelling of foot or hand caused by exposure to cold, mostly affecting the young.

BURNING OIL, TEST FOR:

Heat water in a pot on the fire to 120 degrees Fahr. Take a tin and put in it a table-spoonful of the oil you wish to test, place the tin containing the oil in the hot water, let it cool down to 112 degrees Fahr.; when at this point, approach a light very cautiously towards the oil, and if it takes fire before the light touches it you will be safe in rejecting it.

BURNS, CURE FOR:

Of all applications for a burn, we believe that there are none equal to a simple covering of common wheat flour. This is always on hand, and while it requires no skill in using it, it produces most astonishing effects. The moisture produced upon the surface of a slight or deep burn is at once absorbed by the flour, and forms a paste which shuts out the air. As long as the fluid matters continue flowing they are absorbed and prevented from producing irritation, as they would do if kept from passing off by oily or resinous applications; while the greater the amount of those absorbed by the flour, the thicker the protective covering. Another advantage of the flour covering is that next to the surface it is kept moist and flexible. It can also be readily washed off, without further irritation in removing. It may occasionally be washed off very carefully, when it has become matted and dry, and a new covering be sprinkled on.

BUSINESS INFORMATION:

(1) Demand notes are payable on presentation without grace, and bear legal interest after a demand has been made, if not so written. The presentation or demand must be made at the place where the note is payable, if stated; if not stated, at the maker's place of business, within business hours; should he have no place of business, then at his residence.

(2) An indorser on a demand note is holden only for a limited time variable in different States.

(3) If time or payment is not stated in a note, it is held payable on demand.

(4) A negotiable note must be made payable either to bearer or be properly indorsed by the person in whose order it is made. If the indorser wishes to avoid responsibility, he can indorse "without recourse."

(5) A joint note is one signed by two or more persons, who each become liable for the whole amount.

(6) Three days' grace is allowed on all time-notes after the time for payment expires; if not then paid, the indorser, if any, should be legally notified, to the holden.

(7) Notes falling due Sunday or on a legal holiday must be paid the day previous.

(8) Notes dated Sunday are void.

(9) Notes given by minors are void.

(10) Altering a note in any manner by the holder makes it void.

(11) The maker of a note that is lost or stolen is not released from payment if the amount and consideration can be proven.

(12) Notes obtained by fraud or given by an intoxicated person cannot be collected.

(13) An indorser has a right to action against all whose names were previously on a note indorsed by him.

BUTTER, CREAM, AND MILK, TO PRESERVE:

Butter, cream, milk and flour are peculiarly liable to absorb effluvia(1), and should, therefore, never be kept in moldy rooms or placed where there are sour liquids, aromatic vegetables, such as onions, cabbage, and turnips, or smoked fish or bacon, or, indeed, any kind of food or those of strong odor, lest they lose their flavor. But, alas! how much more essential is it that the utmost care be used in the prohibition of bed-side food and drink in the nursery and sick-room, a practice fraught with constant danger to the sick and of spreading disease to the well.

BUTTER, HOW TO MAKE GOOD:

Milk should never be set for butter in a dark, damp cellar, as is the practice with some butter-makers, as the cream is thereby molded before it has had time to rise, which gives the butter a moldy taste. The milk is allowed to stand too long before being skimmed which gives it a cheesy taste. The cream is kept too long before it is churned, after it is skimmed, which gives it a cheesy taste. The cream is kept too long before it is churned, after it is skimmed, which gives the taste of the other two, and also a sour taste.

The butter should never be washed in water, because it takes away the beautiful aroma so essential in good butter. It should never be taken in a person's warm hands as the heat melts a certain portion of the globules, which gives it an oily taste, and makes it become rancid very soon.

The milk should be set in good clear tin or earthen pans, in a dry, open, airy, and shady place, above ground if possible although a cellar may be so built and ventilated as to answer the purpose. It should never be set over 24 hours in warm weather, and for a dairy of 3 cows or over the cream should be churned every morning and never be kept over 48 hours in warm weather; in cold weather it may be kept longer.

(1) Disagreeable odors.

BUTTER, TO COLOR:

As a rule it is absolutely essential in the winter to color butter in order to make it marketable, or at all attractive as an article of table use at home. There may be a possible exception to this rule in cases where cows are fed largely upon yellow corn, pumpkins, carrots, etc., but this does not lessen the importance of the rule. Of the various substances used in coloring butter, we think that carrots (of the deep yellow variety) give the most natural color and most agreeable flavor. Annatto(1), however, is principally used, and with most satisfactory results. If carrots are used, take two large-sized ones, clean them thoroughly, and then with a knife scrape off the yellow exterior, leaving the white pith; soak the yellow part in boiling milk for 10 or 15 minutes; strain boiling hot into the cream; this gives the cream the desired temperature, colors it nicely, and adds to the sweetness of the butter.

BUTTERFLIES AND MOTHS:

Butterflies and moths, however pretty, are the worst enemies one can have in a garden; a single insect of this kind may deposit eggs enough to overrun a tree with caterpillars; therefore they should be destroyed at any cost of trouble. The only moth that you must spare is the common black and red one; the grubs of this feed exclusively on groundsel(2), and are therefore a valuable ally of the gardener.

BUTTERFLY, TO TAKE AN IMPRESSION OF:

Having taken a butterfly, kill it without spoiling its wings, which contrive to spread out as regularly as possible in a flying position. Then, with a small brush or pencil, take a piece of white paper, wash a part of it with gum-water a little thicker than ordinary, so that it may easily dry. Afterward, laying your butterfly on the paper, cut off the body close to the wings, and, throwing it away, lay the paper on a smooth board with the fly upward, and laying another paper over that, put the whole preparation into a screw press and screw down very hard, letting it remain under that pressure for half an hour. Afterward take off the wings of the butterfly, and you will find a perfect impression of them, with all their various colors marked distinctly, remaining on the paper. When this is done, draw between the wings of your impression the body of the butterfly, and color it after the insect itself.

(1) A reddish yellow dye from the pulp of tropical fruit seeds.
(2) A composite plant with pinnatifid leaves and small yellow flowers which grow as weeds in gardens.

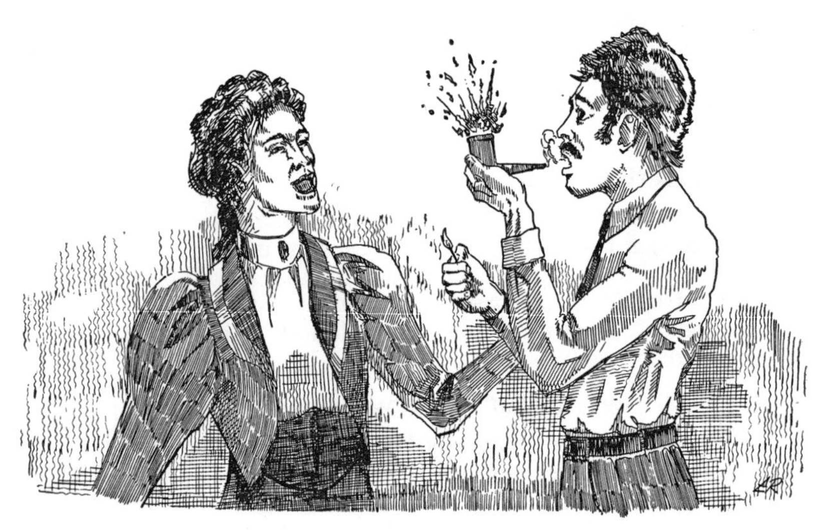

C

CABBAGE, VALUE OF:

This vegetable, so staple an article of food among out-of-door workers, has fallen into general disuse with some on account of the disagreeable odor it emits in cooking, permeating every corner of an ordinarily constructed house from garret to cellar. The best way to prevent this is to keep the vessel in which it boils closely covered, to drop in a bit of red pepper-pod and a pinch of soda, to allow it just time enough to cook and no more, and, lastly, for the cook to pour off the cabbage-water as soon as she lifts the cover and sends it to table. Wash the head nicely—one large head makes a good dish—and put it on in boiling water, slightly salted, after having cut it into quarters, and allow it 40 minutes in which to cook over a brisk fire.

Dressed as cauliflower, with drawn-butter sauce, it may be almost as delicate. Most persons, however, preferring it with some sort of salt meat, we give the direction for cooking it in that way thus: Having your ham, chine(1), or middling(2) nearly ready for dinner, take out enough of the liquor in which it has been cooling to cover the cabbage, which had better be cooked in a separate stew-pot, and treat it otherwise just as if it were plain water; drain from the liquor, and having put your joint of meat in the center of a large meat-dish, put the cabbage all around, and you have before you the daily and favorite dish of country people, with the addition of a plentiful supply of hot corn bread. More elegantly, the cabbage is frequently sent to table, however separately, in a covered vegetable dish, where it may be kept hot longer.

CABBAGE APHIS:

Early in June the cabbage aphis makes its appearance on young cabbage plants, and before long becomes very numerous. Tobacco-smoke or infusion will destroy them.

CABBAGE FLY:

An ash-gray insect. The thorax has 3 indistinct black streaks on the back; the wings are clear, like glass; the abdomen is linear, with black stripes on the back of the male, or entirely ash-gray on the female; the length is 3 lines(3). The larva much resembles that of the onion fly, but is

1) Cut of meat containing a part of the backbone.
2) Bacon or pork from between the shoulder and ham.
3) One twelfth of an inch; 3 lines is 3 twelths or 1/4 of an inch.

thicker. To diminish this pull up sometimes and carry away the plants attacked by the larvae, which may be known by their dull lead color and the withering of their leaves in the sunshine.

CAKED UDDER OF COW:

For swollen or caked udder or bag of a cow wash and rub thoroughly with water as hot as you can bear your hand; then rub with a dry cloth; then apply hog's lard, or, what is better, grate good yellow carrot fine and simmer it in the lard to an ointment, and apply and rub as above.

CALICO, TO WASH:

Infuse 3 gills(1) of salt in 4 quarts of water. Put in it the calico while the solution is hot, and leave until the latter is cold. It is said that in this way the colors are rendered permanent and will not fade by subsequent washing.

CALLAS, TREATMENT OF:

For blooming callas use the soil from the hennery, and on cold mornings pour hot water in the saucers.

CAMPHOR AND ITS USES:

Camphor is not a very steady stimulant, as its effect is transitory, but in large doses it acts as a narcotic abating pain and inducing sleep. In moderate doses it operates as a diaphoretic(2) and antispasmodic increasing the heat of the body, allaying irritation and spasm. It is used externally as a liniment when dissolved in oil, alcohol, or acetic acid, being employed to allay rheumatic pains, and it is also useful as an embrocation in sprains, bruises, chilblains, and, when combined with opium, it has been advantageously employed in flatulent colic and severe diarrhea, being rubbed over the bowels.

When reduced to a fine powder by the addition of a little spirit of wine and friction it is very useful as a local stimulant to indolent ulcers, especially when they discharge a foul kind of matter; a pinch is taken between the finger and thumb and sprinkled into the ulcer, which is then dressed as usual. When dissolved in oil of turpentine, and a few drops are placed in a hollow tooth and covered with jewelers' wool or scraped lint, it gives almost instant relief to toothache. Used internally it is apt to excite nausea and even vomiting, especially when given in the solid form.

As a stimulant it is of service in all low fevers, malignant measles, malignant sore throat, and running small-pox, and when with opium and bark it is extremely useful in checking the progress of malignant estrus and

(1) One forth pint.
(2) Causing perspiration.

gangrene. As a narcotic it is very useful, because it allays pain and irritation without increasing the pulse very much. When powdered and sprinkled upon the surface of a blister it prevents the cantharides acting in a peculiar and painful manner upon the bladder. Combined with senna it increases its purgative properties and it is also used to correct the nausea produced by squills(1), and irritating effects of drastic purgatives and mezereon(2).

Dose: From 4 grains to 1 scruple, repeated in short intervals when used in small doses and long intervals when employed in large doses.

Caution: *When given in an overdose it acts as a poison, producing vomiting, giddiness, delirium, convulsions, and sometimes death.*

CAMPHOR ICE:

Spermaceti, $1^{1}/_{2}$ ounces; gum camphor, three-fourths ounce; oil of sweet almonds, 4 table-spoonfuls. Set on the stove in an earthen dish till dissolved; heat just enough to dissolve it; when warm pour into small molds, if desired to sell then paper and put into tinfoil. Used for chaps on hands or lips.

CAMPHOR TABLETS:

Melt tallow, and add a little powdered camphor and glycerine, with a few drops of oil of almonds to scent. Pour in molds and cool.

CANADA THISTLE:

This is the most troublesome of all the weeds. As soon as the pests appear in the spring strike them off with a sharp hoe below the lower leaf or even with the solid earth; repeat every time a sprout starts, and they will be almost totally eradicated the first season. A few may appear the second year after this treatment; if so, repeat the cutting of the stalks, and if thoroughly done sure death is the result.

CANARIES, CARE OF:

Especial care must be taken to keep the canary scrupulously clean. For this purpose the cage should be strewed every morning with clean sand, or rather fine gravel, for small pebbles are absolutely essential to life and health in cage birds; fresh water must be given every day, both for drinking and bathing, the latter being in a shallow vessel, and during the moulting season a small bit of iron should be put into the water for drinking.

The food of a canary should consist principally of summer rape-seed; i.e., of those small brown rape-seeds which are obtained from plants sown in the spring and which ripen during the summer; large and black rape-seeds, on the contrary, are produced by such plants as are sown in autumn

(1) A drug produced from the bulb of genes Scilla; used as a stimulant, expectorant and diuretic.
(2) A small shrub (Daphne Mezereum) with poisonous red berries used as a cathartic & the leaves as a vesicant.

and reaped in spring. A little chickweed in spring, lettuce-leaves in summer, and endive in autumn, with slices of sweet apple in winter, may be safely given, but bread and sugar ought to be generally avoided. Occasionally, also, a few poppy or canary seeds, and a small quantity of bruised hemp-seed, may be added, but the last very sparingly.

CANARIES, TO REMOVE RED MITES FROM:

Put into the cage as a perch one or more hollow sticks, with holes cut into them at short distances, as in a cane pipe. The insects crawl into these, and can easily be knocked or shaken out, or destroyed by letting hot water run through the sticks. This should be done every day till the bird is relieved. Hang a piece of new white flannel in the cage at night next the perch, so that it shades the bird from the light. In the morning you will find the mites on the flannel; wash, or put in a new piece the following night, and continue doing so until they are removed. It is also well to scald the cage. The perches should be of red cedar wood.

CANCERS, METHODS OF RELIEF:

(1) Gastric juice has effected remarkable cures. External applications must be made 3 times a day for about 20 days. The first application causes much pain, but this may be lessened by the use of almond oil.

(2) Several cases of cancer and other malignant tumors have been speedily cured by the application of acetic acid. In some instances of cure by this prescription the cancers and tumors had been of long standing.

(3) Take an egg, pour out the white, retaining the yelk in the shell; put in salt and mix with the yelk so along as it will receive it; stir them together until the salve is formed; put a portion of this on a piece of sticking-plaster, and apply to the cancer about twice a day.

(4) The exquisite pain which belongs to open cancer is found to be best relieved by the stramonium(1) ointment which is employed in London.

The following is the formula: 1/2 lb. of fresh stramonium leaves and 2 lbs. of lard.; mix the bruised leaves with the lard and expose to mild heat until the leaves become friable, and strain through lint. The ointment thus prepared is spread upon lint, and the dressing changed 3 times a day.

CARD-CASE FOR A WATCH:

Take two pieces of card 16 in. long and 3 1/2 in. wide, and cut the

(1) A dangerous narcotic made from the dried flowers and leaves of the jimson weed.

ends pointed. Cover both pieces with velvet or silk, and embroider a vine of flowers on one end, or, if preferred, paint in water-colors. Overhand the two pieces together and finish the edge with gilt cord. Make a ring of twisted cord at the top. Bend the card up at 3 in. to form the rack, and fasten at the sides with cord and tassels. Twist a large hook with gilt wire and sew an inch below the ring at the top, for the watch.

CARD-PLAYING, ETHICS OF:

Never bet. Nothing is more demoralizing than gambling, and betting small sums or articles at first has always been the way the passion commenced. Guests should never propose card-playing.

Even if you take little pleasure in cards some knowledge of the etiquette and rules belonging to the games in vogue will be useful, unless you object upon principles. If a fourth hand is wanted at a rubber, or if the rest of the company sit down to a round game, do not refuse to join. New and clean cards should be kept in readiness. Married ladies and elderly gentlemen are allowed precedence at the card-table over single young ladies and young men. Ladies of a "certain age," if single, can also claim the privilege. It is rude to urge the request to play on those declining, as many have conscientious scruples. To finger the cards while they are being dealt is a breach of manners.

Partners should never signal to each other. Never be guilty of cheating; if you observe others doing it keep cool, and endeavor to stop it. Never start a conversation that would lead to argument in the pauses of the game. Small talk or chit-chat is admissible.

To play cards with an air of weariness is rude. Strive to appear interested. Avoid argument upon points in playing. Even if you are right it is courteous to yield. Do not show feeling at being beaten. Those who are successful should not crow. Be considerate of poor playing, even if it partially spoils the game. It is a breach of good manners to hurry others who are playing,. It is the duty of those who play to make themselves proficient. Those who play much together should not play with each other in company.

CARDS, VISITING, ETIQUETTE OF:

A visiting card should be a piece of plain white card-board, not glazed, and the name should be engraved in script. Some people still cling to the old Roman letters, to old English, and now and then to a fac-simile of the handwriting. These are not, however, in the highest fashion, which reduces all things to the simplest form. A lady's card should be larger than a gentleman's, and should have her full address and also her residence in the left-hand corner, or the right hand if she prefer it. The latter is the most convenient if she wishes to use her visiting card, as many do, for invitations to 5 o'clock tea. Gentlemen's cards almost invariably have the address in the left-hand corner. In leaving cards the lady of the house leaves her own, her husband's, with those of her sons and daughters who are visiting, on families whom she knows or wishes to know.

If this is a first call, the civility should be returned within a week. In giving an entertainment a lady incloses her husband's card to all who are invited for the first time. It is equivalent to a call on his part. In calling after a dinner or a party the lady also leaves her husband's card, as he is generally too busy (in this country) to make calls.

The custom of calling on all one's acquaintances in a crowded city has become an impossibility; therefore, society women have a day, a few reception days in a month, thus seeing all their friends once a year. If it is impossible to reach them on these occasions, send a card for every member of the family invited, and one's duty is over for the year. When young ladies leave their mother's card there is the same respect expressed as if the mother called in person. Many ladies who are elderly or invalid, or who are disinclined for society, leave all this work for those who are young and strong. It is a great pity that so many American mothers retire from their social duties, but if they do the card is still all-powerful and the lady visited must be content.

A lady never leaves her card on a gentleman. She sends the card of her husband or her son, if she chooses, when she asks him to dinner. Cards should be left for guests visiting at a house if the lady who calls knows of their presences. This, of course, is not always possible; but if a lady is invited to meet a stranger she should call on her immediately. Calls made on a reception day should be emphasized by leaving a card on the hall table; none need be left after that. A gentleman need leave but two cards, be the family ever so large. It is an unkind thing for a family to give a ball, to invite half their friends, and to merely send cards to the rest. It is a mutilated civility, and the cards would better be left out.

A card is the beginning and the end of social intercourse, the alpha and omega. Cards to inquire for a person during illness must be left in person, not sent by post. Christening cards, cards to inquire for the newly arrived little stranger, cards of congratulation, all must be left in person. A card should be left at the door soon after a death, with inquiries for the family. One card is as good as a half dozen.

When returning visits of ceremony, as the first visit after a letter of introduction or as announcing one's arrival in town, or one's departure, one may leave a card at the door without inquiring for the lady. A card sent by post would have been considered in the past insulting, but it has become so much the custom now that it is not to be so considered. There is, however, something cold-blooded in it, unless there be very good reason for it. A visitor should try to call in person at least once a year.

CARMINATIVE[1], DALBY'S:

Magnesia, 3 drams; oil peppermint, 3 drams; oil nutmegs, 7 drops; oil anise, 9 drops; tincture of castor, $1\frac{1}{2}$ drams; tincture of assafœtida[2], 45 drops; tincture of opium, 18 drops; essence pennyroyal[3], 50 drops; tincture of cardamoms, 95 drops; peppermint water, 7 ounces; mix.

CARNATIONS FROM CUTTINGS:

Carnations are easily rooted from slips. Take off the small side shoots when about 2 in. long. If your plants are in pots, plant them around the edge, pressing the soil very firmly about the portion inserted. Do not water them only when the parent plant requires it. If they are cultivated in the ground, plant them in the same bed, taking the same precaution to make the earth compact about the slips, so they will not dry up instead of rooting. If the ground is slightly moist it is enough for them, but if very dry sprinkle occasionally.

CARPETS:

Rag: To make a nice rag carpet you should have the pattern you wish it wove in your mind, to guide you in arranging the colors, and the number of balls you may want of each. Care should be taken in cutting and tearing the rags, so that they will be even-sized threads in the filling; for if the texture of the carpet is uneven it will wear out more easily. The more wool there is, both in warp and woof, the longer the carpet will retain a new, clean look.

(1) A carpet may have a plain stripe of one color, either black, brown, or gray, and the fancy stripe can have the other colors, such as red, blue green, or yellow, etc.; squares can be made in the fancy stripes by cutting two colors equal lengths, and sewing together alternately. A hit-and-miss stripe can be made by sewing all colors together. Two colors can be twisted together; e.g., red and white, or blue and white, which has a very pretty effect. For 20 yds. of carpet it will take 30 lbs of rags and 3 balls of yarn to make that number of yards $1\frac{1}{2}$ yds. wide.

(2) For 33 yds. of carpet get 25 lbs. of brown chain and 15 of orange, and 91/2 lbs of white. A pretty stripe for the rag is: 4 threads of red, 3 of white on each side of the red, and 3 of black on each side of the white; then 4 threads of blue on each side of the black; put all the colors of rags between the stripes.

Selection of: A carpet should always be chosen as a background upon which the other articles of furniture are to be placed, and should be adapted to the room for which it is chosen. The surface of a carpet serving as a ground to

(1) Substances which act as a stimulant to the stomach, causing expulsion of flatulence and allaying pain.
(2) A smelly gum resin.
(3) A prostrate plant growing in pools, the essence used as a popular diaphoretic and emmenagogue.

support all objects should be quiet and negative, without strong contrast of either form or color. The leading forms should be so composed as to distribute the pattern over the whole floor, not pronounced either in the direction of breath or length. The decorative forms must be flat, without shadow or relief whether derived from ornament or direct from flowers or foliage. Small rooms need no borders; wide borders suit large apartments. French moquette and body Brussels are the best carpets to wear. Aubusson, Axminster, and Turkey are equally good, but their price is, of course high.

Tapestry Brussels is not as desirable, as when the gay figures wear off there is nothing left but hemp. On this account an ingrain (two-ply) will often outwear a tapestry. The most durable carpets are closely woven and thick, soft and pliable. In body Brussels the colors can be distinguished on the wrong side. Ingrain carpets, worn beyond repair, should be cut into lengthwise strips and woven the same as a rag carpet. It is unnecessary to sew the ingrain cuttings, weavers generally preferring to overlap the strips as they weave. Mats and carpets assume quite a Persian look when made in this way, and are very durable.

CARPETS, FADED, TO RESTORE:

Dip the carpet in strong salt and water. Blue factory cotton or silk handkerchiefs will not fade if dipped in salt-water while they are new.

CARPETS, TO BRIGHTEN:

A slightly damp cloth rubbed over a dusty carpet brightens it wonderfully, and gathers all the dust. This is an excellent way to cleanse the floor of an invalid's room where noise and dust are objectionable. Carpets should be thoroughly beaten on the wrong side first, and then on the right, after which spots may be removed by the use of ox-gall or ammonia and water.

CARPETS, TO CLEAN:

(1) A few drops of carbonate of ammonia put into a small quantity of warm rain-water will prove a safe and easy antacid, and will change, if carefully applied, discolored spots upon the carpets, and indeed all spots, whether produced by acids or alkalies. If you have a carpet injured by a whitewash this will immediately restore it.

(2) The following mixture is recommended for taking grease out of carpets: Aqua ammonia, 2 ounces; soft water, 1 quart; saltpeter, 1 teaspoonful; shaving-soap, 1 ounce, finely scraped. Mix well, shake, and let it stand a few hours or days before using, to dissolve the soap. When used pour on enough to cover any grease or oil that has been spilled, sponging and rubbing well, and applying again if

necessary; then wash off with clear cold water. It is a good mixture to have in the house for many things; is sure death to bed-bugs if put in the crevices which they inhabit; will remove paint where oil was used in mixing it, and will not injure the finest fabrics.

CARPETS, TO PATCH:

If you have an old carpet badly worn, cut a patch to cover the holes, taking care to match figure or stripe perfectly, paste it on with flour paste, and iron on very tight with a hot iron.

CARPETS, TO PUT DOWN:

All housekeepers understand the difficulty of putting down carpets, and especially where they require considerable stretching. All people have not carpet-stretchers, so I will give you a plan within reach of all, which is far better, as there is no danger of tearing the carpet. Tack one end of the carpet down firmly; then put on a pair of common rubbers, step short, lift your feet as little as possible from the carpet, and scuff across to the opposite side, and stand still while somebody nails it for you. You will be astonished at the ease and quickness with which your work is accomplished, no matter how much stretching your carpet requires. See that the rubbers are not worn too smooth upon the bottoms. Always work the way of the breaths of the carpet, not across them.

CARPETS, TO REMOVE INK FROM:

Take up as much as possible with a spoon, pour cold sweet milk upon the spot and take up with a spoon until the milk is only faintly tinged with ink; then wash with cold water and wipe dry. The writer has in this way removed nearly half a pint of ink from a delicate cream-colored carpet without leaving a stain.

CARPETS, TO RESTORE:

Take 1 pail of warm water add 1 pint of ox-gall(1); dip a soaped flannel into the mixture, and rub well the surface of the carpet, piece by piece, rinsing it as you proceed with clean cold water, taking care not to make the carpet too wet, and finish off by rubbing with a dry coarse cloth. The carpet, of course, must be well beaten before it is operated upon. This process is simple and surprisingly effective in renovating the colors. The only drawback is the effluvium given off by the gall; but this is soon remedied by exposure to the air or by opening the windows if the carpet be laid down.

CARRIAGES, CARE OF:

More injury is done to carriages and wagons by greasing too much than the reverse. Tallow is the best lubricant for wood axles, and castor oil

(1) Bile from the liver of an ox.

for iron. Lard and common grease are apt to penetrate the hub, and work their way out around the tenons of the spokes and spoil the wheel. For common wood axles just enough grease should be applied to the spindle to give it a light coating. To oil an iron axle, first wipe clean with a wet cloth with turpentine, and then apply a few drops of castor oil near the shoulder and end. One tea-spoonful is enough for the wheels. Carriages are sometimes oiled so much that their appearance is spoiled by having the grease spattered upon their varnished surfaces. When they are washed in that condition the grease is sure to be transferred to the chamois from the wheel, and from thence on to the panels.

CARRIAGE-TOPS, CARE OF:

Enamel leather tops should be first washed with castile soap and then warm water, then oiled with neat's-foot oil or sweet-oil and a coat of enamel varnish put on; the leather will look like new. Dashes may be cleaned in the same manner, but varnish color is not very beneficial to patent leather; however, when old and cracked, it may be colored to improve the appearance.

CARROTS, WILD, TO DESTROY:

The carrot is one of the most troublesome weeds with which the farmer has to contend. It is so hardy and prolific that in some of the States laws have been passed for its suppression. If neglected it will spread over pastures and meadows, and take possession of the roadsides. They do not show themselves much in the early part of the season, but after the mowing in June and July they shoot up rapidly, and show their white blossoms in every direction.

Some farmers seek to destroy them by pulling them up by the roots, an effectual, but very expensive process. The plant is biennial, and if it is not permitted to scatter its seeds can just as surely be eradicated by mowing, while in blossom, or any time before it drops its seeds. There is little danger of leaving it until August or early in September. If cut before seeding, the plants may be left upon the ground. If later, gather into heaps and burn, or put into a compost heap.

CARVING:

It is not difficult to learn to carve well, and housekeepers are wholly inexcusable for not acquiring the art, and it is a most graceful accomplishment. The first requisite in carving is a very sharp suitable-sized knife; all efforts or unnecessary exertions are in bad taste, as they show one of two things; the toughness of the meat or the awkwardness of the one carving. Dexterity and address in the manner of using the knife, and not strength, is what is requisite to carve well. The seat should be sufficiently high for the carver to have complete command over the joints before him, and the dish should be of good size, placed sufficiently near the foot of the table. For ham, or any large thick joint, a long sharp-pointed knife is the most suitable, while for poultry or game a short knife is better.

Fish: In carving fish, care should be taken to avoid breaking the flakes. In serving salmon, long slices cut from the backbone and along the flank are the best. Mackerel and shad should be carved so as to raise one side of the meat from the bone; the upper end is considered the best. The roes are much liked by epicures.

Turkey: In carving a turkey, cut off the wing nearest first, then the leg and second joint; then slice from the breast, after which insert the knife between the bones and separate them. The side bone lies beside the rump, and the desired morsel can be taken out without separating the whole bone.

Ducks and Chickens: Ducks and chickens should be placed on the dish with the breast uppermost, and the fork should be put into it, taking off the wings and legs first, without turning the fowl; then the "wishbone" should be cut out so as to leave the well-browned skin over it, and a portion of the meat. Then the side bone should be cut off, and the fowl which is left, in two, from the neck down; the joints may be divided also.

Partridges: Partridges may be carved like other fowls, but the breast and wings are not divided.

Beef: A sirloin of beef should be placed on a dish with the tenderloin underneath. Thin cut slices should be taken from the side next the carver first, then turned over to cut the tenderloin.

Mutton: A shoulder of mutton should be cut across to the middle of the bone first, and then from the thickest part till it comes to the gristle.

Lamb: In a fore quarter of lamb, separate the shoulder from the ribs, then divide the ribs.

Pork: A roast pig should be split down the middle before coming to the table, then the shoulder should be separated from the body on one side, and then the leg removed and divided, as also the ribs.

Veal: To carve a loin of veal, begin at the small end and separate the ribs. A fillet of veal should be cut first from the top. In a breast of veal, the brisket and breast must be separated and then cut in pieces.

Venison: In carving a leg of venison, it should be cut down deep into the bone, in order that the juices may run freely, then large thin slices may be taken from the broad end. In carving a saddle of venison, thin even slices must be cut form the tail toward the upper part of each side. Care should be taken to have the plates warm in cold weather for venison and mutton, as they are best served hot.

Ham: A ham may be carved in several ways. First, by cutting long, delicate slices through the thick fat in the center down to the bone; or by running the point of the knife in the circle of the middle, and cutting thin circular slices, thus keeping the ham moist; and lastly, by beginning at the knuckle and slicing upwards.

CASINO, THE GAME OF:

The game of Casino is played with an entire pack of cards, generally by 4 persons, but sometimes by 3, and often by 2.

Terms used in Casino:

- Great Casino: The ten of diamonds, which reckons for 2 points.
- Little Casino: The two of spades, which reckons for 1 point.
- The Cards: When you have a greater share than your adversary, and reckons for 3 points.
- The Spades: When you have the majority of that suit, and reckons for 1 point.
- The Aces: Each of which reckons for 1 point.
- Lurched: When your adversary has won the game before you have gained 6 points.

In some deals at this game it may so happen that neither party wins any thing, as the points are not set up according to the tricks, etc., obtained; but the smaller number is constantly subtracted from the larger, both in cards and points; and if they both prove equal the game commences again, and the deal goes on in rotation. When 3 persons play at this game the 2 lowest add their points together, and subtract from the highest; but when the 2 numbers together either amount to or exceed the highest, then neither party scores.

Laws of Casino: The deal and partners are determined by cutting, as at whist, and the dealer gives 4 cards by 1 at a time to every player, and either regularly as he deals, or by 1, 2, 3, or 4 at a time, lays 4 more face upward upon the board, and after the first cards are played, 4 others are to be dealt to each person, until the pack be concluded; but it is only in the first deal that any cards are to be turned up. The deal is not lost when a card is faced by the dealer, unless in the first round, before any of the 4 cards are turned up upon the table; but if a card happens to be faced in the pack before any of the said 4 be turned up, then the deal must begin again.

Any person playing with less than 4 cards must abide by the loss; and should a card be found under the table, the player whose number is deficient is to take the same. Each person plays 1 card at a time, with which he may not only take at once every card of the same denomination upon the table, but likewise, all that combine therewith; as, for instance, a ten takes not only every ten, but also nine an ace, eight and deuce, seven and three, six and four or two fives; and if he clear the board before the conclusion of the game he is to score a point, and whenever any player cannot pair or combine, then he is to put down a card.

The number of tricks are not to be examined or counted before all the cards be played; nor may any trick but that last won be looked at, as every mistake must be challenged immediately. After all the pack be dealt out, the player who obtains the last trick sweeps all the cards then remaining unmatched upon the table.

CASTOR OIL, TO ADMINISTER:

If it is necessary to administer castor oil to a child there is no need of sickening him by forcing him to take it clear. Put a little cold water in a wine-glass, then drop the oil in; it will form one large globule; have the child wet his mouth with water, and then drink from the wine-glass rapidly, keeping his mouth closed for a minute or two after, and he will never know by the taste what he has taken. Even cod-liver oil can be taken in this way, and the patient need never be disturbed by the taste.

CAT AND MOUSE, THE GAME OF:

The players stand in a circle, holding each other's hands, excepting one, who acts "the mouse," and who, standing outside the circle, touches one of the players and then runs under the arms of the others. The player thus touched becomes "cat," and must pursue the "mouse" until he catches him; but in doing this he must be careful to pass in and out of the circle under the arms of the same persons passed by the "mouse," who is thus enabled to lead this pursuer a pretty chase. When the cat is agile and the mouse cunning the game can be made to yield a good deal of fun. A "mouse" who has been caught becomes "cat," while the cat who has caught him takes his place in the circle.

CATERPILLARS:

The varieties of caterpillars are innumerable. Many of them feed on leaves; some species are restricted to a single kind of plant; those which infest flowers and garden-plants can only be kept away by watering the plants copiously and frequently, and by examining them often during the spring and summer and destroying the caterpillars. A garden syringe or engine, with a cap on the pipe; full of very minute holes, will wash away these disagreeable visitors very quickly. You must bring the pipe close to the plant, and pump hard, so as to have considerable force on, and the plant, however badly infested, will soon be cleared without receiving any injury. Every time that you use the syringe or garden engine you must immediately rake the earth under the trees and kill the insects you have dislodged, or many will recover and climb up the stems of the plants.

CATS, CARE OF:

It is generally supposed that cats are more attached to places than to individuals, but this is an error. They obstinately cling to certain places because it is there they expect to see the persons to whom they are attached. The cat will return to an empty house, and remain in it many weeks. But when at last she finds that the family does not return she strays away, and if she chances then to find the family she will abide with them. The same rules of breeding which apply to dogs apply also to cats. They should not be over-fed, nor too frequently. Cats are liable to the same diseases as dogs, though they do not become ill so frequently. A little brimstone in their milk occasionally is a good preventive. The veterinary chemist will also prescribe for the serious diseases of cats.

CEILINGS, SMOKY, TO CLEAN:

Ceilings that have been smoked by a kerosene lamp should be washed off with soda-water. Grained wood should be washed with cold tea.

CEILINGS, TO DECORATE:

A country house may oftentimes be so prettily decorated as to be a joy to its possessor and a home not in the least behind city homes in tasteful arrangement. In fact, so many more people in the country own their homes than do city people that it seems almost as if they, as a matter of course, must take a pride in decorating and adorning them. We will not speak of roofs and verandas and vines, etc., which all come outside, and concerning which the male members of the family must be more or less consulted before change can be made, but of the internal arrangements of the wall and wood-work and ceiling. Generally we find the plain, whitewashed ceiling in the country house. But it is no more needful there than in the city. It can be painted any color with contrast well with the wood-work and paper of the walls.

Then with a stepladder, paint, brush, and stencil-plate any lady can decorate her ceiling to suit herself. If she feels that she has not the skill—though it does not take much—she can purchase exceedingly pretty paper for ceiling, designed in artistic patterns and colors, for moderate cost. This, however, needs care in putting on, that it may be straight and smooth, and the pattern not twisted awry. I think the paint and stencil-plate far easier to manage, and if a simple design has been chosen it ought not to be considered a very great task to put it on.

CELERY AS A MEDICINE:

Celery boiled in milk and eaten with the milk served as a beverage is said to be a cure for rheumatism, gout, and a specific in case of small-pox. Nervous people find great comfort in celery.

CELLAR, HOW TO COOL A:

A great mistake is sometimes made in ventilating cellars and milk-houses. The object of ventilation is to keep the cellars cool and dry, but this object often fails of being accomplished by a common mistake, and instead the cellar is made both warm and damp. A cool place should never be ventilated unless the air admitted is cooler than the air within, or is at least as cool as that or a very little warmer.

The warmer the air the more moisture it holds in suspension. Necessarily, the cooler the air the more this moisture is condensed and precipitated. When a cool cellar is aired on a warm day the entering air, being in motion, appears cool, but as it fills the cellar the cooler air with which it becomes mixed chills it, the moisture is condensed and the dew is deposited on the cold walls, and may often be seen running down them in streams. Then the cellar is damp and soon becomes moldy. To avoid this the windows should only be opened at night, and late—the last thing before retiring. There is no need to fear that the night air is unhealthful; it is as pure as the air of midday, and is really drier. The cool air enters the apartment during the night and circulates through it. The windows should be closed before sunrise in the morning and kept closed and shaded through the day.

If the air of the cellar is damp it may be thoroughly dried by placing in it a peck of fresh lime in an open box. A peck of lime will absorb about 7 lbs., or more than 3 quarts, of water, and this way a cellar or milk-room may soon be dried, even in the hottest weather.

CELLAR, THE HYGIENE OF:

One of the most important apartments in the house is the cellar, and withal one that often receives insufficient attention. "Out of sight, out of mind," is exemplified here, and the result may frequently be traced in the impaired health of those who live above the underground lumber-room.

Old packing-boxes, newspapers, broken utensils, rotting fruit and vegetables, and in some cases such garbage as potato-parings, lemon and orange skins, bones, etc., that should of right be consigned to the swill-pail, are suffered to accumulate from one months end to the other. The unwholesome and unpleasant odor that rises like a cloud whenever the cellar door is opened is hastily attributed to the mustiness popularly supposed to be an inseparable adjunct to the underground regions. Slight but persistent unhealthiness in the family is disregarded, and a sharp attack of diphtheria or typhoid fever is perhaps needed to arouse the household to the danger in which they dwell.

The cellar is more readily kept clean if it is cut up into several small rooms, instead of being left in one great, undivided chamber. Where it is not thus arranged it should at least be partitioned off one side by bins to hold the various stores, in place of letting them lie in heaps and corners. When bins are out of the question barrels or large packing-boxes form tolerable substitutes. The coal is usually kept in the vaults provided for that purpose.

It is a great aid in the endeavor to obtain proper neatness in the cellar if the room is well lighted and ventilated. The windows may be kept shut in the day-time, but should always be left open at night to allow the fresh air to enter, except when the weather is so cold that there is danger of freezing the supplies of food kept there. Even then the sashes should be unclosed night and morning long enough to permit a sluice of air to gain admittance. By carefully following this plan much of the musty and earthy odor common to cellars may be banished. Wire netting should be nailed over the outside of the window in a way that may exclude the flies without hindering the opening of the sash. There should be a spring attached to the door that will prevent its being left ajar and a free passage to flies furnished by careless servants.

If there are no separate vaults provided for the coal, and it must be kept in the common cellar, large bins for this are indispensable. The coal should never be dumped into one corner of the cellar, whence its grimy dust will be tracked to the upper floor by every one coming up from below. Nor should the wood, large and small, be thrown into an indiscriminate stack, but neatly piled, the kindling in one place, the logs intended for the open fires in another, and chips, sawdust, and shavings swept together and emptied into a basket or box.

Vegetables, above all, should never be heaped on the floor. They rot more easily there, besides being unsightly, and invariably leaving dirt for some one to sweep up. Barrels of boxes may hold them as well as apples or pears. Both vegetables and fruit should be picked over often, and rotten ones thrown away. The good ones will keep twice as long if this is done. The work may seem tedious, but it is almost essential, especially toward spring, when vegetables begin to decay rapidly. Health demands this as well as economy. Many a case of spring illness has been traced to a harmless-looking barrel in the cellar, where disease germs are fostered in a mass of putrid vegetable matter.

The idea that the cellar is an *omnium gatherum* for useless articles of all sorts should be diligently combated. Whatever is not worth keeping in the certain hope of putting to service at some future time should be thrown away without hesitation. The cellar cannot look neat with a heap of lumber and old iron disfiguring it. Broken packing-cases and staveless barrels may be sent here to be split up and converted into kindlings as speedily as possible, while any boxes that may possibly be put to use are much better kept in the attic out of the damp.

A cellar floor should always be laid in cement. An earth flooring holds the dampness, and is, moreover, very hard to keep clean. The cement can be swept, and even scrubbed, with out trouble. The walls and ceilings should be whitewashed, not only to make the room lighter, but as a means of disinfection. The whitewashing should be repeated at least once a year. The floor should receive its weekly brushing with the rest of the house, and at the same time the cobwebs should be dislodged and all collections of rubbish removed.

The cellar must be supplied with shelves. Swing-shelves are preferable to those set in the wall, as there is less danger with the former of rats and mice having a chance to attack the provisions. One shelf should be kept for the milk, and wiped clean every day after the cream is skimmed. Deposits of sour milk are always unsavory. The meats, vegetables, cakes, etc., stored on the other shelves should always be protected by covers of wire netting.

With all the care one may take, a fly or two will sometimes succeed in effecting an entrance, and the mischief they can do even in a short time renders the precaution worth while. A piece of gauze of mosquito-netting stretched over each pan of milk may also save a fly from involuntary suicide and the milk from waste. Poultry and meat that are hung up for a day or two should be incased in stout brown paper, or, better still, unbleached muslin. All shelves should be scrubbed off every week with a mixture of washing soda and water, then wipe dry.

It is a great convenience to the housewife if she can have a closet partitioned off and well stocked with shelves, where she can keep her pickles, preserves, jellies, and jams. Up-stairs cupboards are seldom cool enough, except when they are in so exposed a position that there is risk of their contents freezing in the bitterest winter weather. Here, too, can be placed the choice fruit, the box of oranges or lemons, the barrel of pineapples and other delicacies, that keep better in a cold place than in ordinary pantry. The semi-gloom also helps preserve canned goods.

Drain-pipes frequently traverse the cellar, and are likely, from the obscurity of the place, to receive less attention than is their due. They should often be examined for leaks, and any such promptly checked. If there are open drains they should be washed down with a strong solution of copperas and water. Should the odor from the drains refuse to yield to this and to chloride of lime or potash they must be inspected by a practical plumber and the matter rectified without delay.

CELLARS, DAMPNESS IN, TO TEST:

Take a thermometer, a glass tumbler filled with water, and a piece of ice, then notice how the thermometer, when placed in the tumbler, has to sink before any moisture begins to show itself on the outside of the vessel of cold water; the lower the temperature to which the thermometer has to sink before moisture is precipitated the less there is of it in the moisture of the cellar.

CELLARS, DRY-ROT IN:

This in cellar timbers, can be prevented by coating the wood with whitewash to which has been added enough copperas to give the mixture a pale yellow hue.

CELLARS, FREEZING IN:

Paste the walls and ceiling over with 4 or 5 thicknesses of newspapers, make a curtain of the same material, paste over the window at the top of the cellar, paste the papers to the bare joist overhead, leaving an air-space between them and the floor; it is better to use a coarse brown paper; whatever paper is employed, sweep down the walls thoroughly, and use a very strong size to hold the paper to the stones; it is not necessary to press the paper down into all the depressions of the wall; every air-space beneath it is an additional defense against the cold.

CELLARS, MOLD IN:

(1) Put some roll brimstone(1) into a pan and set fire to it; close the doors, making the cellar as nearly airtight as possible for 2 or 3 hours, when the fungi will be destroyed and the mold dried up; repeat this operation every 2 or 3 months and the cellar will be free from parasitical growth.

(2) Pour 2 parts of concentrated sulphuric acid over 1 part of common salt; during the process all openings must be closed so as to prevent any escape of the gas, and the greatest care exercised not to enter the cellar after the operation until it has been thoroughly ventilated.

CHAMOIS SKIN, TO CLEAN:

Chamois may be cleaned in a solution of weak soda and warm water; rub plenty of soft-soap into the leather and allow it to remain in soak for two hours, then rub it well until it is quite clean. Afterward rinse it well in a weak solution composed of warm water, soda, and yellow soap. If rinsed in water only it becomes hard when dry, and unfit for use. The small quantity of soap left in the leather allows the finer particles of the leather to separate and become soft like silk. After rinsing wring it well in a rough towel and dry quickly; then pull it about and brush it well, and it will become softer and better than most new leather.

CHAMOMILE AND ITS USES:

The flowers of the chamomile are tonic, slightly anodyne, antispasmodic, and emetic. They are used externally as fomentations in colic, face-ache, and tumors, and for unhealthy ulcers. They are used internally in the form of infusion, with carbonate of soda, ginger, and other stomachic

(1) Sulfur

remedies, in dyspepsia, flatulent colic, debility following dysentery, and gout. Warm infusion of the flowers acts as an emetic, and the powdered flowers are sometimes combined with opium or kino and given in intermittent fevers.

Dose: Of the powdered flowers, from 10 grains to 1 dram, twice or thrice a day; of the infusion, from 1 to 2 ounces, as a tonic, three times a day; and from 6 ounces to 1 pint as an emetic; of the extract, from 5 to 20 grains.

CHAMOMILE TEA TONIC:

Into a common china teapot put about 25 good-sized chamomile flowers, and pour over them 1 pint of boiling water. Let the infusion stand half an hour, then pour it off into a wine-bottle, and, if desired, sweeten it with a little sugar or honey. It is best unsweetened. A wine-glassful should be taken three times a day before eating.

CHANDELIER, TO RENEW:

To renew a dusty and discolored chandelier, apply a mixture of bronze powder and copal varnish. The druggist of whom they are purchased will tell you in what proportion they should be mixed.

CHAPERONE, DUTIES OF:

The duties of a chaperone are tiresome. They call for great unselfishness. She must accompany her young charge into society. She must sit in the parlor when gentlemen are calling. She must, especially after the young lady is "engaged," go everywhere with her. A chaperone should be an intelligent woman. Society requires a certain amount of handling, which only the social expert understands. Some women have this tact, and a great many more have it not. It is a sort of genius. No very young flirtatious married woman, bent on amusing herself, should be selected for a chaperone for young girls. She is no protection to the charge, and she lacks the first requisite of a care-taker, a sense of propriety, and the second requisite, which is unselfishness. If any woman would have a spotless record it should be the chaperone. No harm will come to a girl from the companionship of a nice and good chaperone.

CHAPPED LIPS AND HANDS:(1)

(1) *A good salve may be made in this way:*

Take 2 ounces of white wax, 1 ounce of spermaceti, 4 ounces of almonds, 2 ounces of English honey, 1/4 ounce of essence of bergamot or any other perfume. Melt the wax and spermaceti, then add the honey, and melt all together, and when hot add the almond oil by degrees, stirring it till cold. This is superior to glycerine for chapped hands, sunburns, or any roughness on the skin.

(1) See "Camphor Ice."

(2) *The following is a well-tested, excellent remedy for chapped hands and sores of this nature:*

Put together equal weights of fresh, unsalted butter, tallow, beeswax, and stoned raisins; simmer until the raisins are done to a crisp, but not burned. Strain, and pour into cups to cool. Rub the hands thoroughly with it, and though they will smart at first they will soon feel comfortable and heal quickly.

(3) Instead of washing the hands with soap employ oatmeal, and after each washing take a little dry oatmeal, and rub over the hands, so as to absorb any moisture.

CHARADES, HOW TO PLAY:

Although the acting of charades is by no means an amusement of very recent invention, it is one that may be always so thoroughly attractive, according to the amount of originality displayed, that most young people, during an evening's entertainment, hail with glee the announcement that a charade is about to be acted. It is not necessary that any thing great should be attempted in the way of dressing, scenery, or similar preparation. Nothing is needed beyond a few old clothes, shawls, and hats, and a few clever, bright, intelligent young people, all willing to employ their best energies in contributing to the amusement of their friends.

The word charade derives its name from the Italian word *Schiarare*, to unravel or to clear up. The simplest charades, that require little if any previous preparation, are apt to furnish the most amusement. A little practice makes one quite expert in getting up charades, and the success of one or two good ones will suggest others equally bright.

We give a few simple ones that can be done by any body and almost anywhere. A man or a boy enters with his hat on his head. Man-hat-tan. An ax with several potatoes on it. Commentators on Acts. A gentleman enters. He is greeted by one of the performers with the salutation, "How do you do, doctor?" The answer is, Met-a-physician. And here is another that is somewhat newer. One says, "How do you do, Doc?" and the other says the same. This makes them, of course, A Par-a-dox.

CHARCOAL, TO MAKE:

Make a foundation of earth with a slightly convex surface slightly raised above the natural surface, drive a long, stout stake down in the middle, and round this pile the wood cut into lengths of 3 ft. or so. When the heap is finished cover the pile with 2 in. of dry earth, covered with sod, grass side in. The stake may then be drawn out and the cavity filled with shavings and chips. The hole in the top must be closed as soon as the fire is fairly started. Ventilation spaces must be left at the base till the fire is well established.

CHATTING AT MEALS:

When the stomach is satisfying its appetite the mind should not only be free from any painful emotion, but in a state of gentle and cheerful excitement. “Chatted food,” according to the old proverb, “is half digested.” This suggests the advantage of social eating, than which nothing is more conducive to the enjoyment as well as the digestion of food. With the sociability of a mixed dinner company there comes just the degree of mental liveliness required. The mind is distracted from its own preoccupations by the common talk to which each one contributes, without making an exhaustive draught upon his resources. Thus there is general animation without any individual fatigue. The whole nervous system is by this agreeable means, stirred to a gentle excitement which is favorable to the performance of every bodily function, and especially to that of digestion.

CHECKS:

Bank checks are orders drawn by individuals or firms on a bank or banker, payable either to “bearer” or to “order.” When payable to “bearer” they are usually paid to the holder on presentation; if to “order,” although properly indorsed, strangers cannot draw money on them without being identified.

CHEESE, COLORING FOR:

The coloring for cheese is, or at least should be, Spanish annatto; but as soon as coloring became general a color of an adulterated kind was exposed for sale in almost every shop. The weight of an ounce of real Spanish annatto is sufficient for a cheese of 50 lbs. weight. If a considerable part of the cream of the night’s milk be taken for butter, more coloring will be requisite. The leaner the cheese is the more coloring it requires. The manner of using annatto is to tie up in a linen rag the quantity deemed sufficient, and put it into 1/2 pint of warm water over night. This infusion is put into the tub of milk in the morning with the rennet infusion, dipping the rag into the milk and rubbing it against the palm of the hand as long as any color runs out. The yelk of egg will color butter.

CHEESE, TO KEEP FROM MOLD:

Dissolve a spoonful of bruised pepper, two tea-spoonfuls of salt, and the same quantity of boracic acid in 1/4 pint of brandy for a few days; then filter the fluid through a cloth and dilute with an equal quantity of water. Some of the preparation is introduced into the cracks of the cheese by means of a feather, or, better, with a small glass syringe. If places which have been nibbled by mice are rubbed with the liquid no mold will form. It will put “jumpers” to flight.

CHEMICALS, HOUSEHOLD:

Of chemicals for household use there should be 3 acids in every country cupboard; acetic acid, muriatic acid, and oxalic acid. Vinegar can be used in many cases instead of acetic acid, but vinegar contains coloring matters which stain delicate fabrics, and so is better to use the principal acid. If soda has been spilt on black silk, an application of acetic acid will usually restore the color. Many of the bright blue flannels owe their brilliant shades to an acid compound of a coal-tar color, and as soon as they are washed in soap or ammonia the alkali neutralizes the acid, and the color becomes pale and faded in appearance. If acetic acid or vinegar is added to the second rinsing water, the bright color is in all such cases restored. This fact is worth remembering. Of course, not all shades of blue are made with this compound, hence not all faded blues can be restored. It is well to test a bit of the cloth before washing the whole garment.

Muriatic acid is useful in a multitude of ways. Large stains of wet iron rust can be removed from blue cambric and other thin fabrics. Lay the cloths where the spots are over a large bowl half-filled with hot water, and touch the stains with a drop of the acid, and as soon as the iron dissolves plunge the cloth into the water and wash it out before there is any injury to the cloth. Then the cloth should be rinsed in several waters, and finally in water containing a little ammonia, which neutralizes any trace of the acid. This process is by far the best to remove rust-iron stains from white cloth.

CHERRIES, TO DRY:

(1) Stone, spread on a flat dish, and dry in the sun or a warm oven; pour whatever juice may run from them over them, a little at a time; stir them about, that they may dry evenly. When perfectly dry, line boxes or jars with white paper and pack close in layers; strew a little brown sugar, and fold the top of the paper over them, and keep in a dry, sweet place.

(2) Take large cherries, not too ripe; remove the pits; take equal weights of cherries and sugar; make a thick syrup of the sugar, put in the cherries and boil them a minute, and spread them on an earthen platter till the next day; strain the syrup; boil it down thick; put the cherries in and boil 5 minutes; spread on a platter as before; repeat the boiling 2 more days; then drain; lay them on wire sieves and dry in a nearly cold oven.

CHEWING-GUM:

Take of prepared balsam of tolu, 2 ounces; white sugar, 1 ounce; oatmeal, 3 ounces; soften the gum in water bath and mix in the ingredients; then roll in finely powdered sugar or flour to form sticks to suit.

CHEWING OR MASTICATION:

By this act food not only becomes comminuted, but mixed with the saliva and reduced to a form fit for swallowing. It has been justly regarded by the highest authorities as the first process of digestion, and one without which the powers of the stomach are overtasked, and often performed with difficulty. Hence the prevalence of dyspepsia and bowel complaints among persons with bad teeth, or those who bolt their food without chewing. It may not be necessary to count the movements of one's jaws, but better do that than not masticate properly. Food needs to be thoroughly mixed with saliva as well as to be crushed and softened and torn apart by the teeth. If it is not sufficiently chewed the stomach needs either to be overloaded in order to extract sufficient nutriment by imperfect processes, or, if only an ordinary quantity is eaten, it cannot provide nutriment enough. Food that is bolted irritates the stomach and impairs the digestive organs, so that the victim falls ill as a dyspeptic or worse.

Those who masticate their food too little and bolt it in bulk almost always aid the unnatural process by drinking copiously, so as to wash the food down their throats. Let those who do so pause a moment and consider what they are doing. Not only do they offer the digestive organs more than they can manage in unmasticated food, but, in addition, they fill the stomach with fluid which dilutes the gastric juices and still further obstructs digestion.

Of all the mistakes men make in eating, dressing, sleeping, or exercising, not one that we shall speak of is more hurtful than this peculiarly American 10-minutes-for-refreshments vice of washing meals down with water, (usually ice-water). It is often the cause of abnormal fatness, of that jelly-like bloating we see so much of among men in these days. Such men are unfitted for hard work, for proper exercise, and if disease attacks them they easily succumb. As for dinner, no matter how simple or unostentatious, give it all the consequence that the circumstances will allow. Make much of it. Treat it lovingly, and dwell upon it. It is the time when the cares of life can best be put aside, and a little refreshment be served to the faculties through unrestrained social intercourse and mental entertainment. Eat slowly, and, if best, little, but talk much and joyously. Doubtless that function which Chauncey M. Depew calls a circus, by which he means a lively flow of fun with his family at table, is what we ought all to copy.

CHICKEN CHOLERA:

For chicken cholera mix a good supply of salt in the dough when feeding. Keep plenty of fresh water and a clean house for them.

CHICKEN LICE, TO DESTROY:

The first signs of lice are with early setting hens. From their nest soon a whole house will be overrun with pests. Chicks show the presence of lice very quickly, and lice are certain death to them if they are not protected. Have all the nests movable, and change the contents frequently. With setting hens' nests be sure to have the nest clean and the box and surroundings whitewashed before she is placed. Whitewash and the dust-box are the surest preventatives of lice. Put 2 or 3 coats of whitewash on every interior spot in the building; the lice harbor in the crevices of the rough sidings, and on the under side of the perches.

Let the fowl-house have a dust-box. Mix hot ashes with the dust occasionally to dry it. Do all this early in the year, before spring laying and setting. Kerosene and lard when applied is a sure cure, but they are too often dangerous in their effects. A little castor-oil on the head and under the wings of setting hens is very effective. Don't keep a brood hen in a little coop without a dust wallow. If you want your fowls to be free from lice you must keep their habitation clean. The best way to do that is by occasional change of the nest contents, and thorough whitewashing of the apartment.

CHICKEN-POX:

This is a harmless but an annoying disease. And it resembles modified small-pox, or varioloid, the doctor should be called upon to decide which it is. Keep the patient in the house and other children away.

CHICKENS, GAPES IN:

This very common and fatal complaint in chickens may readily be cured by giving them some small pills of dough thoroughly impregnated with soft-soap.

CHICKENS, TO FATTEN:

The birds must be shut up; the pen or cage must not be too large, and it should not be tight and close. For a dozen birds a coop of 3 ft. wide or deep, 4 ft. long, and 2$^1/_2$ ft. high is large enough. The whole coop may properly be made of slats, except the roof. The floor should be so made as to allow the droppings of the birds to fall through. Birds that will agree peaceably only should be cooped up in a fattening-pen. If one is cross and masterful turn him or her out, and keep the fattening ones quiet.

Give as much food as they will eat up clean in a trough or basket in front of the cage, and give water after the feed is eaten. As a change, give some sand or gravel, or powdered charcoal, once a day. Keep the coop out in a airy place, but not where cold winds will blow through it. Feed rather sparingly than otherwise the first 2 or 3 days; afterward give as much as they will eat. This continued for 2 weeks should give you good, fat fowls; if they are not fat something is wrong and they should be let out. Fowls will fatten after 2 weeks' feeding, but they will not be so good to eat. Three weeks is long enough if all is right.

CHICKENS, YOUNG, FOOD FOR:

A writer in the Poultry Yard, who believes that chickens are often injured by corn-meal, would not let them have corn in any form until they are 3 or 4 weeks old, unless it be a little scalded or cooked meal, fed occasionally; and the principal food should be stale bread crumbled fine or moistened with milk, with wheat screenings, (when they get old enough to eat), scalded oatmeal, and cottage cheese, made from sour milk. This is not a very expensive method of feeding, as the chickens, being so small, will not consume much of it daily, while the best results have invariably followed such a system of feeding and management. It is far better to go to a little extra expense than to stand the chance of losing a number of valuable birds.

CHICORY:

This is the dried and roasted root of a plant allied to the dandelion, and it is found by almost unanimous testimony to be an agreeable flavorer of coffee. Dr. Hassall denounces the use of chicory, but with no sufficient reason. He states it to be "diuretic and aperient"—qualities which we declare to be in its favor, for it is the prevailing defect of our food that it is too astringent and heating, and the fact that chicory finds such general approbation we believe rests in the very qualities which Dr. Hassall condemns. We know a respectable grocer who, before legislation, took the matter up from conscientious motives, ceased to mix the chicory with coffee; the immediate effect was the falling-off of his coffee trade, his customers declaring that his coffee was not so good as previously; and he was compelled again to mix chicory with it to meet their taste.

CHILBLAINS(1):

First, insist on the patient wearing large shoes which do not compress the feet; touch the toes with nitrate of silver; liniment of aconite(2) is recommended; an ointment of lard and dry mustard rubbed in before the fire for 20 minutes will cure the trouble after a few applications: paint the affected parts with flexible collodion to protect them from the air; bathing in very hot water is efficacious; a strong solution of acetate of lead (20 grains to 1 ounce of water) is highly recommended; sulphurous acid is useful in mild cases; a local application of a thick paste composed of slaked lime, moistened with a very little water, and common oil, is recommended as a good remedy; laudanum(3), taken internally in very small doses of from 2 drops for young children, night and morning, up to 6 or 8 for adults, will also cure chilblains; anoint the affected part with either of the following formulae:

(1) A painful swelling of hand or foot caused by exposure to cold.
(2) Made from the poisonous dried root of the blue monkshood plant.
(3) Opium in alcohol; tincture of opium.

(1) Tincture of iodine, 1 ounce; Labarraque's mixture of chlorinated soda, 2 ounces: mix; dry the foot before the fire.

(2) Alcohol, 4 ounces; glycerine, 1 ounce; carbolic acid, 1 scruple; mix and make an ointment; anoint chilblains thoroughly 2 or 3 times a day.

Another very good remedy is to place red-hot coals on a pan, throw a handful of corn-meal over them, and hold the suffering feet in the dense smoke. Severe weather may produce a recurrence of the trouble at intervals, but persistent use of this remedy will prevent it as well as cure it. It has been known to effect very marked cures where the persons were unusually exposed, and when all other remedies were useless. There are local applications which sometimes afford relief, if a person can strike on the right one. Turpentine is to many a great blessing. Glycerine is a good thing to rub into the hands before washing with castile soap and tepid water. Warm vinegar sometimes avails. Kid gloves, lined with wool, are recommended, and, in general, care must be taken to keep the hands and feet from wet and cold.

Chilblains or Chapped Hands, Ointment for: Sweet oil, 1 pint; Venice turpentine, 3 ounces; hogs' lard, 1/2 lb.; beeswax, 3 ounces. Put all into pipkin(1) over a slow fire, and stir it with a wooden spoon till the beeswax is all melted and the ingredients simmer. It is fit for use as soon as cold, but the longer it is kept the better it will be. It must be spread very thin on the soft rag, or (for chaps or cracks) rubbed on the hands when you go to bed. A visitor to a large poor district has never know this to fail.

CHILDREN, CARE OF:

Early Food of Children: The nursing child finds its earliest and best food in the mother's milk. In most cases nothing more is needed until the first teeth appear. If the mother's milk is not sufficient, diluted milk from the cow may be used to supply the lack. If the mother does not nurse the child, cow's milk may be substituted. In such case the milk should consist for the first month of milk 1 part and water 2 parts, with about a half tea-spoonful of pure sugar to a half tumbler of the diluted milk. Condensed milk may be used instead, in which case the proportion should be 1 part of condensed milk and 10 parts water. Experience shows this mixture to be the best first food next to the mother's milk.

Early Diet: As a rule the child should be weaned when from 10 to 12 months old. Except in case of teething the time should not extend beyond that period, and may terminate at the age of 8 months. The nursing should not cease at once, as the abruptness of such change might prove unhealthful. It is well to wean the child first from day nursing, late from night nursing. Food may

(1) A small earthen boiler.

now be given, consisting of milk and sweetened water, with a little bread or cracker soaked therein. If convenient, arrowroot or rice flour, sage, or weak gruel of oatmeal may be added. It is best that the early food be neither cold nor hot—"milk-warm" is better. No tea or coffee or highly seasoned food should be given. A little tender meat, finely divided, or a little beef-tea, may be given once a day after the teeth for masticating food appear.

Exact Time for Weaning: Between the dentition of the 4 anterior molar teeth and the canines there is an interval of several months. This interval is recommended by that distinguished French medical professor and author, Foussagrives, as the most favorable time for weaning. All mothers should know this fact, and, when possible, weaning should be deferred until the child has 12 teeth. This rule is infinitely better than any one founded on age. Forced weaning at the time of dentition leads to disorders of the digestive passages. Hence it is dangerous to begin weaning during a teething crisis.

Regular Meals for Children: Later, as well as earlier, these meals should be as regular as possible, and the children should not be allowed to eat "between meals." The younger the child the more frequently should the meals be given. The habit of regularity cannot too strongly be insisted upon. And yet not one mother in ten observes this rule. The exercise of a little care with a little common sense will early enable the mother to arrange the plan of regular meals and keep it.

Baths for Children: For convenience, and to prevent chilliness, the child from the first should be washed in a small tub, with the body except the head immersed in milk-warm water. For thorough cleansing this should be done every morning and every evening. Not only is such a bath healthful in itself, but it also accustoms the child to the water. The warm bath should be used until 1½ or 2 years old, when a cool bath should be substituted. The bath should be very brief—at first not more than 2 minutes. The child's body should be quickly wiped dry and quickly clothed. No wet or soiled napkins should be allowed to remain on the child.

Clothing for Children: The clothing should be warm and light. As a rule, let long clothes be worn for about 6 months; then change, not to short clothes, but to those half way between short and long; later, when the child should learn to walk, to short clothes. Great care should be taken to keep the feet warm and dry. It is well to have fine soft flannel worn next to the skin. This should always be loose.

Sleep of Children: The best-informed medical advisers tell us that when in health children for the first month should sleep two thirds of the time, and then a little less, and so on until about 15 months old, when their sleep should be about 12 hours in 24. A child should be encouraged as long as possible to take a nap in the middle of the day, though after the age of 2 yrs. it will be found difficult in many cases to induce a continuance of the habit. Parents should insist that their children go to bed at regular hours. The earlier the hour the better, and nothing, neither callers at home nor company away from home, should allow interruption to the rule.

"Knock-knees," and How to Prevent Them: "Knock-knees," a common deformity, the physician ascribes to a common childish habit—that of sleeping on the side with one knee tucked in the hollow behind the other. He has found that where one leg has been bowed inwardly more than the other, the patient has always slept on one side, and the uppermost member has been that most deformed. Here the preventive is to pad the inside of the knees, so as to keep them apart, and let the limbs grow freely their own way.

Exercise for Children: They should be much in the open air, and for this purpose the baby carriages, now largely introduced into all large towns, are a great boon to society. All violent exercise should be avoided. Tossing up and down or jolting in a chair is not well, especially during the first months. In carrying the child around in the arms or carriage it should be kept in a horizontal position.

CHILDREN, COOKERY FOR:

Food for an Infant: Take of fresh cow's milk 1 table-spoonful, and mix with 2 table-spoonfuls of hot water; sweeten with loaf-sugar as much as may be agreeable. This quantity is sufficient for once feeding a new-born infant; and the same quantity may be given every 2 or 3 hours, not oftener, till the mothers's breast affords natural nourishment.

Milk for Infants Six Months Old: Take 1 pint of milk, 1 pint of water, boil it, and add 1 table-spoonful of flour. Dissolve the flour first in half a tea-spoonful of water; it must be strained in gradually, and boiled hard 20 minutes. As the child grows older, 1/2 water. If properly made, it is the most nutritious, at the same time the most delicate, food that can be given to young children.

Broth: Broth, made of lamb or chicken, with stale bread toasted and broken in, is safe and healthy for the dinners of children when first weaned.

Milk: Milk, fresh from the cow, with very little loaf-sugar, is a good and safe food for young children. From 3 yrs. old to 7 pure milk, into which is crumbled stale bread, is the best breakfast and supper for a child.

For a Child's Luncheon: Good sweet butter with stale bread is one of the most nutritious, at the same time the most wholesome, articles of food that can be given children after they are weaned.

Milk Porridge: Stir 4 table-spoonfuls of oatmeal smoothly into a quart of milk; then stir it quickly into a quart of boiling water, and boil up a few minutes till it is thickened; sweeten with sugar. Oatmeal, where it is found to agree with the stomach, is much better for children, being a fine opener as well as a cleanser; fine flour in every shape is the reverse. Where biscuit-powder is in use, let it be made at home; this, at all events, will prevent them getting the sweepings of the baker's counters, boxes, and baskets. All the left bread in the nursery, hard ends of stale loaves, etc., ought to be dried in the oven or screen, and reduced to powder in the mortar.

Meats for Children: Mutton, lamb, and poultry are the best. Birds and the white meat of fowls are the most delicate food of this kind that can be given. These meats should be slowly cooked, and no gravy, if made rich with butter, should be eaten by a young child. Never give children hard, tough, well-worked meats of any kind.

Vegetables for Children.—Eggs, etc.: Their rice ought to be cooked in no more water than is necessary to swell it; their apples roasted, or stewed with no more water than is necessary to steam them; their vegetables so well cooked as to make them require little butter, and less digestion; their eggs boiled slow and soft. The boiling of their milk ought to be directed by the state of their bowels; if flatulent or bilious, a very little curry-powder may be given in their vegetables with good effect; turmeric and the warm seeds (not hot peppers) are particularly useful in such cases.

Potatoes and Peas: Potatoes, particularly some kinds, are not easily digested by children; but this is easily remedied by mashing them very fine and seasoning them with sugar and a little milk. When peas are dressed for children, let them be seasoned with mint and sugar, which will take off the flatulency. If they are old let them be pulped, as the skins are perfectly indigestible by children's or weak stomachs. Never give them vegetables less stewed than would pulp though a colander.

Rice-pudding with Fruit: In a pint of new milk put 2 large spoonfuls of rice well washed; then add 2 apples, pared and quartered, or a few currants or raisins. Simmer slowly till the rice is very soft, then add 1 egg beaten, to bind it. Serve with cream and sugar.

Puddings and Pancakes for Children: Sugar and egg browned before the fire, or dropped as fritters into a hot frying-pan without fat, will make a nourishing meal.

To prepare Fruit for Children: A far more wholesome way than in pies or puddings is to put apples sliced, or plums, currants, gooseberries, etc., into a stone jar, and sprinkle among them as much sugar as necessary. Set the jar in an oven on a hearth., with teacupful of water to prevent the fruit from burning, or put the jar into a saucepan of water, till its contents are perfectly done. Slices of bread or some rice may be put into the jar to eat with the fruit.

Rice and Apples: Core as many nice apples as will fill the dish; boil them in light syrup; prepare 1/4 lb. of rice in milk with sugar and salt; put some of the rice in the dish, and put in the apples and fill up the intervals with rice, and bake it in the oven till it is a fine color.

A Nice Apple-cake for Children: Grate some stale bread and slice about double the quantity of apples; butter a mold, and line it with sugar paste, and strew in some crumbs mixed with a little sugar; then lay in apples with a few bits of butter over them, and so continue till the dish is full; cover it with crumbs or prepared rice, season with cinnamon and sugar. Bake it well.

Fruits for Children: That fruits are naturally wholesome in their season if rightly taken no one who believes that the Creator is a kind and a beneficent Being can doubt. And yet the use of summer fruits appears often to cause most fatal diseases, especially in children. Why is this? Because we do not conform to natural laws in using this kind of diet. These laws are very simple and easy to understand. Let the fruit be ripe when you eat it, and eat when you require food.

Fruits that have seeds are much healthier than the stone fruits. But all fruits are better for very young children baked or cooked in some manner, and eaten with bread. The French always eat bread with raw fruit. Apples and winter pears are very excellent food for children, indeed, for almost any person in health; but best when eaten for breakfast or dinner. If taken late in the evening, fruit often proves injurious. The old saying, that apples are gold in the morning, silver at noon, and lead at night, is pretty near the truth. Both apples and pears are often good and nutritious when baked or stewed for those delicate constitutions that cannot bear raw fruit. Much of the fruit gathered when unripe might be rendered fit for food by preserving in sugar.

Ripe Currants: Ripe currants are excellent food for children. Mash the fruit, sprinkle with sugar, and with good bread let them eat of this fruit freely.

Blackberry Jam: Gather the fruit in dry weather; allow 1/2 lb. of good brown sugar to every pound of fruit; boil the whole together gently for an hour, or till the blackberries are soft, stirring and mashing them well. Preserve it like any other jam, and it will be found very useful in families, particularly for children—regulating their bowels, and enabling you to dispense with cathartics. It may be spread on bread or on puddings instead of butter; and even when the blackberries are bought it is cheaper than butter. In the country every family should preserve at least, 1/2 peck of blackberries.

To make Senna and Manna(1) Palatable: Take 1/2 ounce when mixed, senna and manna; put in 1/2 pint of boiling water; when the strength is abstracted pour into the liquid form a 1/4 to 1/2 lb. of prunes and 2 large table-spoonfuls of W. I. molasses. Stew slowly until the liquid is nearly absorbed. When cold it can be eaten with bread and butter without detecting the senna, and is excellent for costive children.

CHILDREN'S DISEASES, TREATMENT OF:

In the case of a baby not yet being able to talk it must cry when it is ill. The colic makes a baby cry loud, long, and passionately, and shed tears, stopping for a moment and beginning again. If the chest is affected it gives one sharp cry, breaking off immediately as if crying hurt it. If the head is affected it cries in sharp piercing shrieks, with low moans and wails between. Or there may be quiet dozing, and startings between. It is easy enough to perceive, where a child is attacked by disease, that there is some change taking place; for either its skin will be dry and hot, its appetite gone; it is stupidly sleepy or fretful and crying; it is thirsty or pale and languid, or in some way betrays that something is wrong.

When a child vomits or has a diarrhea, or is costive and feverish, it is owing to some derangement and needs attention. But these various symptoms may continue for a day or two before the nature of the disease can be determined. A warm bath, warm drinks, etc., can do no harm, and may help to determine the case. On coming out of the bath and being well rubbed with the hand, the skin will show symptoms of rash if it is a skin disease which has commenced. By the appearance of the rash the nature of the disease can be learned. Measles are in patches, dark red, and come out first about the face. If scarlet fever is impending, the skin will look a deep pink all over the body, though mostly so about the neck and face.

Chicken-pox shows fever, but not so much running as the nose and appearance of cold, as in measles, nor is there so much of a cough. Besides the spots are smaller and do not run much together, and are more diffused over the whole surface of the skin and enlarge into little blisters in a day or two.

Let the room where a child is sick be shady, quiet, and cool. Be careful not to speak so suddenly as to startle the half-sleeping patient, and handle it with the greatest tenderness when it is necessary to move it. If it is lungs that suffer, have the little patient somewhat elevated upon the pillows

(1) Laxative.

for easier breathing, and do every thing to soothe and make it comfortable, so as not to have it cry and to thus distress its inflamed lungs.

If the child is very weak do not move it too suddenly, as it may be startled into convulsions. In administering a bath the greatest pains must be taken not to frighten the child. It should be put in so gradually, and so amused by something placed in the water on purpose, as to forget its fear; keep up a good supply of fresh air at a temperature of about 66 degrees Fahr.

If a hired nurse must be had, select, if possible, a woman of intelligence, gentle and loving disposition, kind and amiable manners, and of a most pacific, unruffled, and even temper. If a being can be got possessed of these angelic qualities, and we believe there are many such, you will be quite safe in intrusting to her care and the management of your sick child, or yourself either, in case of sickness. She should not be under 25 or over 55, as between these two ages she will, if healthy, be in her full strength and capacity.

CHILDREN TEETHING:

The pain of teething may be almost done away with and the health of the child benefited by giving it fine splinters of ice, picked off with a pin, to melt in its mouth. The fragment is so small that it is but a drop of warm water before it can be swallowed, and the child has all the coolness for its feverish gums without the slightest injury. The avidity with which the little things taste the cooling morsel, the instant quiet which succeeds hours of fretfulness, and the sleep which follows the relief are the best witnesses to this magic remedy. Ice may be fed to a 3 months' old child this way, each splinter being no larger than a common pin, for 5 or 10 minutes, the result being that it has swallowed in that time a teaspoonful of warm water, which, so far from being a harm, is good for it, and the process may be repeated hourly as often as the fretting fits from teething begin.

CHIMNEY, TO CLEAN:

To clean a chimney place a piece of zinc on the live coals in the stove. The vapor produced by the zinc will carry off the soot by chemical decomposition.

CHIMNEYS, SMOKING:

(1) Large fire-places are apt to smoke, particularly when the aperture of the funnel does not correspond in size; for this a temporary remedy may be found in opening a door or window—a permanent cure by diminishing the lower aperture; the best method of cure is to carry from the air a pipe under the floor and opening under the fire. The chimney may only smoke when the wind is in a particular quarter, connected with the position of some higher building, or a

hill, or grove of trees; the common turn-cap, as made by tin and iron men, will generally be found a fully adequate remedy.

(2) Use a screen or blower of fine wire gauze, from 36 to 40 wires to the inch, immediately in front of the fire and about 2 in. therefrom.

CHINA, CARE OF:

When fine china is put away in the china closet pieces of paper should be placed between them to prevent scratches on the glaze or painting; the china closet should be in a dry situation, as a damp closet will soon tarnish the gilding of the best crockery. In a common dinner-service it is a great evil to make the plates too hot, as it invariably cracks the glaze on the surface, if not the plate itself; when the glaze is injured, every time the "things" are washed the water gets to the interior, swells the porous clay, and makes the whole fabric rotten.

CHINA, TO MEND:

China may be mended by a paste made of the white of an egg mixed with flour. The article so mended will not hold water, but for vases, lamp-shades, and similar purposes answers a good purpose and is handy.

CHINTZ, TO WASH:

Take 2 lbs. of rice and boil it in 2 gallons of water till soft; when done pour the whole into a tub, let it stand till about the warmth you in general use for colored linens; put the chintz in and use the rice instead of soap. Wash the chintz in this till the dirt appears to be out; then boil the same quantity as above, but strain the rice from the water and mix it with warm water. Wash it in this till quite clean; afterward rinse it in the water the rice was boiled in. This will answer the end of the starch, and no wet will affect it, as it will be stiff when it is worn. If a gown it must be taken to pieces, and when dried hang it as smooth as possible; after dry rub it with smooth stone, but use no iron.

CHIP DIRT FOR FRUIT TREES:

Many farmers do not know that they have a mine of wealth—a small one—in the very door-yard. Chip dirt is the very best material to mix with the soil in setting out young trees. It is full of the elements of plant food and retains moisture. If you are setting out a new orchard plow up and utilize the soil from the old wood-pile.

CHLORIDE OF LIME A DISINFECTANT:

This is very useful to counteract disagreeable smells and as a disinfectant. It should be put into small earthen pans and set where needed. Of course it will require occasional renewing. This useful disinfectant should be kept in every house to purify a sick-room, and to remove all unpleasant smells. Tainted garments may be rendered harmless by sprinkling them with a weak solution of it; and a piece of sponge dipped in this solution and held to the nose will enable any one with comparative safety to enter a foul sewer.

CHOKING, WAYS TO RELIEVE:

(1) Do not lose an instant. Force the mouth open with the handle of a knife or a long spoon; push the thumb and fingers deep down into the throat beyond the root of the tongue, and feel for the foreign body. If the obstruction cannot be grasped, a hair-pin bent into a hook and guided by the left hand will often bring it out. If this fails get some one to press against the front of the chest, or support it against the edge of a table, and strike several hard, quick blows with open hand on the back between the shoulder-blades. Further treatment must be applied by a physician, who should have been immediately sent for.

(2) To prevent choking break an egg into a cup and give it to the person chocking to swallow. The white of he egg seems to catch around the obstacle and remove it. If one egg does not answer the purpose, try another. The white is all that is necessary.

(3) A smart blow with the flat of the hand on the back, just below the neck, will often relieve the windpipe. If it does not, send for the doctor at once.

(4) Foreign bodies lodged in the throat can be removed by forcibly blowing into the ear. The plan is so easily tried and so harmless that we suggest its use.

CHOLERA, RULES FOR THE PREVENTION OF:

We urge the necessity in all cases of cholera of an instant recourse to medical aid, and also under every form and variety of indisposition; for all disorders are found to merge in the dominant disease.

- Let immediate relief be sought under the disorder of the bowels especially, however slight. The invasion of cholera may thus be readily prevented.
- Let every impurity, animal and vegetable, be quickly removed to a distance from the habitations, such as slaughter-houses, pig-sties, cess-pools, necessaries, and all other domestic nuisances.
- Let all uncovered drains be carefully and frequently cleansed.
- Let the grounds in and around the habitations be drained so as effectually to carry off moisture of every kind.

- Let all partitions be removed, from within and without habitations, which unnecessarily impede ventilation.
- Let every room be daily thrown open for the admission of fresh air; this should be done about noon, when the atmosphere is most likely to be dry.
- Let dry scrubbing be used in domestic cleaning in place of water cleaning.
- Let excessive fatigue and exposure to damp and cold, especially during the night, be avoided.
- Let the use of cold drinks and acid liquors, especially under fatigue, be avoided, or when the body is heated.
- Let the use of cold acid fruits and vegetables be avoided.
- Let a poor diet and the use of impure water in cooking or for drinking be avoided.
- Let the wearing of wet and insufficient clothes be avoided. Let a flannel or woolen belt be worn around the belly.
- Let personal cleanliness be carefully observed. Let every cause tending to depress the moral and physical energies be avoided.
- Let crowding of persons within houses and apartments be avoided.
- Let sleeping in low or damp rooms be avoided.
- Let fires be kept up during the night in sleeping or adjoining apartments, the night being the period of most danger from attack, especially under exposure to cold or damp.
- Let all bedding and clothing be daily exposed during winter and spring to the fire, and in summer to the heat of the sun.
- Let the dead be buried in places remote from the habitation of the living. By the timely adoption of simple means such as these, cholera or other epidemic diseases will be made to lose their venom.

CHOLERA INFANTUM, REMEDY FOR:

Toast a half-slice of stale bread very brown, break in a goblet, and fill with water; put in as much soda as you can hold on a three cent piece; let the little one drink a little at a time. If the stomach is very irritable give only a tea-spoonful at a time. In some cases, with the advice of a physician put a tea-spoonful of paregoric in the gobletful.

CHROMOS(1), TO MOUNT:

Take common bleached muslin, (heavily starched is best), make a thick flour paste, cook till clear, then strain. Saturate the cloth with the paste, lay the chromo on the cloth face up, turn over and smooth out all the wrinkles and air puffs. Have a stretch-frame prepared of the proper size made of three eights in. soft wood, mitered and well nailed. Lay the chromo on the frame—back on frame. Commence in center of frame and drive a tack on each side, drawing the canvas gently, but not too tight, both sidewise and endwise of the frame; this obviates the difficulty of puckering on the corners. The end is not so particular only to draw quite tight. If it is not smooth when first finished it will be all right when it dries. You can varnish with best white varnish after it is dry.

CIDER BARRELS, TO CLEANSE:

Pour in lime-water and then insert a trace-chain through the bung-hole, remembering to fasten a strong cord on the chain so as to pull it out again. Shake the barrel until all the mold inside is rubbed off. Rinse with water and finally pour in a little whisky.

CINDERS IN THE EYE, TO REMOVE:

A small camel's hair brush dipped in water and passed over the ball of the eye on raising the lid. The operation requires no skill, takes but a moment, and instantly removes any cinder or particle of dust or dirt without inflaming the eye.

CISTERNS, WATERPROOFING:

To make cisterns and tanks waterproof paint thickly on the inside with a mixture composed of 8 parts of melted glue and 4 parts of linseed oil, boiled with litharge. In 48 hours after the application it will have hardened so that the cistern or tank can be filled with water.

CISTERN WATER, TO CLEAR:

(1) Never allow a mudhole to remain about a well. If the water is muddy and impure throw in a peck of lime to purify it; if animalculae(2) appear in the water throw in $^1/_2$ gallon of salt to make them settle to the bottom.

(2) Add 2 ounces of powered alum and 2 ounces of borax to a 20-barrel cistern of rain-water that is blackened or oily, and in a few hours the sediment will settle, and the water be clarified and fit for washing.

(1) Chromolithograph, a colored picture printed with the lithograph process.
(2) Microscopically small animals.

CISTERN WATER, TO KEEP SWEET:

To prevent cistern water from becoming impure, have the supply pipe run nearly to the bottom of the well, where the purest water is always to be obtained.

CLAP! CLAP!:

This game may be played in or out of the house.

Example:

Mary puts her hand under her pinafore, cloak, or cape, holds up a finger inside it, and of course out of sight, and says,

"Mingledy, mingledy, clap! clap! How may fingers do I hold up?"

The others guess 1, 2, 3, or 5, as they think most likely to be right; but it is very rarely that the guess proves correct. If not, the guesser pays a forfeit, and the player (changing the number of fingers) begins again. When a little girl guesses rightly, it becomes her turn to play and the former pays a forfeit.

CLEANING COMPOUND:

Mix 1 ounce of borax and 1 ounce of gum camphor with 1 quart of boiling water. When cool add 1 quart of alcohol; bottle and cork tightly. When wanted for use shake well and sponge the garments to be cleaned. This is an excellent mixture for cleaning soiled black cashmere and woolen dresses, coat-collars, and black felt hats.

CLEANING MIXTURE:

To clean coat-collars, to take out grease from floors or carpets, and to clean paint or white walls, (kalsomined), take half a bar of washing soap, and a lump of saltpeter and sal soda each as large as a walnut; add 2 quarts boiling soft water, stir well, and let it stand till cool, then add 3 ounces of ammonia: bottle and cork tight. Will keep good a year. It is best to bottle when lukewarm and add the ammonia at any time.

CLEANLINESS:

The proper healthfulness of cities and dwellings depends upon personal cleanliness, household cleanliness, and municipal cleanliness. All the legislation conceivable will be of no service in preserving the health of a city unless the first of these is observed, and it is there that the work should commence.

Free baths, with whatever of compulsion is necessary to make that class of citizens use them who need them most, and which class is most adverse to their use, are the first importance. Bodily cleanliness is the first step toward household neatness, for no clean family will live in a filthy house. For methods see *BATHING*.

The cleansing of dwellings does not depend alone on the use of water. Dry dirt is preferable to moist and moldy cleanliness. Scrubbing is good sanitation only when followed by thorough drying and ventilation. Dry dirt, even on a kitchen floor is far more tolerable, hygienically, than slops and rotten beams under the floor. Moist and mildewed papers held to sodden walls by putrid paste will originate diseases which could have no existence in a dry atmosphere.

These evils are often intensified by the addition of sewer-gases escaping from defective joints. Tear off sodden paper, carry off from the roofs the rain which permeates the walls, and put down kitchen floors that are impermeable to water.

To properly cleanse streets and alleys is to remove the filth, by scraping and sweeping it up and carting it away; by leaving the streets as dry as may be except from the most superficial sprinkling; by removing all the slops and garbage from the alleys, and using disinfectants at all offensive localities. A model street is one composed of a smooth, not slippery, hard material, impermeable to moisture, having its dust and accumulations swept or washed away at night.

CLINKERS IN STOVES, TO REMOVE:

When the firebricks have become covered with clinkers which have fused and adhered they may be cleaned by throwing oyster or clam shells into the fire-box when the fire is very hot, and allowing the fire to go out. The clinkers will generally cleave off without the use of much force the next morning. From 1 quart to 1 peck will be sufficient for most stoves, and the operation can be repeated if some of the clinkers still adhere. Salt sprinkled on clinkers adhering to fire-brick will also loosen them.

CLOCKS TO CLEAN:

Take the movement of the clock to pieces. Brush the wheels and pinions thoroughly with a stiff, coarse brush; also the plates where the trains work. Clean the pivots well by turning in a piece of cotton cloth held tightly between your thumb and finger. The pivot-holes in the plates are generally cleansed by turning a piece of wood into them, but I have always found a strip of cloth or a soft cord drawn tightly through them to act the best. If you use two cords, the first one lightly oiled and the next dry, to clean the oil out, all the better. Do not use salt or acid to clean your clock—it can do no good, but may do a great deal of harm. Boiling the movement in water, as is the practice of some, is also foolishness.

To Oil Properly: Oil only, and very lightly, the pallets of the verge, the steel pin upon which the verge works, and the point where the loop of the verge wire works over the pendulum wire. Use none but the best watch oil. Though you might be working constantly at the clock-repairing business, a bottle costing but 25 cents would last you 2 yrs. at least. You can buy it at any watch-furnishing establishment.

A Defect to Look After: Always examine the pendulum wire at the point where the loop of the verge wire works over it. You will generally find a small notch or at least a rough place worn there. Dress it out perfectly smooth, or your clock will not be likely to work well. Small as this defect may seem, it stops a large number of clocks.

CLOSETS, DAMP, TO PURIFY:

In damp closets and cupboards generating mildew a tray full of quicklime will be found to absorb the moisture and render the air pure. Of course it is necessary to renew the lime from time to time as it becomes slaked. This remedy will be found useful in safes and strong-rooms, the damp air of which acts frequently most injuriously on the valuable deeds and documents contained therein.

CLOTH, TO FASTEN ON WOODEN SURFACES:

The following is a German process for fastening cloth to the top of tables, desks, etc.:

Make a mixture of $2^1/4$ lbs. of wheat flour, 2 table-spoonfuls of powdered resin, and 2 table-spoonfuls of powdered alum; rub the mixture in a suitable vessel, with water, to a uniform, smooth paste; transfer this to a small kettle over a fire, and stir until the paste is perfectly homogeneous—without lumps. As soon as the mess has become so stiff that the stirrer remains upright in it, transfer it to another vessel and cover it up, so that no skin may form on its surface.

This paste is applied in a very thin layer to the surface of the table; the cloth, etc., is then laid and pressed upon it and smoothed with a roller. The ends are cut after drying. If leather is to be fastened on, this must first be wet. The paste is then applied and the leather rubbed smooth with a cloth.

CLOTH, TO MAKE WATER-PROOF:

To make cloth water-proof dissolve 8 lbs. oleic acid in 6 quarts of alcohol; add gradually 20 lbs. sulphate of alumina; leave 24 hours to settle; carefully pour off the liquid and save the remaining deposit; filter this through flannel and press it into a cake. Dissolve 1 lb. of this in 15 to 20 gallons of water, strain, saturate the fabric thoroughly, remove, and let dry. The fabric is water-proof without having its ventilating qualities destroyed.

CLOTHES, WASHING:

To Clean a White Lace Veil: Put the veil into strong lather of white soap and very clear water, and let it simmer slowly for $^1/4$ hour. Take it out and squeeze it well, but be sure not to rub it. Rinse it in 2 cold waters, with a drop or two of liquid blue in the last. Have ready some very clear gum arabic water, or some thin starch, or rice water. Pass the veil through it, and clear it by clapping. Then stretch it out even and put it to dry on a linen cloth, making the edge as straight as possible, opening out all the scallops and fastening each with pins. When dry, lay a piece of thin muslin smoothly over it, and iron it on the wrong side.

Fine Colored Fabrics: To wash colored stockings, or any delicate colored fabrics, table-linen, lawns, or cambrics, etc., dissolve 1 table-spoonful of sugar of lead in 1 gallon water; soak the articles thoroughly in the solution; then dry.

Merino Stockings: Boil the soap to make a lather, wash them in this warm, and rinse in a second lather. If white, mix a little blue. Never rinse in plain water, or use cold water.

Colors Stand in Delicate Hose: Turn the stockings right side out, and wash in a lather of lukewarm water and white castile soap; then wash the wrong side. If very much soiled, two waters will be required. Rinse in lukewarm water and then in cold water; dry as soon as possible by heat, not by sun. It is better not to iron them, but when nearly dry, smooth and pull them into shape by hand.

Chintz: Boil 2 lbs. of rice in 2 gallons of water till soft, and pour it into a tub; let it stand until it subsides into a moderate warmth; put the chintz in and wash it, without using soap, until the dirt disappears; then boil the same quantity of water and rice as before, but strain off the rice and mix it in warm water. Wash the chintz in this till quite clean; afterward rinse it in the water the rice was boiled in; this will answer for starch and dew will not affect it.

Prints: To a sufficient quantity of hot water for washing a dress add a table-spoonful of ox gall. Let the dress remain in this a few minutes, then cool enough to wash out like other prints. Rinse immediately in cold water and dry as quickly as possible in the open air. If there are spots to be removed apply soap when dry.

Woolen Clothing: Articles of woolen washed in ordinary soap and water not only shrink, but acquire a peculiar fatty odor, due to the decomposition of the soap by the lactic and acetic acids present in the perspiration and consequently precipitation of the greater part of the fat of the soap in the fiber of the wool. To prevent these effects steep the articles for several hours in a warm, moderately concentrated solution of washing-soda; then, after the addition of warm water and a few drops of ammonia, wash and rinse them in luke-warm water.

Table Linen: Put a tea-spoonful of sugar of lead into two thirds of a pail of water, and when dissolved soak the table-linen in it 15 or 20 minutes. Be careful in wringing the article from this water that there is no cut or sore on the hands, as the sugar of lead is poisonous. Every thing that is liable to fade must be washed quickly, and not allowed to soak in suds or rinsing-water, and hung in a shady place to dry.

- Never wash flannel, silk, or colored things on a wet or cloudy day, but lay them aside for a fair day; and when washing such articles, do not let them stand and soak, but wash, rinse, starch,(if needed), and hang out each thing as fast as possible, and then take the next.

CLOTHING:

The object of our clothing should be threefold; warmth in winter, coolness in summer, and health and comfort at all times. Our clothes have no power to manufacture or impart heat. Heat is generated within our bodies, and what is termed warm clothing is that made from materials that are bad conductors of it, and which consequently retain the natural heat of our bodies; and cool clothing is made from materials that are good conductors of heat, and hence convey it away from the body or allow it to escape. Linen is a good conductor of heat, and is hence largely worn in summer and in tropical or warm climates. Cotton is not so good a conductor of heat, and hence is warmer than linen. Silk and wool are bad conductors of heat, and are hence much warmer and consequently better suited for winter clothing and for colder climates. Furs and feathers are very bad conductors of heat, and much used for wraps of various kinds.

All kinds of clothing near the skin absorb more or less of insensible perspiration, and should be frequently changed. Clothing worn through the day should be laid off and a night-dress used for sleeping in. India rubber, when worn continuously, is injurious and unhealthy, on account of interrupting and retaining the insensible perspiration. All wearing apparel of this kind should be laid off upon entering the house.

All persons should wear thick or thin flannel next the skin winter and summer; it absorbs the perspiration and does not chill the body by coming in contact with it, as cotton and linen garments do. The feet should at all times be kept warm and dry, and the shoes and boots should be made of substantial material and with thick soles. Clothing should be made to fit the form.

We should not attempt to torture the body into some unnatural form to suit the foolish caprice of fashion. The dress of children should favor to the fullest extent the natural and unrestrained development of the body. Many poor infants are cruelly tortured, deformed, or permanently injured for life by tight and misshaped dresses. The practice of dressing infants in long clothes is objectionable when continued too long or beyond severe weather, for besides being injurious to health, it cramps the action of the limbs, and by so doing prevents their proper development.

CLOTHING AND HEALTH:

Healthy Clothing: The most healthful clothing for our climate the year around is that made of wool. If worn next the skin by all classes, in summer as well as winter, an incalculable amount of coughs, colds, diarrhea, dysenteries, and fevers would be prevented, as also many sudden and premature deaths from croup, diphtheria, and lung diseases. Winter maladies would be prevented by the ability of a woolen garment to keep the natural heat about the body more perfectly, instead of conveying it away as fast as generated, as linen and flaxen garments do, as also cotton and silk, although these are less cooling than Irish linen, as any one can prove by noticing the different degrees of coldness on the application of a surface of 6 in. square of flannel, cotton, and linen to the skin the moment the clothing is removed. The reason is that wool is a bad conductor of heat.

Flannel in Summer and Winter: The benefit and comfort of wearing flannel next the body, in summer as well as winter, cannot be overestimated. Flannel is not so uncomfortable in warm weather as many believe. Frequent colds and coughs are almost unknown when flannels are worn. Some women object to them because they are bulky about the waist. This objection can be obviated by shaping them in tight sack fashion, or cutting them out like waists and buttoning them behind. The sudden and frequent changes of our climate are scarcely felt, and certainly do very little injury to those persons who wear flannels constantly. Above all, mothers should clothe the tender bodies of their little ones with under-garments of this material. Warmth is almost as necessary to healthful development as food, and parents should endeavor to clothe their children so as to secure the greatest amount for them.

Insufficient Clothing: One of the great evils induced by fashion is the unequal distribution of clothing upon the person. One part over-clothed and another not half clad is a very common condition, especially among women and children. Women are governed by fashion, children are governed by women, and it is the great resource of fashion to produce new effects by piling on the textures, now here and now there, and by leaving other parts exposed. If the declared purpose were to induce disease, no surer or more effectual way could be found to do it than this. The derangement of the circulation is direct and immediate; its healthy equilibrium is destroyed, the thinly dressed parts lose blood to the more vascular, and internal derangements give rise to various chronic bodily ailments.

High-heeled Boots and Shoes: Says the Journal of Chemistry: "We shall not quarrel with the little jaunty hats of the ladies, for they are indeed pretty and no harm results from them, as of all parts of the body the head needs the least clothing. But, to pass to the other extremity, we have to say that the detestable high heels to boots and shoes, running, as they do, almost to a point, are spoiling the gait and ruining the ankle-joints of children and young misses. We are careful to order our shoemakers to remove such heels from shoes before permitting them to be brought into our dwelling. Heels of moderate height and good breath are of great service in elevating the feet so as to avoid direct contact with moist earth, and they also give support and add firmness to the step. Why should fashion push good devices to absurd extremes? We must aid the dethroning of the tyrant when her decrees lead to the physical or moral injury of the race."

Newspapers as Protectors from Cold: A newspaper folded several times and laid across the chest during a cold walk or ride is a most excellent protector. If the bed-clothing is not sufficiently warm, especially at hotels, 2 or 3 large newspapers spread on the bed between the blankets will secure a comfortable night, as far as cold is concerned. A thin shawl may be made warm by folding a paper inside it. The paper is impervious to the wind and cold air from outside, and prevents the rapid escape of warm air from beneath it. If you suffer from cold feet on a journey, fold a piece of newspaper over your stockings; this is better than rubbers.

Under-clothing: All under-clothing should be suspended from the shoulders in order to relieve the waist, and it is needless to say corsets should be abandoned. To do this, the two principal articles should be joined, forming a garment something like children's night-drawers, but fitting closer to the body. The petticoats and skirts should be hung from the shoulders by straps made of muslin or other light material.

Garters: One of the most frequent and flagrant causes of obstruction in the circulation is the ordinary elastic garter. Children should never wear them at all, as the stockings can be perfectly well kept up by attachment of elastic straps to the waistband. If garters are worn, it is important to know how to apply them with the least risk of harm. At the bend of the knee the superficial veins of the leg unite and go deeply into the under part of the thigh beneath the hamstring tendons. Thus a ligature below the knee obstructs all the superficial veins, but if the constriction is above, the hamstring tendons keep the pressure off the veins which return the blood from the legs. Unfortunately most people, in ignorance of the above facts apply the garter below the knee. Elastic bands are the most injurious. They follow the movements of the muscles and never relax their pressure upon the veins. Non-elastic bands, during muscular exertion, become considerably relaxed at intervals, and allow a freer circulation of the blood.

Muffling the Throat: There is nothing that makes the throat delicate and sensitive more than muffling it closely in wraps of woolen and fur. The rule is that the neck should be kept as cool as comfort will allow. Tight collars frequently cause diseases of the throat and lungs. The neck should be dressed lightly. From the many movements which are made by the larynx in speaking it is inferred that it is a matter of great importance that the neck in health should be always loosely dressed. Tight cravats(1) are sure to obstruct the proper function of this organ and bring on irritation, which may lead to bronchitis or consumption.

An eminent physician, who devotes his whole attention to the throat and lungs, says that about three fourths of all throat diseases would get well by wearing very loose collars and no neck-tie at all. He also adds: "If you have a disease of the throat, let nature do the curing, and the physician just as little as possible."

CLUB-FOOT:

A disease common to cabbage grown in moist mucky land. It is caused by a maggot or worm that infects the fine rootlets of the plant, and produces a thickening of the root. Salt, applied 2 or 3 times during the season is recommended as a remedy. An application of lime to the soil will prove of benefit, or the use of sulphur is good. Another remedy is to boil leaves and twigs of the scarlet-berried alderberry to a strong decoction, and pour 1 gill, cold, on the center of the plant; 1 application is generally sufficient. On heavy soil it may be necessary to loosen the earth about the stem of each plant. As a preventive, water the plants once or twice with the decoction after setting out.

COAL, HOW TO BURN:

A writer in the Journal of Health offers the following suggestions concerning the economical combustion of coal:

A very common mistake is made and much fuel wasted in the manner of replenishing coal fires both in furnaces and grates. They should be fed with a little coal at a time, and often; but servants, to save time and trouble, put on a great deal at once, the first result being that almost all of the heat is absorbed by the newly put on coal, which does not give out heat until it has itself become red-hot. Hence for a while the room is cold, but when it becomes fairly aglow the heat is insufferable. The time to replenish a coal fire is as soon as the coals begin to show ashes on their surface; then put on merely enough to show a layer of black coal covering the red. This will soon kindle, and as there is not much of it an excess of heat will not be given out.

Many almost put out the fire by stirring the grate as soon as fresh coal is put on, thus leaving all the heat in the ashes when it should be sent to the new supply of coal. The time to stir the fire is just when the new coal laid on is pretty well kindled. This method of managing a coal fire is

(1) Silk, muslin, etc., worn about the neck.

troublesome, but it saves fuel, gives a more uniform heat, and prevents the discomfort of alterations of heat and cold above referred to.

COCKROACHES, WAYS TO DESTROY:

The disagreeable odor which the cockroach emits, and which soon permeates all places that it inhabits, proceeds from a dark-colored fluid which it discharges from the mouth. The cockroach loves warmth and moisture, hence its populousness in kitchens, where fire and water are almost ever present. It is a night prowler and swarms out from its secret lairs on the departure of daylight.

(1) For the destruction of the cockroach we recommend a mixture containing a table-spoonful of red lead, the same amount of Indian meal, with molasses enough to make a thick batter. Set this on a plate at night in places frequented by the insects, and all that eat of it will be poisoned.

(2) Another preparation is composed of 1 tea-spoonful of powdered arsenic with a table-spoonful of mashed potato. Crumble this every night where the insects will find it. This will be found to be an effectual poison. Great care should be exercised in the use of such dangerous agents. An innocent method of destroying cockroaches is to place a bowl or basin containing a little molasses on the floor at night. A bit of wood, resting one end on the floor and the other on the edge of the vessel, serves as a bridge to conduct the insects to the sweet deposit. Once in the trap its slippery sides prevent retreat, and thus cockroaches may be caught by the thousands.

(3) *The following is said to be effectual:* These vermin are easily destroyed simply by cutting up green cucumbers at night and placing them about where roaches commit depredations. What is cut from the cucumbers in preparing them for the table answers the purpose as well, and three applications will destroy all the roaches in the house. Remove the peelings in the morning and renew them at night.

(4) Common red wafers, to be found at any stationer's, will answer the purpose. The cockroaches eat them and die. Also, sprinkle powdered borax plentifully around where they congregate most and renew it occasionally; in a short time not a roach will be seen. This is a safe and most effectual exterminator.

(5) Take some pieces of board, spread them over with a thin coat of molasses, shake powdered borax over the molasses, and place the boards in their haunts. Gum camphor is a speedy remedy to clear the house of cockroaches.

COCKTAIL, THE PERNICIOUS:

The late Dr. Willard Parker, the elder, used to say of that great American drink, the cocktail, that cocktails instead of being a stimulant are an irritant; they are like a whip and spur to a horse instead of like oats. Cocktails are essentially bad. They not only contain liquor in a concentrated form, but the bitters in them are apt to have properties that are irritating rather than stimulating. A very bad point about cocktails is that they are apt to be drunk hastily and on an empty stomach. Spirits should always be well diluted, slowly imbibed, and taken with food, or after eating.

Alcohol temporarily stops the action of the gastric juices and irritates the coating on the stomach in such a way as to stimulate hunger, but not by the production of a true appetite. It is a false appetite and not a healthy one that is thus brought about, and in the meantime digestion is retarded. The cocktail drinker is very apt to become a victim of catarrh(1) of the stomach, and, like all alcohol tipplers, soon finds his liver seriously affected. The drunkard's or whisky liver is what doctors call this form of disease, which consists of a chronic inflammation of that organ.

COFFEE-POTS, TO CLEANSE:

Musty coffee-pots and teapots may be cleaned and sweetened by putting a good quantity of wood ashes into them and filling up with cold water. Set on the stove to heat gradually till the water boils. Let it boil a short time, then set aside to cool, when the inside should be faithfully washed and scrubbed in hot soap-suds, using a small brush, that every spot may be reached; then scald 2 or 3 times and wipe till well dried. It must be a desperate case if the vessels are not found perfectly sweet and clean if this advice is strictly followed.

Pots and pans or plates that have been used for baking and grown rancid may be cleansed in the same way. Put the plates into a pan with wood ashes and cold water, and proceed as above stated. If no wood ashes can be had, take soda. If cooks would clean their pie-plates and baking-dishes after this fashion after using they would keep sweet all the time.

COFFEE vs. TEA:

Coffee or tea (they are substantially the same) must be considered to be a good thing. They are both a food and a stimulant. Of course, as a stimulant they may be too strong for the nerves even of some men who are physically strong. In such cases they cannot be used. But the majority of persons who find that they cannot drink them will probably think otherwise if they drink them without cream or sugar, for these are generally at the bottom of the trouble. To enjoy coffee thoroughly it is not necessary to put more than 1 part to 3 or 4 or 5 of hot milk.

Some look upon coffee as a poison. But, as Voltaire says, "If it be so

(1) Inflammation of the nose or throat.

it is a very slow poison." He had drunk it for 80 yrs. Coffee is adulterated with chicory, roasted beans, peas, and acorns, but chiefly by chicory. Having your own mill, buy the roasted beans; find out a respectable grocer, ascertain his roasting-days, and always buy from a fresh roast. If you like the flavor of chicory, purchase it separately, and add to taste. Chicory in small quantities is not, as has been represented, injurious, but healthful; because the "taraxacum" root has been used medicinally, and its name has found a place in pharmacopœias, it has been vulgarly set down as "physic," and thrown to the dogs. The tonic hop might be discarded upon the same pretext. Chicory is a healthful addition to coffee, but you need not pay the coffee price for it. Bring your coffee and mix with chicory for yourself.

The Cup of Black Coffee: A cup of black coffee after dinner mainly serves the purpose of gratifying the fancy, but it is not the injurious agent that some have made it out to be. Of course, if a man's nerves are not adapted to coffee, that is another thing; but, as an additional application of heat and a stimulant to the stomach, it can be regarded favorably.

To Boil Coffee:

(1) To make 2 quarts take $^1/_2$ lb. of ground coffee, put it into a coffee-pot that will hold a gallon, the best shape being one with a broad base and narrow mouth. Pour the right quantity of water upon it, which should be fresh and boiling at the time. Stir well, and let it boil up twice; when it rises near the brim stir it repeatedly to prevent its running over; pour out some, but return it to the pot, repeating this 3 times, in order to clear the spout. Put it on the fire again, and when it boils dash a gill of cold water into it; take it off instantly, and let it stand a few minutes to clear itself. Have a little cap fitted over the top of the coffee-pot spout, attached to it by a little chain.

(2) Grind a tea-cupful of coffee in the evening, and, having first seen that your coffee-pot has been thoroughly cleansed and scalded, put in your ground coffee, with a little white of egg and a crushed egg-shell, if it has not been already glazed with egg, and pour over it 3 pints of fresh cool spring water. Cover up, excluding every particle of air, and in the morning, about half an hour before breakfast, set the pot back on part of the stove, and let it come to a boil only just when you are ready to send it to the table.

COLD BATHS, VARYING VIEWS:

Not every one can take cold baths. Stout men are apt to enjoy them more than slender men, but there are plenty of stout fellows whose breaths shorten or whose hearts are violently affected by the sudden, intense, and all-enveloping cold. One of the best men in the Harvard crew of 1869, who had nothing the matter with his heart or lungs, never could take a cold bath.

One recognized way of taking a cold bath is to remain in the water $1^1/2$ minutes and then go back to bed dripping wet, there to remain until you are dry, which will follow in 10 or 15 minutes. A great many persons find it impossible to take the time required for a cold bath in the morning, and a great many others cannot stand the shock of taking one.

Those who find running water too chilling should remember that the best advice we have obtained favors water that has stood in a well-aired bedroom over night. It is not necessary to take the time for using a regular bath. The English custom of using a tub takes less time. Soap is necessary with a morning bath. It dissolves the fatty matter left by perspiration. This resists water without soap. The soap should be rubbed on with a hand-brush. The morning bath must necessarily be viewed differently according to the subject's circumstances. The time consumed in taking it is the most important consideration to most persons.

It is only the well-to-do who can step from a bedroom into an adjoining bath-room without any longer delay than it takes to fill the bath; without that if they have a valet. Men in ordinary dwellings and boarding-houses are often obliged to wait their opportunity to use the only bath-tub. Then, again, they are obliged to clothe themselves from head to foot in order to make the journey to and from the bath-room, all of which consumes valuable time.

COLD DISHES:

The list of cold dishes that are at once appetizing and nutritious is a very long one. Any meat that is good hot is good also cold; so of eggs cooked in many ways; so of most kinds of bread, and of many kinds of pudding and pies and other desserts; so also of many kinds of vegetables. Potato salad is a standing and very popular dish in our restaurants; pork and beans are served cold; so are macaroni and rice and the varieties of mush.

Cold food should be eaten slowly, so that the warmth of the body be communicated to it and it be raised to the temperature of the body before it reaches the stomach. If it enters the stomach cold it will not digest until it reaches 98 degrees Fahr. A quick bolting of a cold meal will invariably be followed by heaviness and often by indigestion, which slow mastication *(Gladstone's 32 bites to a mouthful)* and reasonable intervals between mouthfuls would have been entirely prevented. Large draughts of ice-water will delay digestion, as the ice-water reduces the temperature of the stomach below the point at which digestion begins. A cup of hot chocolate or of hot water will lend sufficient heat to make a cold meal very palatable so far as temperature is concerned.

COLDS:

Sudden warming when cold is dangerous as well as the reverse. There is ordinarily little, if any, danger to be apprehended from wet clothes so long as exercise is kept up, for the "glow" about compensates for the extra cooling by evaporation. Nor is a complete drenching more likely to be injurious than wetting of one part. But never sit still wet, and in changing rub the body dry. When over-heated or drenched with perspiration put on a warm garment before resting still. Except in localities where malignant miasmata prevail, and that only in warm weather, persons who are out of doors the most take and feel cold least.

How to Avoid: Some people may not know that when exposed to a severe cold a feeling of warmth is really created by repeatedly filling the lungs to their utmost in this manner:

Throw the shoulders well back and hold the head well up. Inflate the lungs slowly, the air entering entirely through the nose. When the lungs are completely filled, hold the breath for 10 seconds or longer, and then expire it quickly through the mouth. After repeating this exercise while one is "chilly," a feeling of warmth will be felt over the entire body, and even to the feet and hands. It is important for all to practice this exercise many times each day, and especially when in the open air. If the habit ever becomes universal, then consumption and many other diseases will rarely, if ever, be heard of.

Not only while practicing the "breathing exercise" must the clothing be loose over the chest, but beginners will do well to remember, in having their clothing fitted, to allow for the permanent expansion of the chest of 1, 2, and even 3 in., which will eventually follow. One might with propriety say that too many people choke or stifle the skin by an excess of clothing, and, as a consequence, take cold easily. Some impurities are thrown out of the system by the skin, as others are by the lungs, the bowels, the kidneys. It is absolutely essential to health that the emanations from the skin pass easily through the clothing. This—which is called "transpiration"—may be interfered with by excess of clothing, or by clothing of a very close texture. All who wear India rubber coats know how uncomfortable they cause them to feel after they have been on a short time.

On the accession of Leo X. to the papacy there was a grand procession at Florence in his honor. A little girl was made to personate the golden age, by being coated from head to foot with gold leaf. Before the day was over she died in convulsions, killed because "transpiration," or, in other words, because carbonic acid gas(1) and dead, worn-out matter, which should have been thrown out by her skin, were shut up in her system by the metallic covering.

Ordinary clothing will not of course, prevent transpiration, but an excess will interfere with it, and when too much clothing is worn the same soon becomes foul unless the outside air can freely mingle with the gases from the body and so dilute them. Some wear the thickest and heaviest un-

(1) Carbon dioxide.

dervests which they can buy, and such people are very generally the victims of frequent colds. Following the rule of light clothing they would be much safer from the dangers of exposure, were they to wear two light undervests instead of one very thick and heavy.

Seven Important Remedies: A cold, like measles or mumps, or other similar ailments, will run its course of about 10 days in spite of what may be done for it, unless remedial means are employed within 48 hours after its inception. Many a useful life will be spared to be increasingly useful by cutting a cold "short off" before it has taken firm hold on the system.

The following are safe, simple, and authenticated remedies:

(1) On the first day of taking a cold there is a very unpleasant sensation of chilliness. The moment you observe this, go to your room and stay there; keep it at such a temperature as will entirely prevent this chilly feeling, even if it requires 100 degrees of Fahr. In addition, put your feet in hot water, half a leg deep, as hot as you can bear it, adding hot water from time to time for a quarter of an hour, so that the water shall be hotter when you take your feet out than when you put them in; then dry them thoroughly, and then put on warm, thick woolen stockings, even if it be summer, for summer colds are the most dangerous, and for 24 hours eat not an atom of food, but drink as largely as you desire for any kinds of warm teas, and at the end of that time, if not sooner, the cold will be effectually broken without any medicine whatever.

(2) *Dio Lewis's remedy is the use of cold water as follows:* "Eat no supper. On going to bed drink 2 tumblers of cold water. On rising in the morning drink freely of cold water. For breakfast eat a piece of dry bread as large as your hand. Go out freely during the morning. For dinner eat about the same as you ate at breakfast. During the afternoon take a sharp walk, or engage in some active exercise which shall produce a little perspiration. Go without your supper and retire early, drinking, before you jump into bed, as much cold water as you can swallow."

(3) Many colds are from over-eating or eating gross food. Strong persons with large lungs, who exercise a great deal and breathe much, can dispose of a large quantity of food, but the feeble and sedentary must eat moderately or break down early; for this kind of a cold one preventive is worth a dozen cures, viz., cut off the supplies.

(4) Dr. Paillon, of France, announces what he considers to be a new method of curing a cold in the head. It consists in inhaling through the nose the emanations of ammonia contained in a smelling-bottle. If the sense of smell is completely obliterated, the bottle should be kept under the nose until the pungency of the volatile alkali is felt.

The bottle is then removed, but only to be re-applied after a minute; the second application, however, should not be long, that the patient may bear it. This easy operation being repeated 7 or 8 times in the course of 5 minutes, but always very rapidly, except the first time, the nostrils become free, the sense of smell is restored, and the secretion of the irritating mucus is stopped. This remedy is said to be peculiarly advantageous to singers.

(5) Borax has proved a most effective remedy in certain forms of colds. In sudden hoarseness or loss of voice in public speakers or often obtained by slowly dissolving and partially swallowing a lump of borax the size of a garden pea, or about 3 or 4 grains, held in the mouth for 10 minutes before speaking or singing. This produces a profuse secretion of saliva, or "watering" of the mouth and throat, probably restoring the voice or tone to the dried vocal cords, just as "wetting" brings back the missing notes to a flute when it is too dry.

(6) *The following is an excellent and safe remedy for children:*

Take onions, slice thin, and sprinkle loaf-sugar over them; put in the oven and simmer until the juice is thoroughly mixed with the sugar. It makes a thick syrup, very nice. Give a tea-spoonful as seems to be needed, 4 or 5 times a day.

(7) *Dr. George M. Beard, (allopathist)*(1), *a well-known medical lecturer and writer, strongly recommends the following formula or prescription, suggested originally by one of his patients, and since often given by Dr. B.:*

Take of camphor, 2 parts; powdered opium, 1 part; carbonate of ammonia, 2 parts. Dissolve the camphor to the thickness of cream, and then add the opium and ammonia. Let it be prepared by the druggist. Keep the bottle tightly corked, and take a dose just before retiring at night. Dose, from 3 to 6 grains in a little water. The druggist who puts up the powder will show the buyer the quantity to be taken. It should be kept on hand at all times, and should be first taken immediately after being chilled through, and should be repeated the following night.

COLIC:

Violent shooting, griping pains, with a sense of twisting around the lower part of the belly; the skin of the belly drawn into knots, obstinate constipation; sometimes nausea and vomiting.

Treatment: If there is evidence that the pain arises from any thing eaten, empty the stomach with an emetic of a large tea-spoonful of laudanum or chloroform in some peppermint-wafer or ginger tea; or give 1/4 grain of sulphate of morphia in the arm by hypodermic

(1) Remedies which produce results different or opposite than that of the disease.

injection; apply a large mustard poultice over the entire belly; repeat the landanum or morphia hourly, till the pain is subdued.

Bilious: The paroxysms(1) are sometimes caused by the passage of stones through the gall duct, and relief is only obtained when these reach the intestines; sometimes they appear to be the result of the irritant action of acrid, unhealthy bile.

Treatment: The continued use of chloroform or opium, or both, is necessary, with hot fomentations(2), to relieve the pain; 5 grains of bicarbonate of soda with 1/2 grain of calomel, once in 4 hours, and a large blister over the right abdominal region, may be beneficial where symptoms of inflammation of the bowels set in.

Painters': Caused by exposure to the poisonous influences of lead; the belly is shrunken and hard, and sometimes the intestines may be felt contracted into knots; the pain is lessened by pressure; there is obstinate constipation; and the suffering is most intense.

Treatment: The pain should be relieved by full doses of chloroform, or some forms of opium, and mustard poultices and hot fomentations. When an attack comes on suddenly give a full dose of laudanum, 1/2 to 1 tea-spoonful, with 2 or 3 table-spoonfuls of dilute sulphuric acid, or of the aromatic acid, (elixir of vitriol), added with large warm injections and hot fomentations repeated as may be necessary. The iodide of potash will eliminate the lead from the system, and may be used in doses of 5 to 10 grains 3 or 4 times daily, for this purpose. The regular use of weak sulphuric acid lemonade, 1/4 to 1/2 tea-spoonful of the acid to 1 pint of sweetened water, is a preventive, the bowels being kept open by an occasional laxative.

COLIC, REMEDIES FOR:

(1) For the violent internal agony termed colic take a tea-spoonful of salt in a pint of water; drink and go to bed. It is one of the speediest remedies known. It will revive a person who seems almost dead from a heavy fall.

(2) Phares's method of treating colic consists in inversion—simply in turning the patient upside down. Colic of several days' duration has been relieved by this means in a few minutes.

(3) Dr. Tepliashin has recommended a thin stream of cold water from a tea-pot lifted from 1 to 1 1/2 ft. from the abdomen in cases of colic. He has seen it relieve pain when opium and morphia had failed.

(4) A loaf of bread hot from the oven, broken in two, and half of it placed

(1) Any sudden and violent action or fit; a convulsion; a spasmodic affection.
(2) Treatment with warm liquids, such as water by means of a flannel steeped in the liquid.

upon the bowels, and the other half opposite it upon the back, will relieve colic from whatever cause almost immediately.

COLLODION, USES OF:

This is gun-cotton dissolved in ether. It is very useful for many purposes; especially is it useful in photography. Those who take pleasure in striking cuttings of tender plants in Waltonian cases, or under small glasses in the house, will find it of great assistance in the case of the cutting which enters the ground, with a camel-hair brush dipped in collodion. This will materially hasten the formation of the callus, which is necessary before any roots can be formed.

COLOGNE WATER:

A very fair article, that will improve with age, may be made as follows:

1 pint of alcohol, add 12 drops each of oils of bergamot, lemon, neroli, orange-peel, rosemary, and 1 dram of cardamom seed.

Another recipe: 1 pint of alcohol, 60 drops of lavender, 60 drops of bergamot, 60 drops of essence of lemon, 60 drops of orange-water. To be corked up and well shaken. This also is better for considerable age.

COMFORTABLES, TO RENOVATE:

After washing and thoroughly drying bed-quilts, fold and roll them tight, then give them a beating with the rolling-pin to liven up the batting, and make them soft and new.

COMIC CONCERT, THE:

In this performance the company for the time imagine themselves to be a band of musicians. The leader of the band is supposed to furnish each of the performers with a different musical instrument. Consequently a violin, a harp, a flute, an accordion, a piano, a Jew's-harp, and any thing else that would add to the noise are all to be performed upon at the same time. Provided with an instrument of some description himself, the leader begins playing a tune on his imaginary violoncello, or whatever else it may be, imitating the real sound as well as he can both in action and voice. The others all do the same, the sight presented being, as may well be imagined, exceedingly ludicrous, and the noise almost deafening.

In the midst of it the leader quite unexpectedly stops playing, and makes an entire change in his attitude and tone of voice, substituting for his own instrument one belonging to some one else. As soon as he does this the performer who has been thus unceremoniously deprived of his instrument takes that of his leader, and performs on it instead. Thus the game is continued, every one being expected to carefully watch the leader's actions, and to be prepared at any time for making a sudden change.

CONSTIPATION, CAUSE AND CURE:

Over-indulgence in animal food is a frequent cause of constipation. No nation consumes such quantities of flesh meats, and so many times a day, as the American. Dyspepsia and constipation result. The rapidity with which we eat, and which causes dyspepsia, is equaled by the carelessness, the hurry, and the neglect which we inflict upon the colon and rectum. A neglect of a regular and proper hour to evacuate the bowels often induces constipation. Abstain from tea and coffee, eat plenty of fresh vegetables, drink a glass of water immediately after rising in the morning, eat slowly, and masticate the food well, avoid salt meats and salt fish, and take 1 tablespoonful of sulphur every other night upon retiring.

CONTAGION, TO PREVENT:

Among diseases liable to be spread by the distribution of organic poisons may be mentioned scarlet fever, typhus fever, typhoid fever, yellow fever, measles, small-pox, diphtheria, infectious ophthalmia, hydrophobia, erysipelas(1), cholera, and glanders(2). The walls of hospitals should be glass-lined the better to prevent contamination, and means should be used to destroy the contagious matter by chemical agents. Solar light and great heat are other powerful disinfectants.

Thoroughly disinfect all fecal discharges, and if in the country they should be taken at least 200 ft. from any well. Under no circumstances should they be disposed of in an open out-house. In the city, in case the drainage is good, it is safe to use the sewer. Contagion is largely propagated by means of clothing. This should be placed in a box or a closet maintained at a temperature of 220 degrees, dry, for perhaps an hour. Carbolic acid(3) will not permanently destroy the effect of vaccine virus. People are far more liable to contract diseases on an empty than on a full stomach.

CONVALESCENCE:

With convalescence come manifold dangers that must be guarded against with jealous care. A single act of imprudence then may render unavailing all the watchful anxiety of the previous weeks. An invalid is peculiarly liable to take cold when first allowed to sit up. The room should be slightly warmer than usual, the chair or couch on which he is to sit, covered with a blanket, and he himself well wrapped in blankets and shawls. If possible close-fitting flannels should be worn, and the feet must be covered with stockings. He should not be allowed to remain too long out of bed the first time, and it is well to have it warmed before he returns to it.

No visitors should be admitted, and all excitement should be avoided

(1) Inflammation of the skin, usually a deep red color spreading rapidly.
(2) An often fatal disease communicated to man by glandered animals (enlargement and induration of the glands of the lower jaw).
(3) Phenyl alcohol, phenol, phenic acid, coal-tar creasote.

until he has had time to rest after the exertion. Except those actually engaged in the care of the sufferer not more than one friend at once should ever be allowed to enter the sick-room. In some cases quiet is absolutely essential to recovery, and it is always desirable. The visitor should wait where the invalid can see without being obliged to turn his head; he should enter and leave the house and move about the room quietly; carry a cheerful face and speak cheerful words, but tell no lies to be cheerful; do not fall into gay and careless talk in the attempt to cheer the patient; don't ask questions, and thus oblige the patient to talk; talk about something outside, and not about the disease and circumstances of the patient; tell the news, but not the list of the sick and dying; never whisper in the sick-room; if possible carry with you something to please the eye and to relieve the monotony of the sick-room—a flower, or even a picture; if desirable, some little wholesome delicacy to tempt the appetite will be well bestowed; but is most unkind kindness to tempt the sick to eat too much of rich cakes, preserves, sweetmeats, etc.

The weakness and languor inseparable from long illness render convalescence sometimes a very tedious and trying time. The small stock of strength is unequal to the demands made upon it, and it should be husbanded in every possible way. At night the invalid should have something to take the last thing before going to sleep; any light nourishment will answer—a cup of cocoa, beef-tea, or thin custard; a delicate sandwich, and, if stimulant is ordered, a glass of wine taken then will prevent exhaustion during sleep. At the early morning hours, from 3 to 5, the powers of life should be re-enforced by food, as they are considered then to be at their lowest ebb. If it is impossible to heat any thing, a cold drink is better than nothing. Half a pint of milk with the white of 1 egg beaten up in it may be given. There is usually little appetite at this early hour, and something must be chosen that can be easily taken.

During convalescence properly regulated exertion is highly serviceable; but it should never be carried so far as to produce exhaustion, and should be pursued for some time indoors, before it be attempted in the open air; the latter, at first, should always take place in a carriage that can be opened or closed at will; the patient may then attempt short walks in the open air; but in all cases it is of importance that he is not unduly fatigued.

CONVENIENCES, LITTLE:

There are women who for years have done the daily cooking for a family, and never a pot-lifter in the whole time. They lifted hot utensils about with a damp dish-cloth, or a handful of their dress skirt, or any thing that came handy, as the scars on their hands and wrists testify. Think of the pain, ill-temper, and scorched aprons and dresses a few pot-lifters might have saved. And they are so simply made. You need only to make a cushion of 2 circular pieces of some strong, heavy fabric—I prefer bed-ticking, or unbleached or colored canton flannel—about 8 in. in diameter, filled with batting.

A good pattern is made by laying a small dinner-plate on the cloth and marking around it; your first impression on removing the plate may be that it is going to be large enough for a door-mat, but it takes up wonderfully in sewing and stuffing. Besides, you want it large; a lifter small enough to allow the hand to slip off on a hot handle is a constant vexation of spirit. It should be large enough to protect both hands, if necessary.

Baste the batting to the cover before sewing it together; this keeps it more evenly distributed. When sewing up the opening left for turning the holder right side out insert a loop of tape by which to hang it up. Make several. Then do not hang them in the closet or the furthest end of the pantry, but over the baking table or behind the stove, just where they will be at hand when needed.

Another article equally indispensable is a board upon which to set pots while taking up the contents. It is inconvenient to do the "dishing-up" from the stove, to say nothing of the extra polishing we thereby make ourselves, while to ruin the paint or oilcloth on a table, or the bottom of an inverted plate, as I have seen done, by setting a hot pan or skillet on it, is something the majority of us cannot afford. These boards—"crock-covers," we call them—are very useful for covering jars; but the one used for pot-stand should be used for that exclusively. Nail a strip of leather to hang it by, for in a model kitchen all such things are hung up and not strewn around.

While one is attending to the pot-lifters it is a good time to see to the supply and condition of her iron-holders. They are most convenient oblong, about 4 in. by 7, and the most suitable material is bleached canton flannel. Iron-holders should never be of colored cloth. Many a smirch on some fine, white garment comes from dropping a dark or soiled holder upon it. These are not to be hung up, but kept with the ironing-sheets in a closet. As they are needed only once a week, and must not be soiled, they can be put away more carefully than frequently used articles.

In our list of homely little housekeeping necessities is found "feather brooms." Turkey wings are very useful to brush up hearths, while these brooms, made of single stiff turkey feathers bound together, are superior to whisk-brooms for use on fine rugs and carpets. Often a chamber that is not in need of a thorough sweeping looks the better for being "brushed up," and such a broom is found to do it nicely. Once made, they never "go-a-begging" for a job.

COOK-STOVE, CARE OF THE:

"Why is it that I burn out so many sets of stove linings?" some one asks. Let me tell you. Use a little more care than you have been using; watch and see that a clinker is not allowed to form on the linings, and if one does form, remove it carefully with the poker. At night the fire-box should be evenly full of coal after raking out all the dead cinders and ashes in the range; never fill your stove with coal above the top of the linings. Never use a shaker when it is possible to avoid it; instead, use the poker freely and you will have a better fire and use less coal. Shaking the fire brings it down into a solid mass, and the air cannot circulate through.

When the fire from any cause becomes dull, do not stir it over the top or put in wood, but rake out the cinders and open drafts. At night do not close the drafts as soon as the coal for the night is put on, but let it burn a short time, or, as one man expresses it, "until you think the coal is warm all through." There is then very little danger of gas, even if the stove is a poor one.

The ashes should never accumulate in the ash-pan until they reach the grate. If this happens even once the grate will usually be burned out. Always run the range so that you can get all the heat needed without having the top red-hot, as this will warp the covers and centers, and if a little water should happen to fall on the stove while so hot the top of the range is very apt to crack. Keep the stove well blacked; if the lids get covered with grease turn them over and let the top of the lid come next the fire until the grease is all burned off. If the covers are red and the blackening does not adhere, let them get wet, so that they will rust a little, and then black them.

When buying a range, buy one that is moderately heavy and made of the best quality of iron. All the joints of a heating stove or range should fit well, because if they do not, when the range has been used a short time you will notice gas escaping, and will not be able to tell where it comes from.

CO-PARTNERSHIPS:

Partnerships may be either general or special. In general partnerships money invested ceases to be individual property. Each member is made personally liable for the whole amount of debts incurred by the company. The company is liable for all contracts or obligations made by individual members. Special partners are not liable beyond the amount contributed. A person may become a partner by allowing people generally to presume that he is one, as, by having his name on the sign, or parcels, or in the bills used in the business.

A share or specified interest in the profits or loss of the business as remuneration for labor may involve one in the liability of a partner. In case of bankruptcy the joint estate is first applied to the payment of partnership debts, the surplus only going to the creditors of the individual estate. A dissolution of partnership may take place under express stipulations in the articles of agreement, by mutual consent, by the death or insanity of one of the firm, by award of arbitrators, or by court of equity in cases of misconduct of some member of the firm. In case of death the surviving partners must account to the representatives of the deceased.

COPYING PAPER, TO MAKE:

To make black paper, lamp-black mixed with cold lard; red paper, Venetian red mixed with lard; green paper, chromo green mixed with lard; blue paper, Prussian blue mixed with lard. The above ingredients to be mixed to the consistency of thick paste and to be applied to the paper with a rag; then take a flannel rag and rub till all color ceases to come off. Cut your sheets 4 in. wide and 6 in. long, put four sheets together, one of each color, and sell for 25 cents per package. The first cost will not be over 3 cents.

Direction for writing: Lay down your paper upon which you wish to write; then lay on the copying paper, and over this lay any scrap of paper you choose; then take any hard-pointed substance and write as you would with a pen.

CORAL, TO CLEAN:

Soak it in soda and water for some hours. Then make a lather of soap, and with a soft hair-brush rub the coral lightly, letting the brush enter all the interstices. Pour off the water and replenish it with clean constantly, and then let the coral dry in the sun.

CORN, TO PREVENT BEING DESTROYED:

To prevent the corn being destroyed or eaten by chickens, birds, or insects before it grows through the surface of the soil, prepare the seed before planting by sprinkling a sufficient portion of coal-tar, procured at the gas manufactory, through it, stirring so that a portion will adhere to each grain; then mix among the corn some ground plaster of Paris, which will prevent the tar from sticking to the fingers of those who drop the corn, and vegetation will be promoted thereby. The tar and plaster will not injure the corn so as to prevent its growing, by being kept some days after it is so mixed together.

CORN-CRIBS, RAT-PROOF:

Take posts 10 or 11 ft. long and 8 in. square; mortise 2 ft. from one end; for end-sills, 2 in. mortise with tusk. Taper posts from sill to the end by hewing off inside until the end is reduced to 4 in. diameter; make smooth with the draw-knife, and nail on tin, smooth half way to the end below the sill. Let sills be 8 in. square, also end-tie them and the rafter-plates strong with moderate inter-ties. Brace well and lath up and down with three quarters in. lath; dove-tail or counter-sink joints crosswise; lay the floor and board up the ends with ungrooved boards; let each bin be 12 ft. long, 6 ft. wide at the sill, and $7^1/_2$ ft. at plate; and if full to peak it will hold 250 bushels. If preferred, lay the floor with lath or narrow boards, with room for ventilation. Each post should stand on stone and be about 3 in. from the ground, and each stone have a foundation 3 ft. square and below the frost.

CORNER CLOSETS:

A bedroom that is without a closet is very inconvenient. But closets can be improvised with small outlay and a little ingenuity. In one corner of the room have strips 1^1/2 and 2 ft. long, and ^{1}/2 in. thick, nailed to the wall on each side 5^1/2 ft. from the floor. Have a shelf made that will rest on these strips. It will, or course, be triangular in shape. On the under side of this shelf put in a dozen or more screw-hooks, and put holes also in the strips supporting the shelf. These hooks will furnish support for articles of clothing. Three feet from the floor nail other strips, put hooks in them also, and on these hang shoe-bags and short articles of clothing. Across the edge of the shelf tack a curtain that shall fall to the floor or nail strips near the ceiling and attach the curtain by a rod to the ends of these strips.

In another corner of the room have 2 or 3 triangular shelves put in, resting on strips above described. The upper shelf should be at the height of a washstand, and the one below allow space for the ewer to stand. From side-strips above the upper shelf, brackets may be suspended holding the various requisites for the toilet. Hooks put in these strips afford a place to hang splashers as well as towels. A third shelf near the floor may be added if desired. A curtain opening in the middle should be fastened near the ceiling and fall to the floor. Facilities should be fastened near the ceiling and fall to the floor. Facilities for looping it back when the toilet shelf is used should be provided. When one uses a bedroom as a sitting-room these corner closets are very great additions to the comfort and elegance of the room.

CORN FOR SEED:

Always select even-rowed ears and ears whose rows are straight and regular on the cob. Ears that taper are the best, because better protected by the husks, and then, too, the silk—the female part of the plant—remains alive longer. The reason for selecting the top ear for seed is that it is always more fully developed, more uniform and more vigorous in its germination, having been better fertilized when in the silk.

CORNS, HOW TO PREVENT AND HOW TO REMOVE:

For prevention of corns use daily friction of cold water between the toes. For their removal, the following suggestions are given:

(1) Hard corns may be carefully picked out by the use of a small, sharp-pointed scalpel or teuolomy knife, and if well done the cure is often radical, always perfect for the time.

(2) They may be equally successfully removed by wearing over them for a few days a small plaster made by melting a piece of stick diachylon and dropping on a piece of white silk. The corn gradually loosens from the adjacent healthy skin, and can be readily pulled or picked out.

(3) Soft corns require the use of astringents, such as alum dissolved in white of egg, or the careful application of tincture of iodine.

(4) A simple cure for both hard and soft corns, which rarely fails, is a poultice of bread dipped in cider vinegar and applied every night until cured.

(5) Lemon juice effects only a temporary cure, unless applied before the corn has gained ground firmly.

(6) A large cranberry or raisin split open and bound to the toe is very good.

(7) The strongest acetic acid (vinegar) applied night and morning with a camel's hair brush to either soft or hard corns will remove them in one week's time.

(8) The heart of a potato boiled in its skin, placed on a corn, and left there for 12 hours will give temporary relief.

(9) Apply a good coat of gum arabic mucilage over them every evening on going to bed.

(10) Apply castor oil, after paring closely, every night before going to bed.

(11) Take a little sweet-oil on getting up in the morning and before retiring at night, and rub it on the corn with the tip of the finger, keeping the corn well pared down. This relieves the friction, which causes corns, and will cure them in a short time.

(12) Apply with a brush morning and evening a drop of a solution of the perchloride of iron.

(13) After removing the stocking at night, with the nails of the thumb and forefinger loosen the corn at the edges, and gradually peel it across until it comes off. This is done with entire ease when the toe is not inflamed and sore, and if the corn hardens again in a few weeks, as it will be apt to, the process is easily repeated. The main point is, don't pinch the feet with tight shoes.

(14) Soak the feet well in warm water, then with a sharp instrument pare off as much of the corn as can be done without pain, and bind up the part with a piece of linen or muslin, thoroughly saturated with sperm oil, or, what is better, the oil which floats upon the surface of the pickle or herring or mackerel. After three or four days the dressing may be removed, and the remaining cuticle removed by scraping, when the new skin will be found of a soft and healthy texture, and less liable to the formation of a new corn than before.

COSTIVENESS(1), TO CURE:

Common charcoal is highly recommended for costiveness. It may be taken either in tea- or table-spoonful, or even larger doses, according to the exigencies of the case, mixed with molasses, repeating it as often as necessary. Bathe the bowels with pepper and vinegar. Or take 2 ounces of rhubarb, add 1 ounce of rust of iron, infuse in 1 quart of wine. Half a wine-glassful every morning. Or take pulverized blood-root, 1 dram; pulverized rhubarb, 1 dram; Castile soap, 2 scruples.(2) Mix and roll into 32 pills. Take one morning and night. By following these directions it may perhaps save you from a severe attack of piles or some other kindred disease.

COUGHS, HOW TO RELIEVE SEVERE—SEVEN GOOD RECIPES:

(1) The paroxysm of coughing may often be prevented or cured by using a little dry salt as a gargle. Let those who doubt try it. It will relieve the tickling in the throat.

(2) Equal parts of horehound(3), elecampane(4) root, comfrey(5) root, spikenard(6), and wild-cherry bark. Boil in 1 gallon soft water down to 1 quart; strain, and add 1 pound of honey. Take a table-spoonful 3 times a day, or when the cough is troublesome.

(3) Roast a lemon very carefully without burning it; when it is thoroughly hot cut and squeeze it into a cup upon 3 ounces of sugar, finely powdered. Take a spoonful whenever your cough troubles you. It is good and agreeable to the taste. Rarely has it been known to fail of giving relief.

(4) Take 1 quart thick flaxseed tea, 1 pint of honey, 1/2 pint of vinegar, 2 spoonfuls saltpeter. Boil all together in a new earthen pot that is well glazed until it becomes a pretty thick syrup; keep stirring well while boiling with a pine stick; if fresh from a green tree the better. Dose, 1 table-spoonful 3 or 4 times a day.

(5) A medical writer says: "We are often troubled with severe coughs, the result of colds of long standing, which may turn to consumption or premature death. The remedy I propose has been often tried by me with good results, which is simply to take into the stomach before retiring for the night a piece of raw onion, after chewing. This esculent in an uncooked state is very heating, and tends to collect the waters from the lungs and throat, causing immediate relief to the patient."

(1) Constipation.
(2) One third of a gram.
(3) The juice of a bitter plant of the mint family.
(4) A medicine made from the Inula helenium plant.
(5) A plant of the symphytum family with a sweetish taste used to help heal and congeal wounds.
(6) A Himalayan plant whose roots yield an aromatic substance used in perfumery.

(6) Common sweet cider, boiled down to one half, makes a most excellent syrup for coughs and colds for children, is pleasant to the taste, and will keep for a year in a cool cellar. In recovering from an illness the system has a craving for some pleasant acid drink. This is found in cider which is placed on the fire as soon as made, and allowed to come to a boil, then cooled, put in casks, and kept in a cool cellar.

(7) Take a handful of hops, put it into 3 pints of hot water; let it boil 1/2 hour, or until the strength is out. Strain and add 1 1/2 cups of best kind of molasses, and 1 cup of white sugar. Boil down slowly in a bright dish or enameled kettle to about 1 quart. Then bottle up, and it is ready for use. Drink a little when you cough.

COUNTERPANES(1):

(1) A handsome one is made of satin and lace. Take a square of antique lace and line it with the desired shade of satin; around it sew an insertion of satin of the desired width; around this one of antique lace, and so on until it is of the desired size. Lining each insertion of lace or not; finish with a deep edge of lace.

(2) A pretty and attractive one is made of the old bits of silks lying around. Make squares of crinoline lined with calico of the desired size; on these baste the odd ends of silk regardless of color or shape, turning their edges in neatly; around the edge of each piece work the feather-edge or herring-bone stitches; a flower or any design may be embroidered on the larger pieces of silk; when all the squares are done, place them on a foundation lined with some desired material, and join their edges by some fancy stitch. Tastes differ as to the style of counterpane to be used. The white is always neat, and is in reality the most serviceable, because it may be made to look as good as new by its passage through the hands of the laundress. Indeed, Marseilles spreads, if properly done up, improve with repeated washings.

They lose thus that stiffness which shows a mis-fold nearly as plainly as would a sheet of paper, and renders it all but impossible to draw them smoothly and evenly across the bed. The counterpane should never be spread up over the bolster, but turned back neatly just below this, and the upper sheet folded back over it. By this method the spread may be taken off at night, and the top of the sheet left undisturbed.

COURTSHIP AND MARRIAGE:

Use the same scrutiny and common sense in love affairs as in busi-

(1) Bed coverings or quilts.

ness. Do not suppress true feeling, neither mistake impulse and passion for the flame of love. Courtship should not progress where affection exists but on one side. Avoid a hasty marriage. Never become engaged until you have taken time enough to get thoroughly acquainted. A young man will do well to make up his mind not to marry until he is 25. Girls of good sense will not be ambitious to marry until after their twentieth year. It is generally best for them to seek partners among gentlemen who are a few years older. Do not wait till you have acquired a fortune before you marry, but do not assume the responsibilities of a family without a prospect of being able to maintain one. Men and women should mate with those unlike rather than like each other. Exact rules cannot be laid down for temperaments. People who are not extreme opposite temperaments can safely intermarry.

In paying attention to a lady with a view of marriage do not omit your duties toward others' society. Lovers should remember that the laws of social intercourse are not abrogated when they become engaged. Never take costly presents to a young lady thinking thereby to obtain her favor. Offer her neat trifles, and procure any books that she may express a desire to read. After engagement show your generosity in proportion to your means.

If your intimacy with a lady does not suggest the proper mode to ask her hand, there is no hope for you, unless she loves you so well as to arrange the matter herself. "Popping the question" by rule is absurd. Adapt that mode that seems most natural. After an engagement to marry is entered into in good faith, and it is so understood by the lady's family, no motives of delicacy should prevent her enjoying the society of her lover alone. But neither of them should ever show their fondness in company. An engaged young lady should not encourage her lover to be too loving; she should not be lavish of her carresses nor forward to receive his. A becoming modesty will result in drawing the lover more powerfully. They should study the dispositions and tastes of each other, and endeavor to gratify them.

Engagements made with deliberation and between parties sufficiently long acquainted to understand each other will seldom be broken off. If such a painful necessity occurs, let it be met with firmness, but with delicacy. If you have made a mistake, it is better to correct it at the last moment than not at all.

Immediately after the announcement of engagement there is scope for the display of good breeding, and there are certain rules which must be observed. Members of the gentleman's family should call upon the family of the lady, and they should return the call soon. It is not necessary to be intimate. All that is required is the friendly interchange of visits. If the family of the gentleman does not reside in the same city as that of the lady, the announcement of the engagement should be followed by letters from his parents or nearest relatives to the young lady herself or her parents. Kindly feeling should be the tone of such letters, and they must be answered at once.

It is customary for the gentleman to make some present soon after the engagement; the most elegant is a handsome engagement ring. It is proper for this to be followed by gifts upon birthdays, Christmas, or New Year's, and the lady is at liberty to return the compliment. When once the engagement is allowed, it is the custom to admit the gentleman into the intimate society of his newly adopted relatives. It is well for a young lady to have a settlement of a liberal sum of money by her parents, or by the husband himself, if wealthy, and during the arrangement of pecuniary matters a young lady should endeavor to understand what is going on, receiving it in the right spirit. If she has a private fortune she should, in all points left to her, be generous and confiding; at the same time, prudent and far-seeing.

In case of a quarrel, when calm second thought asserts its sway, both should see which can forgive and apologize the quickest. Do not call too frequently upon your lady; thus avoid the ridicule of her friends and family. Flirtations on either side should be avoided as a matter of etiquette and humanity.

CRACKED LIPS:

Early in the autumn the winds cause fissures or cracks in the lips that are not only extremely unpleasant to look upon, but are exquisitely painful, and by touching them with your tongue you intensify the pain very much. Go to the drug-shop and get there an old remedy, so old that it has charm of novelty. It rejoices in an overpowering Latin name, but when you ask the druggist for it in English, say you want citron cream. Apply this with your fingers or a soft linen cloth, and the cooling and healing result that will follow will convince you that even in medicine sometimes old things are best.

CRAMBO, THE GAME OF:

One player leaves the room, while the rest take their places in a circle. They select a word and call the guesser in. He is then told a word that rhymes with the one chosen, and he then goes on to guess by describing without naming other words to rhyme till he arrives at the right one. For example, the word chosen is "play." The guesser goes round the circle and asks each in turn a question, the answer giving the word he has thought of. He is told that the word chosen rhymes with "say." "Is it the poet's month?" "No; it is not May." "Is it a road to anywhere?" "No; it is not way." And so on, till he ends in guessing rightly, when the last speaker leaves the room, while another word is selected to tax his ingenuity. This is an excellent game, but Dumb Crambo in which the words are acted, is a funnier and more lively pastime.

CRIB-BITING, REMEDY FOR:

Crib-biting is often a habit, but may be caused by disease. Indigestion occasions a constant irritation and uneasiness which may impel the horse to take hold with the teeth and stretch the neck as a means of relief. From this grows the habit of crib-biting and wind-sucking, which ceases when the cause is removed.

As a remedy give the horse in his feed daily, for a few weeks, 1 dram of copperas and 1/2 ounce of ground ginger, and feed him upon cut feed, with crushed or ground grain, and an ounce of salt in each feed. Cribbing is a vice which springs from a habit more than any other cause. It begins frequently from a desire to ease the teeth from inconvenience or perhaps pain at that period when the dentition is perfecting, and then becomes fixed upon the horse as a vice. It is not injurious except when accompanied with wind-sucking, which is a series of deep inspirations by which flatulence and colic are caused. When the habit is fixed on a horse it is difficult to break it, and the only effective method is to use a muzzle, which prevents him from thus using his teeth.

CROCKERY, TO MEND:

Take 4 lbs. of white glue, 1 1/2 lbs. of dry white lead, 1/2 lb. isinglass, 1 gallon soft water, 1 quart alcohol, 1/2 pint white varnish; dissolve the glue and isinglass in the water by gentle heat if preferred; stir in the lead, put the alcohol in the varnish, and mix the whole together.

CROSS QUESTIONS AND CROOKED ANSWERS:

This is a pleasant game that may be enjoyed while sitting in a circle round the fire. The person at either end who is honored by commencing the game must in a whisper ask a question of the player sitting next to him, taking care to remember the answer he receives, and also the question he himself asked. The second player must then do likewise, and so on, until every one in the party has asked a question and received an answer; the last person, of course, being under the necessity of receiving the answer to his question from the first person. Every one must then say aloud what was the question put to him, and what was the answer he received to the question he asked—the two together, of course, making nothing but nonsense, something like the following:

Q. Who is your favorite author? A. Beans and Bacon. Q. Were you ever in love? A. Cricket, decidedly. Q. Are you an admirer of Oliver Cromwell? A. Mark Twain Q. Why is a cow like an oyster? A. Many as time.

Another way of playing this game is for one person to stand outside the circle; then, when all the whispering is finished, to come forward and ask a question of each person, receiving for his replies the answers they all had given to the questions they asked each other. Or what is, perhaps, a still better plan, both questions and answers may be written on different colored paper, and then, after being shuffled, may be read aloud by the leader of the game.

CROUP(1), TREATMENT AND CURE:

There are various remedies for this enemy in the nursery. As in other diseases prevention is better than cure. Children liable to croup should not play out of doors after 3 o'clock in the afternoon. If a woolen shawl is closely pinned around the neck of the patient when the first symptoms of croup appear the attack may be diminished in power. The child struggling for breath naturally throws its arms out of bed to breath through its pores, and thus takes more cold and increases its trouble.

Bichromate of potassa in minute doses—as much as will rest on the point of a pen-knife, given every 1/2 hour till relief is obtained, is the best remedy we have ever tried. Mustard plasters on the ankles, wrists, and chest will draw the blood from the throat and relieve it; cloths wrung from hot water and placed about the throat and chest wrapped in flannel give relief. A tea-spoonful of alum pulverized, and mixed with twice its quantity of sugar to make it palatable, will give almost instant help.

Another remedy is the following: Take equal parts of soda or saleratus(2) and syrup or molasses; mix and give a tea-spoonful for a child 2 yrs. old, larger doses for older children, smaller for nursing babies. Repeat the doses at short intervals until the phlegm is all thrown up, and upon each recurrence of the symptoms; or grate a raw onion, strain out the juice, and to 2 parts sweet lard and 6 parts pulverized sugar, mix thoroughly, and give a tea-spoonful every 15 minutes until relief is obtained. Among the many remedies given we hope that one or more may be available to every mother who needs aid in this matter.

Six Methods of Instant Relief:

- One tea-spoonful of molasses and a tea-spoonful of goose-oil, given to a child inclined to the croup, will generally relieve it at once.
- For speedy relief take a knife or grater, and shave or grate off in small particles about a tea-spoonful of alum; mix it with about twice the quantity of sugar or honey, to make it palatable, and administer as quickly as possible. This will give almost instant relief.
- A lady correspondent of the Main Farmer says the following is an effective remedy for croup: "Half a tea-spoonful of pulverized alum in a little molasses. It is a simple remedy, one almost always at hand, and 1 dose seldom fails to give relief. If it should, repeat it after 1 hour."
- French physicians claim the discovery of a perfect cure for

(1) Inflammation of the respiratory passages.
(2) An impure bicarbonate of potash, formally used in making bread, replaced by baking powders.

croup in flour of sulfur exhibited in water. M. Langauterie gives in croup tea-spoonful doses of a mixture of sulphur and water (a tea-spoonful to a glass of water) every hour with wonderful effects. Seven severe cases were cured in 2 days.

- J. K. Holloway, M.D., in a letter to the Medical and Surgical Journal, describes the successful cure of a very extreme case of croup by causing the patient to inhale the evaporations of lime-water. The patient had been suffering for 36 hours with membranous croup, and without relief from other medicines. No time was to be lost. Lime unslaked was put into a pitcher as to cause inhalation of the free lime vapor. In 20 minutes the patient was fully relieved.

CRYING AND HEALTH:

Probably most persons have experienced the effect of tears in relieving great sorrow. It is even curious how the feelings are allayed by free indulgence in groans and sighs. A French physician publishes a long dissertation on the advantages of groaning and crying in general, and especially during surgical operations. He contends that groaning and crying are two grand operations by which nature allays anguish; that these patients who give way to their natural feelings more speedily recover from accidents and operations than those who suppose it unworthy of a man to betray such symptoms of cowardice as either to groan or cry.

He tells of a man who reduced his pulse from 126 to 60 in the course of a few hours by giving full vent to his emotions. "If people are at all unhappy about any thing, let them go into their room and comfort themselves with a loud boo-hoo, and they will feel 100 per cent. better afterward." Then let the eyes and mouth be regarded as the safety-valve through which nature discharges her surplus steam.

CRYSTALLIZED CHIMNEY ORNAMENTS:

Select a crooked twig of white or black thorn, wrap some loose wool or cotton around the branches, and tie it on with worsted. Suspend this in a basin or deep jar. Dissolve 2 lbs. of alum in a quart of boiling water and pour it over the twigs. Allow it to stand 12 hours. Wire baskets may be covered in the same way.

CURCULIO(1) IN FRUIT TREES, REMEDY FOR:

Sawdust saturated in coal-oil and placed at the roots of the tree will be a sure preventive; or clear a circle around the tree from all rubbish, fill up all little holes and smooth off the ground for a distance of at least 3 ft. each way from the tree, then place chips or small pieces of wood on the

(1) Weevils with heads extending into long snouts.

ground within the circle; the curculio will take refuge in large numbers below the chips, and you can pass around in the mornings and kill them off.

CURRANT WORMS, TO DESTROY:

Put 1 lb. of coarsely ground quassia wood into 10 or 15 gallons of water and, after stirring it 2 or 3 times, apply it with a watering-spout by sprinkling the bushes every morning for several days. The result is a plentiful crop of leaves and fruit of an excellent quality. Water may be added as long as bitterness remains.

CURRY POWDER, TO MAKE:

This is the genuine East India recipe: Take the fennel seed, cummin seed, and coriander seed, each 4 ounces, with 2 ounces of caraway seed, dry them before the fire, then grind and sift them; add to this 2 ounces of ground turmeric and the same of ground black pepper, 1 ounce of ground ginger, and $^1/_2$ ounce of Cayenne pepper. Mix well, and keep dry and well stopped.

CURTAINS:

To those who find lace curtains and the necessary rods and rings too expensive a luxury I would suggest using plain white cheese-cloth curtains trimmed with lace and cretonne. Very pretty and dainty curtains can be made as follows: For 1 window take 6 yds. of plain white cheese-cloth; cut each curtain 3 yds. long. Make a 10-in. hem at bottom of curtain and with woven, knitted, or crocheted cotton lace 5 in. wide ornament the bottom and the entire length of inside of curtain. Across the top of the curtain sew 2 strips of cretonne(1), leaving a 4-in. space between the strips. Sew lace across the lower edge of lower strip and the curtain is complete.

For rods use well-shaped broomsticks, neatly painted with black paint; the ends can be ornamented with the fancy knobs, such as are used on the more expensive curtain rods, and which can be obtained at the furniture stores at a trifling cost. Gilt or scarlet and gilt harness rings can be used, also cornice screws instead of brackets, on which to suspend the rods. Loop the curtains back with bands of cretonne.

CURTAINS, SILK RAG, TO MAKE:

Cut the silk into strips about $^1/_2$ in. wide, (a little more or less makes no difference), either straight or on the bias. Sew the pieces together strongly and roll into balls, keeping each color and shade by itself. Pieces of narrow ribbons, old cravats and sashes, old waists of dresses—in fact, every scrap of silk—can be made use of whether soiled or fresh. After making a number of balls send them to a rag-carpet weaver, who will weave them for about 25 cents a yard. It will take $1^1/_2$ lbs. of silk to make a yard

(1) A cotton fabric with pictorial patterns printed on one side.

of material three-fourths yard wide, which is the width of nearly all looms. If the balls of silk are given to the weaver with directions how to place the colors, and the width of the stripes are desired, the stuff when finished will have a very handsome effect, and is very heavy. It is suitable for portieres, curtains, rugs, or table-cloths.

Bedroom curtains can be made of unbleached muslin sheeting with a simple hem upon the edge. All the trimming required is tally across the top about 2 ft. from the cornice. The light falling through the unbleached muslin gives the fine ecru tone so much in vogue at the present, and it is impossible to detect the nature of the fine twilled India material so much admired when combined with strips of Oriental embroidery. Really beautiful curtains for a parlor can be made of canton flannel in the same way, and the effect produced is that of a rich cream-colored plush or velvet. It is impossible to judge of the beauty of these cheap and novel hangings without having seen them.

CURTAINS FOR BEDROOMS, ETC:

A very stylish and graceful design for sitting-room or bed-room curtains recently originated in the New York art rooms, and full directions are given here for making a pair. The curtains are inexpensive, the full cost for two deep windows being about $3.50. The materials required are 2 yards of cretonne, 10 or 12 yards of cheesecloth, and sufficient lace for finishing the front edges of the curtain and making an insertion across the top of each. Be careful in purchasing the cheesecloth to get a piece which is evenly woven and without black threads. Scrim(1) may be used instead of cheesecloth, if preferred, but it is more expensive. In buying the cretonne get two patterns which harmonize, buying 1 yard of each.

Cut each yard in four pieces lengthwise. Each curtain has two pieces at the top with an insertion of lace in between. One curtain only will be described. Of each pattern of cretonne take one piece, stitch the lace insertion between them, turn down the edge—about 1 in.—of the one intended for the top of the curtain, and stitch the cheesecloth on the other piece with a pudding-bag seam. Make a hem 12 in. deep on the bottom of the curtain. The lace for the curtain should be about 4 in. wide. Lay the straight edge of the lace toward the selvage(2) and the pointed edge turning backward. Stitch it on, fold down the hem on the wrong side, and catch it fast with long stitches. Cut a V-shaped piece out of the lace at the lower corner of the curtain, seam the lace together, and sew it across the bottom of the curtain.

CUT FLOWERS, RULES FOR ARRANGING:

The first thing to be considered in arranging cut flowers is the vase.

(1) Thin canvas.
(2) A woven edge of cloth (to prevent raveling).

If it is scarlet, blue or many-colored, it may necessarily conflict with some hue in your bouquet. Choose rather pure white, green, or transparent glass, which allows the delicate stems to be seen. Brown Swiss-wood, silver, bronze, or yellow straw conflict with nothing. The vase must be subordinate to what it holds. Use a bowl for roses; tall-spreading vases for gladiolus, fern, white lilies, and the like; cups for violets and tiny wood flowers. A flower-lover will in time collect shapes and sizes to suit each group.

Colors should be blended together with neutral tints, of which there are abundance—whites, grays, purples, tender greens—and which harmonize the pink, crimsons, and brilliant reds into soft unison. Certain flowers assort well only in families, and are spoiled by mixing. Of these are balsams, hollyhocks, and sweet-peas, whose tender liquid hues are as those of drifting sunset clouds. Others may be massed with good effect.

In arranging a large basket or vase it is well to mentally divide it into small groups, making each group perfectly harmonious with itself, blending the whole with green and delicate colors. And above all, avoid stiffness. Let a bright tendril or spray of vine spring forth here and there, and wander over and around the vase at its will.

The water should be warm for a winter vase—cool, but not iced, for a summer one. A little salt or a bit of charcoal should be added in hot weather, to obviate vegetable decay, and the vase filled anew each morning. With these precautions your flowers, if set beside an open window at night, will keep their freshness for many hours even in July, and reward by their beautiful presence the kind of hand which arranged and tended them.

CUTS, HOW TO TREAT:

There is nothing better for a cut than powdered resin. Get a few cent's worth, pound it until it is quite fine, put in a cast-off spice-box, with perforated top; then you can easily sift it on the cuts. Put a soft cloth around the injured member and wet it with water once in a while. It will prevent inflammation or soreness.

D

DAISY-CHAINS, TO MAKE:

Gather the daisies with long stems, make a loop in a stem, put the head of another daisy through it, then tighten the loop so as to hold the daisy; or push the stem through the daisy's "eye" or flower, and thus unite them. Daisy means "day's eye," because it opens when the sun rises, and shuts up or goes to sleep when he sets.

DANDRUFF, TO REMOVE:

(1) Wash the head thoroughly and often with pure soft water, and brush it vigorously until the hair is dry.

(2) The white of an egg rubbed well into the hair with the fingers, and then washed out with plenty of tepid water, is good.

(3) Borax removes the dandruff quickly and perfectly, but it is apt to make the hair dry and stiff.

(4) Ammonia and all other alkalies should be avoided.

(5) A simple and effectual remedy. Into a pint of water drop a lump of fresh quicklime[1] the size of a walnut; let it stand all night, then pour the water off clear from the sediment or deposit, add $^1/_4$ pint of the best vinegar, and wash the head with the mixture. Perfectly harmless; only wet the roots of the hair.

DAUGHTERS, WHAT TO TEACH OUR:

At a social gathering some one proposed this question: "What shall I teach my daughter?" The following replies were handed in:

- Teach her the library.
- Teach her to arrange the parlor and the library.
- Teach her to say "no," and mean it, or "yes" and stick to it.
- Teach her how to wear a calico dress, and to wear it like a queen.
- Teach her how to sew on buttons, darn stockings, and mend gloves.

(1) Unslaked lime.

- Teach her to dress for health and comfort as well as for appearance.
- Teach her to cultivate flowers and to keep the kitchen garden.
- Teach her to make the neatest room in the house.
- Teach her to have nothing to do with intemperate or dissolute young men.
- Teach her that tight lacing is uncomely as well as injurious to health.
- Teach her to regard the morals and habits, and not money, in selecting her associates.
- Teach her to observe the old rule, "A place for every thing, and every thing in its place."
- Teach her that music, drawing, and painting are real accomplishments in the home, and are not to be neglected if there be time and money for their use.
- Teach her the important truism that "the more she lives within her income the more she will save, and the further she will get away from the poor-house."
- Teach her that a good, steady, church-going mechanic, farmer, clerk, or teacher without a cent is worth more than 40 loafers or non-producers in broadcloth.
- Teach her to embrace every opportunity for reading, and to select such books as will give her the most useful and practical information in order to make the best progress in earlier as well as later home and school life.

DECANTERS, TO CLEAN:

Roll up in a small pieces some soft brown or blotting paper, wet them and soap them all. Put them into the decanters about one quarter full of warm water; shake them well for a few minutes, then rinse with clear cold water; wipe the outsides with a nice dry cloth, put the decanters to drain, and when dry they will be almost as bright as new ones. This is the best and safest mode of cleaning decanters. Some persons, however, use a little fine sand, and others egg-shells crushed into small pieces, which are shaken about in the glass with cold water; a beautiful polish may be given by this means.

DECANTER-STOPPERS, TO REMOVE:

Stoppers of glass decanters frequently, from a variety of causes, become so fixed that they cannot be removed without danger. Whenever this is the cause place a little sweet-oil with a feather around the stopper and the neck of the decanter, and set it near the fire. When tolerably warm, tap the stopper gently on all sides with a light piece of wood, and it will soon become loose, or the neck of the decanter may be rubbed sharply with a piece of list(1); the friction will expand the glass of the decanter, and in this way set the stopper free. Great care must be taken that the stopper is not broken.

DIAMONDS, TO POLISH:

The plane in use by all the large diamond-cutters is simply a cast-iron disk of good metal, with a vertical spindle run through its center, balanced and turned and faced true in a lathe. The disk revolves at about 1,000 revolutions per minute. With a little diamond-dust and oil the stone is set in a small brass cup filled with common soft solder; it is then screwed up in the clamps and applied to the skive(2) till the facets are formed.

DIAMONDS, TO TEST:

The diamond may be distinguished from every other stone by its peculiar virtue of single refraction. Every other precious stone (with the exception of the garnet, from which it can otherwise be readily distinguished) possesses the quality of double refraction; a double image of a taper or small light being given off when it is viewed through their facets. This results from their inferior refracting, and consequently reflecting, power. It can also be tested by its superior hardness. Further, if any other of the precious or artificial stones are immersed in alcohol, or even water, they lose their luster which the diamond does not.

A simple and ready way of distinguishing precious from artificial stones is to touch them with the tongue—the stone being the best conductor of heat will feel cold, the glass much less so. Sir David Brewster invented an instrument to distinguish real gems, called a lithiscope. The usual mode of estimating its value is by its weight in carats, (about 4 grains). If it is a diamond of the first water, free from flaws, and properly cut, its value is as the square of its weight in carats multiplied by 8; i.e., a diamond of 1 carat is worth $40 ; of 2 carats, $100; of 10 carats, $2,000, and so on. Beyond a certain weight fancy prices step in and human credibility requires a long breath. Uncut diamonds vary from $10 to $25 per carat.

DIARRHEA AND DYSENTERY:

- In all cases of diarrhea, dysentery, etc., perfect rest should be enjoined, which adds more to the removal of the difficulty than the too-frequent use of medicine. A recumbent position is best.
- Parched corn and meal boiled in skimmed milk, and fed

(1) The strengthened edge of a cloth.
(2) A revolving table for lapping diamonds.

frequently to children suffering from summer diarrhea, will almost always cure, as it will dysentery in adults, and often the cholera in its earliest stages.

- Common rice, parched brown like coffee, and then boiled and eaten in the ordinary way, without any other food, is, with perfect quietude of the body, one of the most effective remedies for troublesome looseness of the bowels.
- Put $^1/_4$ lb. of oatmeal, $1^1/_2$ ounces of sugar, $^1/_2$ tea-spoonful of salt, and 3 pints of water into a stew-pan; boil slowly 20 minutes, stir continually. Before serving add 1 pint boiled milk, 1 ounce butter, and a little pounded spice.
- A spoonful or two of pure raw wheat-flour, thinned with water so that it can be easily drunk. Three or four doses taken at intervals of 10 or 12 hours will generally cure any case not absolutely chronic. To make the dose palatable for children it can be sweetened and flavored with some drops, not acid.
- Take 1 gill of rice and place in a spider(1) over the fire, stirring it constantly until thoroughly brown. Do not burn it. As soon as it is thoroughly brown fill the spider with boiling water, and let it boil till the mass is of the consistency of thin paste. If the rice is not cooked perfectly soft add a little more water and let it boil away again. Be careful at the last moment that it does not burn on the bottom. When cooked soft turn into a bowl, sweeten with loaf or crushed sugar, and salt to suit the taste. Eat in milk.
- For diarrhea in children take 1 cup of wheat flour, and tie in a stout cloth and drop in cold water; then set over the fire and boil 3 hours steadily. After it is cold remove the cloth and crust forming by boiling. The ball thus prepared can be kept ready for use for any length of time. To use, grate a table-spoonful for a cupful of boiling water and milk—each one half. Wet up the flour with a very little cold water; stir in and boil 5 minutes. Sweeten to taste. Use a little salt if desired.

DIGESTION:

All of the strength of body and mind, of power to move, to work, to think, comes from proper food well digested. A few hours of effort use up certain elements in the muscles, nerves, and brain which can only be replaced by digested food. Tonics and stimulants may temporarily help the dormant or weak digestive organs, enabling them to digest food, but they do

(1) A kitchen utensil with feet for boiling over a hearth.

not add to the stock of strength. The food in the stomach is moistened and largely liquefied by a fluid supplied from the blood, coming in through myriads of little openings on the inner coating of the stomach. If there is much food to be worked up there must be great flow of blood to supply this digesting fluid, the gastric juice. The blood is then drawn away from other parts of the body. After a heavy meal one feels dull, sluggish, because there is less general circulation of the blood.

If violent or strong exertion of a body or mind is made soon after eating it draws the blood from the stomach and digestion of the food is retarded. If there is more food than the stomach can readily supply gastric juice for, some of it will be imperfectly worked over, and will go into the system in that condition. It will disturb the brain and other organs. It will affect or intensify any local trouble or disease. If one has weak or diseased lungs this imperfectly digested food will irritate and intensify the trouble. To be well digested by the gastric juice the food must first be mixed with a good supply of saliva, by thorough chewing. Eat slowly and keep every portion of food to be swallowed some time in the mouth, to get a full supply of saliva.

DINING-ROOM, CARE OF THE:

The dining-room in every home, be it great or small, should be the brightest and most pleasant room in the house; the table furniture and entire apartment should be scrupulously neat and orderly, while it should be the aim of every housekeeper to study the comfort and taste of the family in the arrangement and preparation of every meal. The table-cloth should always be spotless and fine, and an under cover of white cloth spread on the table gives the linen a heavier, smoother appearance. Napkins should be fine and thick, and should never be starched. The dishes should be well kept and free from cracks, the silver always brightly polished.

At dinings or entertainments no ornament is so attractive as flowers. Beside each plate should be placed as many knives, forks, and spoons as will be needed; a glass for water, and, where wine is used, glasses for it are set near each plate. The napkin neatly folded is placed on each plate, and within its folds a small slice of bread. All plates needed are set out ready. At breakfast the coffee and tea are set before the mistress, with the cream, sugar, cups, and saucers. The meat, with plates, is set before the master. For family use or a small dining one caster is sufficient. Butter is put in two small butter-dishes, with lumps of ice. Honey or syrup is served in saucers.

To clear the table after meals and properly wash the dishes is a very important branch of housekeeping, and if carelessly done causes great annoyance and discomfort to the family. As soon as a meal is over the fragments should all be gathered up, and the plates scraped; the crumbs should be lightly swept. To wash the dishes have clear hot water in the dish-pan; first wash the silver without soap, dry on an old soft towel immediately, then add soap, wash glasses, rinse, and wipe. Next take the cups and saucers, leaving the greasy articles until the last. Always keep clean linen dish-cloths and tea-towels; those for the dining-room should never be used in the kitchen.

By attention to these suggestions and the exercise of good judgement the humblest household may always have a pleasant dining-room and an attractive table. The dining-room should be aired daily as thoroughly as any of the bed-chambers. The odor of stale breakfasts and dinners is extremely unappetizing, and its existence should be rendered impossible by opening the windows and shutting the doors immediately at the close of each meal.

Food should never be left standing on the table after the family have quitted the room. That which is to appear again should be carried at once to the cellar or pantry. The scraps left on the plates should be gathered in one dish and sent immediately to their destination in the garbage pail. The soiled china, glass, and silver should be taken into the butler's pantry and neatly piled at the side of the sink. In hot weather it is well to cover them with water at once, that they may not attract flies. The thorough rinsing of all china that has been used should be an invariable preliminary to the washing of it in scalding suds.

DINNER-PARTIES:

When a lady issues invitations for a dinner to 10 or 20 persons she should do so a fortnight in advance, using the following formula, written or engraved on note-paper:

Mr. and Mrs. James Clyde
request the pleasure of
...... company at dinner on
....
at 7 o'clock

—the blanks filled by the hostess with the name or names of the guests, and the date. The invitations should be answered by the recipient at once, and the engagement, if accepted, kept. If personal illness or death of relatives, or any other imperative reason for absence occurs subsequent to the acceptance, the hostess should be apprised of it as soon as possible.

A gentleman should never be invited without his wife, or a lady without her husband, unless one or the other is merely visiting the city or town where their hostess resides. A previous engagement might warrant either husband or wife in declining the invitation, while the other is free to accept and go alone. A lesser number of guests—4 or 6—may be invited, with less ceremony, within the week, but always in writing.

A pretty informal note is written somewhat as follows:

Dear Mrs. T— — —:

Will you and your husband dine with us Friday evening? Quite by ourselves, except for the Johnsons, who will be with us also. At our usual hour—quarter to eight.

Sincerely yours,
L.S— — —.

A note like this should also be answered immediately, and the same obligation of keeping the engagement, if accepted, observed. The usual hour for dinner-parties is 7 o'clock, but it can well be a little later in order to insure punctuality; for, whatever the hour, the guests must be careful to be punctual to the minute, and no hostess is justified in keeping her dinner waiting, at the risk of its being spoiled, for any delaying guest when all but one are assembled.

When entering the drawing-room, the lady goes first, not on her husband's arm. At elegant dinner-parties frequently the gentleman finds a card in the hall, on which his name and that of the lady whom he is to take in to dinner are written, and also a tiny spray or *boutonnière* of flowers, which he places in his button-hole. At smaller entertainments the hostess indicates to the gentleman in the drawing-room the lady he is to take in, and, in any case, if they are not acquainted, introduces him to her.

When all the guests have arrived, dinner is announced by the servant. Then the host takes the eldest lady—or if a bride is present, or any lady to whom the dinner is given, then that lady—and leads the way to the dining-room; and the others follow, the hostess last and on the arm of the gentleman to whom the entertainers desire to show most honor. French bills of fare sound fine, but when the dishes are divested of their foreign titles they often prove to be some of our old acquaintances in new dresses. A simple menu tastefully served is quite as attractive to the average diner-out.

The dinner *à la Russe*, at which every thing is handed by the servants, is the most popular style. The arrangement of the table is a matter of moment, but with care and taste much expense is not necessary. The table-cloth for dinner should always be of white damask, laid over an under-cover of white Canton flannel. In the center a long mat of colored velvet, wedged with gilt or silver lace, may be laid, but this is not a necessity; the white table-cloth is. Colored cloths are used only for luncheon or tea. The colored centermat may be of velveteen, which will look just as well as the velvet.

A border of flowers arranged all around has a very pretty effect. Flowers all of one color, put in crystal glass, are most effective. Carnations, roses, violets, and ferns are the favorite floral decorations. Heavily scented blooms, tuberoses especially, should not be used; but the dainty fragrance of the rose is never unwelcome.

The substitution of lamps and candelabra for the more glaring yet not more brilliant gaslight is attended with some annoyances. Yet no dinner-table is thought complete in effect without one or two colored lamps and a certain number of candles or the pretty little fairy lamps which adorn a table so beautifully.

At each place should be laid 2 knives, 3 forks, and a soup-spoon, all of silver, if possible; and before each plate a small salt-cellar of some fanciful design. The large dinner-napkins of white damask ought never to be arranged in fancy shapes, as frequently seen in hotels and restaurants. Let each be folded in a three-cornered pyramid, to stand by the plate and hold the roll or piece of bread. Cut-glass tumblers are used in preference to goblets; in either case the glasses or plates should never be reversed in laying the table, but set on in the position they are to be in when in use. Menu or card holders may be placed before each plate to hold the dinner-card and the bill of fare, but these may be dispensed with, and, if decorated or engraved cards cannot be had, the menu and name of the guest can be written on separate cards and laid on each plate.

If the principal dishes are served or carved by the host or hostess, as must be done unless there are two servants to wait on the table, it will be best to have large carving-cloths of fringed butcher's linen laid on the table where the dish is to be placed, to preserve the table-cloth from splashes. These are removed when the desert is served. The sideboard is arranged as tastily as may be, and all the pretty pieces of china and silver not needed on the table can be displayed here. It is well, also, to have a small table at one side upon which the finger-bowls and reserve of plates, forks, and spoons, are to be placed. After the fish has been removed hot plates are brought on for the meats.

The waiter or waitress should be directed to carry a napkin to cover the fingers when serving the meats, and all plates or dishes should be handed or set before the guest from the left. After the coffee has been served (in small cups) the hostess slightly inclines her head to the lady whom her husband led in to dinner, and they both rise, and all then follow to the drawing-room. The English custom of leaving the gentlemen to cigars and their usual accompaniment, which the ladies are not supposed to care for, has in a great measure been ignored by American hostesses, and it is a most excellent invocation on their part.

DIPHTHERIA, PRECAUTIONS WITH:

Cleanliness in and around the dwelling and pure air in living and sleeping rooms are of the utmost importance where any contagious disease is prevailing, as cleanliness tends both to prevent and mitigate it. All filth from cellar to garret and around the house should be removed; drains should be put in perfect repair; dirty walls and ceilings should be lime-washed, and every occupied room should be thoroughly ventilated. Apartments which have been occupied by a person sick with diphtheria should be cleansed with disinfectants, ceilings lime-washed, and wood-work painted; the carpets, bed-clothing, upholstered furniture, etc., exposed many days to fresh air and sunlight. Many articles should be exposed to a high artificial temperature to kill all germs of infection.

When diphtheria is prevailing, no child should be allowed to kiss strange children, nor those suffering from sore throat, nor should it sleep with or be confined to rooms occupied by, or use toys, handkerchiefs, etc., belonging to children having sore throat, cough, or catarrh. If the weather is cold the child should be warmly clad with flannels. The well children should be scrupulously kept apart from the sick in dry, well-aired, rooms, and every possible source of infection rigidly guarded. Every attack of sore throat, cough, and catarrh should be at once attended to; the feeble should have invigorating food and treatment; the sick should be rigidly isolated in well-aired, sun-lighted rooms; all discharges from the mouth and nose should be received into vessels containing disinfectants, as solutions of carbolic acid or sulphate of zinc.

DIPHTHERIA, TO GUARD AGAINST:

Procure from a drug-store 1 lb. of sulphate of zinc. Put into an ordinary waterpail 8 table-spoonfuls with 4 of common salt, and to this add 1 gallon of boiling water. This disinfecting solution is to be kept in the room, and into it should be placed and kept for 1 hour every article of soiled clothing, bedding, handkerchiefs, etc.

DISEASE, PREVENTION OF:

A large proportion of the ills which now afflict and rob us of so much time and enjoyment might easily be avoided. A proper knowledge and observance of hygienic laws would greatly lessen the number of such diseases as pneumonia, consumption, catarrh, gout, rheumatism, scrofula, dyspepsia, etc.

It is a lamentable fact that in densely populated cities nearly one half of the children die before they are 5 yrs. old. Every physiologist knows that at least nine tenths of these lives could be saved by an observance of the laws of health. Prof. Bennett, of Edinburgh, estimated that 100,000 persons die annually in Scotland from diseases easily preventable, and the same testimony could be obtained from the medical profession in this and other countries.

Methods of Prevention: With the advance of medical science the causes of many diseases have been determined. Vaccination has been found to prevent or mitigate the ravages of small-pox. Scurvy, formerly so fatal among sailors that it was deemed "a mysterious infliction of divine justice against which man strives in vain," is now entirely prevented by the use of vegetables or lime-juice. Cholera, whose approach strikes dread in the community, and for which no certain specific has been found, is but the penalty for filthy streets, bad drainage, over-crowded tenements, and general filthiness, and it may be controlled, it not prevented, by suitable sanitary measures. The same may be said of that dreadful scourge, the yellow fever. There is no quarantine like cleanliness, good drainage, and ventilation.

Why Medicine is Taken: The first step in the cure of any disease is to obey the law of health which has been violated. If medicine is taken, it is not to destroy the disease, since that is not a thing to be destroyed, but is to hold the deranged action in check while nature repairs the injury and brings the system again into harmonious movement. This tendency or power of nature is the physician's chief reliance. *Vis medicatrix nautre* is the great sheet-anchor, the power of nature to repair the breach made by violated law.

The very best and most skillful physicians have little confidence in medicine itself to cure diseases. The chief physician is nature, and the chief remedy is a resort to hygienic measures. Nature can be assisted by the intelligent employment of proper medicines. The indiscriminate use of patent nostrums and specific preventives and remedies, of whose constituents nothing is known, and which propose to prevent or to cure almost all diseases, cannot be too greatly deprecated. No well educated physician, unless perhaps in some very peculiar case, will refuse to his patient a knowledge of the medicine he prescribes, as well as the nature of its operation. With the need of medicine comes the need of a competent physician to advise its use.

DISHES, HOW TO WASH:

The right way to wash dishes is to have 3 pans, one containing warm soap-suds, another warm clean water, and the other hot clear water.

(1) Wash and wipe the glassware.

(2) The silver, having a plate in the bottom of the pan for the silver to rest on.

(3) Take the dishes, 1 at a time, wash the side you eat off of in the suds, then place them in the warm clear water, where there is a clean dish-cloth, and wash both sides, then rinse them in the hot water and drain off.

DISINFECTANTS, HOW TO PREPARE AND USE THEM:

Charcoal: Powdered charcoal is one of the best of disinfectants. It is very prompt in absorbing affluvia and gaseous bodies, as well as rendering harmless and even useful those bodies which are easily changed. Charcoal powder has long been used as a filter for putrid water. When the impurities are absorbed they come in contact with condensed oxygen gas, which exists in the pores of all charcoal which has been exposed to the air, and in this way become oxydized and destroyed. A layer of pulverized charcoal will prevent the escape of all offensive odor from any decomposing substance.

Copperas: Common copperas, called sulphate of iron, in its crude state can be purchased for 5 cents a pound; this dissolved in 2 gallons of water and thrown over ill-smelling places is one of the cheapest, simplest, and most convenient deodorizers, and is applicable to privies, sinks, gutters, and heaps of offal(1).

Chloride of Lime: To give off chlorine, to absorb putrid effluvia, and to stop putrefaction use chloride of lime; and if in cellars or close rooms the chlorine gas is wanted pour strong vinegar or diluted sulphuric acid upon the plates of chloride of lime occasionally, and add more of the chloride. We have known a large manufactory filled with deadly sewage air cleansed in a single half hour by throwing half a bushel of chloride of lime into the vaults from which the poisonous gas emanated. Chloride of lime is often deleterious in close dwellings because of the chlorine evolved. It may be used safely in the open atmosphere.

Carbolic Acid: A weak solution of carbolic acid may be used in saucers or shallow earthen dishes; or a cloth saturated with it may be hung in the room where the offensive odor is suspected. In large cities the streets in the most densely populated wards have been watered on alternate days with a weak solution of carbolic acid with excellent results. There is no doubt that this excellent antiseptic and disinfectant has been very beneficial. The inhabitants of those streets have often expressed satisfaction at the freshness and removal of disagreeable smells which this acid produces, and they regard it as an addition to their comfort.

Disinfecting Mixture: Common salt, 3 ounces; black manganese, oil of vitriol, of each 1 ounce; water, 2 ounces. Carry this mixture in a cup through the apartments of the sick.

Coffee as a Disinfectant: Experiments with roasted coffee prove it to be a powerful means of rendering harmless and destroying animal and vegetable effluvia. A room in which meat in an advanced state of decomposition has been kept can be instantly deprived of all smell by simply carrying through it a coffee-roaster containing 1 lb. of newly roasted coffee. The best mode of using the coffee is to dry the raw bean, pound it in a mortar, and then roast the powder on a moderately heated iron plate until it becomes a dark brown color. Then sprinkle it in sinks and cesspools, or expose it on a plate in the room to be purified.

(1) Garbage or heaps of discarded waste from the butchering of animals.

Sunflowers as Disinfectants: Experiment in France and Holland have shown that sunflowers when planted on an extensive scale will neutralize the pernicious effects of exhalations from marshes. This plan has been tried with great success in the fenny districts near Rochefort, France; and the authorities of Holland assert that intermittent fever has wholly disappeared from districts where sunflowers have been planted. It is not yet determined what effect the flower produces on the atmosphere—whether it generates oxygen, like other plants of rapid growth, or whether, like the coniferoe, it emits ozone and thus destroys the organic germs of miasms that produce fever.

Boiling after Disinfection: Permanganate of potassa may be used in disinfecting clothing and towels from cholera and fever patients during the night, or when such articles cannot be instantly boiled. Throw the soiled articles immediately into a tub of water in which there has been dissolved an ounce of the permanganate salt to every 3 gallons of water. Boil the clothing as soon as it is removed from this colored solution.

How to Fumigate Rooms: To fumigate and cleanse the air of an apartment there is no more simple way than to heat a common iron shovel quite hot, and pour vinegar slowly upon it. The steam arising from this process is pungent and of a disinfectant character. Open windows and doors at the same time.

Another way is to fumigate with sulphurous acid, thus: Arrange to vacate the room for 12 hours. Close every window and aperture, and upon an iron pipkin or kettle with legs burn a few ounces of sulphur. Instantly after kindling it every person must withdraw from the place, and the room must remain closed for the succeeding 8 hours. If any other kind of fumigation is resorted to, as that by chlorine, bromine, or nitrous acid, a sanitary officer or chemist should superintend the process. Fumigation should be resorted to in dwelling houses only by official orders or permission, as the disinfecting gases are very poisonous.

To Disinfect Water-closets: *To disinfect a water-closet or a quantity of earth that is contaminated by cholera excrement, or liable to be infected, use solution of carbolic acid and copperas mixed as follows:*

To every cubic foot of soil or filth give from 1 to 3 pints of the strong solution. To every privy and water-closet allow at the rate of 1 pint, to be poured in daily at evening, for every person on the premises. This practice should be kept up while cholera is in the country. This method of systematic disinfection would be useful in every household; but when cholera is present in any city or country such thorough application of this means of protection cannot be safely neglected in any city or place to which persons may come from towns where cholera is epidemic. The best sanitary chemists advise that the estimated quantity of the privy and sewer disinfectants required for each person daily, in the presence of cholera should be 1/2 ounce sulphate of iron and 1/2 dram or 1/2 tea-spoonful of carbolic acid.

Heat and Steam: Heat has long been known as among the most efficient of disinfectants. And the use of steam, as a facile means of communicating it against yellow fever especially, was effectually demonstrated as long ago as 1848. Since that time in addition to the common use of steam for the disinfection of vessels, it has been extensively used for the disinfection of personal clothing and bedding and to this end steam disinfection chambers abroad at least, have long since ceased to be a novelty.

The first one constructed in this country was in connection with the New York Quarantine hospitals, where it continues to be a prominent feature. Another new disinfecting compound for purifying the atmosphere of the sick-room has just been presented to the Berlin Medical Society. Oil of rosemary, lavender, and thyme in the portion of 10, 2 1/2 and 2 1/2 parts respectively are used with nitric acid in the proportion of 30 to 1 1/2. The bottle should be shaken before using, and a sponge saturated with the compound and left to diffuse by evaporation. Simple as it is, the vapor of this compound is said to possess extraordinary properties in controlling the odors and effluvia of offensive and infectious disorders.

DOGS, CARE OF:

The best way to keep a dog healthy is to let him have plenty of exercise and not to overfeed him. Let them at all times have a plentiful supply of clean water, and encourage them to take to swimming, as it assists their cleanliness. When you wash them do not use a particle of soap, or you will prevent their licking themselves, and they may become habitually dirty. Properly treated, dogs should be fed only once a day. Meat boiled for dogs and the liquor in which it is boiled thickened with barley meal or oatmeal forms capital food.

The distemper is liable to attack dogs from 4 months to 4 yrs. old. It prevails most in spring and autumn. The disease is known by dullness of the eye, husky cough, shivering, loss of appetite and spirits, and fits. When fits occur the dog will most likely die unless a veterinary surgeon is called in. During the distemper dogs should be allowed to run on the grass, their diet should be spare, and a little sulphur be placed in their water. Chemists who dispense cattle medicines can generally advise with sufficient safety upon the diseases of dogs, and it is best for unskillful persons to abstain from physicking them.

Hydrophobia is the most dreadful of all diseases. The first symptoms are attended by thirst, fever, and languor. The dog starts convulsively in his sleep, and when awake, though restless, is languid. When a dog is suspected he should be firmly chained in a place where neither children nor dogs or cats can get near him. Any one going to attend him should wear thick leather gloves and proceed with great caution. When a dog snaps savagely at an imaginary object it is almost a certain indication of madness; and when it exhibits a terror of fluids it is confirmed hydrophobia.

Some dogs exhibit a great dislike of musical sounds, and when this is the case they are too frequently made sport of. But it is a dangerous sport, and dogs have sometimes been driven mad by it. In many diseases dogs will be benefited by warm baths. The mange is a contagious disease which it is difficult to get rid of when once contracted. The best way is to apply to a veterinary chemist for an ointment, and to keep applying it for some time after the disease has disappeared, or it will break out again.

DOMESTIC SURGERY:

Dressings: Dressings are substances usually applied to parts for the purpose of soothing, promoting their reunion when divided, protecting them from external injuries, as a means of applying various medicines, to absorb discharges, protect the surrounding parts, and securing cleanliness.

Certain Instruments: Certain instruments are required for the application of dressings in domestic surgery, viz., scissors, a pair of tweezers or simple forceps, a knife, needles and thread, a razor, a lancet, a piece of lunar caustic(1) in a quill, and a sponge.

The Materials: The materials required for dressings consist of lint, scraped linen, carded cotton, tow(2), ointment spread on calico, adhesive plaster, compresses, pads, poultices, old rags of linen or calico, and water.

The following rules should be attended to in applying dressings:

(1) Always prepare the new dressings before removing the old one.

(2) Always have hot and cold water at hand, and a vessel to place the foul dressings in.

(3) Have one or more persons at hand ready to assist, and tell each person what they are to do before you commence—it prevents confusion; thus one is to wash out and hand the sponges, another to heat the adhesive plaster to hand the bandages and dressings, and, if requisite, a third to support the limb, etc.

(4) Always stand on the outside of a limb to dress it.

(5) Place the patient in as easy a position as possible, so as not to fatigue him.

(6) Arrange the bed after changing the dressings, but in some cases you will have to do so before the patient is placed on it.

(7) Never be in a hurry when applying dressings; do it quietly.

(1) Nitrate of silver fused at a low heat.
(2) A tuft of wool or the coarse part of hemp or flax.

Poultices: Poultices are usually made of linseed-meal, oatmeal, or bread, either combined with water and other fluids. Sometimes they are made of carrots, charcoal, potatoes, yeast, and linseed-meal, mustard, etc.

Bandages: Bandages are strips of calico, linen, flannel, muslin, elastic-webbing, bunting, or some other substance of various lengths, such as 3, 4, 8, 10, or 12 yds., and 1, $1\frac{1}{2}$, 2, $2\frac{1}{2}$, 3, 4, or 6 in. wide, free from hems or darns; soft and unglazed. They are better after they have been washed. Their uses are to retain dressings, apparatus, or parts of the body in their proper positions, support the soft parts, and maintain equal pressure.

Bandages are simple and compound; the former are simple slips rolled up tightly like a roll of ribbon. There is also another simple kind which is rolled from both ends; this is called a double-headed bandage. The compound bandages are formed by many pieces. Bandages for the head should be 2 in. wide and 7 yds. long; for the leg, $2\frac{1}{2}$ in. wide and 7yds. long; for the thigh, 3 in. wide and 8 yds. long; and for the body, 4 or 6 in. wide and 10 or 12 yds. long.

DON'TS FOR PARENTS:

(1) Don't forget that you brought your children into the world without their knowledge or consent. You have no right to embitter the life you have thus thrust upon them. Parents have been known to make absolute slaves of their children, compelling almost constant attendance under the popular delusion that young limbs are never tired, and like the old slave-master giving nothing in return but food and clothes.

(2) Don't laugh at and deride your children's hobbies. Remember how much brighter life has seemed to you when you could realize some cherished dream, and treat them accordingly.

(3) Don't forget that youth needs amusement. Your children have not only bodies, but minds. Rest for the body and amusement for the mind are demands of nature which too many parents ignore. If you do not provide for your children healthful and sufficient amusement, then thank God for his mercy on you if your children do not take to dangerous or wicked pleasures when they are older.

(4) Don't forget that your children are beginning life, while you, perhaps, are ending it. Give then the benefit of your experience, but don't expect that your experience will serve them in place of an experience of their own.

(5) Don't be impatient with your children when they doubt your estimate of the world's allurements. Remember it is you who have tested these

things, not they. You did not see with your father's eyes, neither should you expect your children to see with your eyes.

(6) Don't demand respect of your children, or endeavor to enforce it by authority. Respect is paid not to those who demand, but to those who deserve it.

(7) Don't neglect your children's friends. Invite them to your house. Show your children that their friends are your friends, and your children's friends will be such as you will approve.

(8) Don't be jealous of your children's friends. If you make your society delightful to your children they will always prefer you to any other companion. If your child prefers every one else to you stop and ponder whether you have not compelled him to seek elsewhere the companionship, love, and sympathy he ought to find in you.

(9) Don't be afraid to let your children see your love for them. Let a child feel that no matter where he goes, or what he does; no matter whether friends forsake or foes slander him, his parents' love and trust will always follow him—and that child is not only safe for all time, but the thought of this love will shine out like a lamp in a dark place, cheering and strengthening him against all odds.

DRESS, HEALTHFUL:

The leading requirement in healthful apparel consists in the equal distribution of warmth over all parts of the body, thus favoring equal circulation, without which health cannot be sustained. To secure this we must have all under-garments with high necks, long sleeves, and leglets reaching to the shoe-top and fitting close inside the stocking. The number of the under-garments of each season, as well as the peculiarities of each individual.

The material best suiting the need of our robust boys and the best manner of "making up" are not so difficult to determine; but for our girls—our delicate country girls, who walk a long distance to and from school through all extremes of weather—how shall we clothe them with equal comfort? The outer waist, with its buttons for all bands to be attached to, can be made from the corset or bustle. Instead of these useless accessories see that each girl is provided with long coats, leggings, mittens, and hood, with arctics and rubbers, all in readiness for their separate need. While the shoes for our girls should be heavy enough for ordinary good walking, there are extremes of wet and cold that must be provided for. If limited in means, the mother must watch over the outlay of money set aside for clothing until the girls are taught that the feather on their cap is not so important, even in lending attraction to the face, as is the healthful glow which attends the well protected feet.

DRILLS, TO TEMPER:

Select none but the finest and best steel for your drills. In making them never heat higher than a cherry red, and always hammer till nearly cold. Do all your hammering in one way, for if, after you have flattened your piece out, you attempt to hammer it back to a square or a round, you spoil it. When your drill is in proper shape heat it to a cherry red, and thrust it into a piece of resin or into quicksilver(1). Some use a solution of cyanuret potassa and rain-water for tempering their drills, but the resin or quicksilver will work best.

DRINK:

- Water enters more largely into the composition of our bodies than all other substances combined. Apart from its immediate invigorating influence, it favors the rapid transformation of tissues, and in this manner facilitates the elimination of deleterious substances from the system. A copious draught of water at retiring will sometimes entirely break up a recent cold. A tumbler of fresh water drank regularly upon rising in the morning will often do more toward overcoming chronic constipation than medicine. In warm weather drink moderately of cold water.
- Chocolate, from its large proportion of albumen, is a nutritive beverage, but at the same time, from its quantity of fat, the most difficult to digest. Its aromatic substances, however, strengthen the digestion. A cup of chocolate is an excellent restorative, and invigorating even for weak persons, provided their digestive organs are not too delicate.
- Tea and coffee do not afford this advantage. Albumen(2) in tea-leaves and legumin in coffee berries are represented in very scanty proportions.
- Buttermilk nearer satisfies all the conditions of a cheap and wholesome summer drink than anything known at present. It is agreeable to all palates, thirst-subduing, and wholesome.
- Lemonade is one of the best and safest drinks for any person, whether in health or not. It is suitable to all stomach diseases and excellent in sickness.
- Alcoholic liquors should be avoided. They are heating as well as stimulating; their use tends to excess and sure reaction.

DRINK, VERY STRENGTHENING:

Beat the yelk of a fresh egg with a little sugar, beat the white to a

(1) Mercury.
(2) Nutritive protein.

strong froth, stir it into the yelk, fill up the tumbler with new milk, and grate in a little nutmeg.

DROPSY(1), REMEDY FOR:

Take 1 pint of bruised mustard-seed, 2 handfuls of bruised horse-radish root, 8 ounces of lignum-vitae(2) chips, and 4 ounces of bruised Indian hemp-root. Put all the ingredients in 7 quarts of cider, and let it simmer over a slow fire until it is reduced to 4 quarts. Strain the decoction, and take a wine-glassful 4 times a day for a few days, increasing the dose to a small tea-cupful 3 times a day. After which use tonic medicines. This remedy has cured cases of dropsy in 1 week's time which have baffled the skill of many eminent physicians. For children the dose should be smaller.

DRUNKENNESS, CURE FOR:

(1) There is a prescription in use in England for the cure of drunkenness by which thousands are said to have been enabled to recover themselves. The recipe came into notoriety by the efforts of Mr. John Vine Hall, commander of the steamship Great Eastern. He had fallen into such habitual drunkenness that his most earnest efforts to reclaim himself proved unavailing; at last he sought the advice of an eminent physician, which he followed faithfully for several months, and at the end of that time he had lost all desire for liquor, although he had been for many years led captive by a most debasing appetite. The recipe, which he afterward published, and by which so many other drunkards have been assisted to reform, is as follows:

Sulphate of iron, 20 grains; magnesia, 40 grains; peppermint, 44 drams; spirits of nutmeg, 4 drams, dose, 1 table-spoonful twice a day.

(2) Let the inebriate begin by taking every 2 hours 1 dram (tea-spoonful) tincture of cinchona, (Peruvian bark), He can increase the dose 6 drams (tea-spoonfuls) without any danger, and take it in that proportion 4 to 10 times a day. It will not destroy his appetite for food. In the course of a few days the antiperiodic properties of the cinchona begin to tell, and he loses not only all taste for the tincture, but also for every thing in the way of alcohol.

(3) *Here is the Peruvian bark remedy, which is said to kill the disease and the inclination to drink at one and the same time:*

Take 1 lb. of best fresh quill red Peruvian bark, powder it and soak it in 1 pint of diluted alcohol. Afterward strain and evaporate it down to 1/2 pint. Dose, a tea-spoonful every 3 hours the first and second days, the

(1) Edema, the accumulation of watery fluid in the areolar tissue or serous cavities.
(2) From the wood of the guaicum officinale tree, very hard and heavy, soft when cut but later hardening. with exposure to air.

tongue to be moistened occasionally between the doses. If the patient has a headache in consequence of taking the medicine reduce the dose. The third day take 1/2 tea-spoonful every 3 hours. Afterward reduce the dose to 15 drops, then to 10, then to 5. To make a cure it takes from 5 to 15 days, and in extreme cases 30 days; 7 days are about the average in which a cure can be effected.

DUCK ON THE ROCK:

The number of players is not limited. A large stone is set up to serve as a "rock," and about 30 ft. from it a line is drawn to mark the goal. Each player provides himself with a good-sized stone, known as a "duck." By one of the many methods of counting out known to all boys one of the crowd is declared "it" and must place his duck on the rock. Now in turn each of the other players from the goal line tosses his duck at the duck on the rock. The aim of the one who is "it" is to "tag" one of the other players, who, under certain circumstances, becomes "it" in his place.

(1) He who is "it" must always keep the duck on the rock. When it is knocked off he must immediately replace it. He cannot tag any one while the duck is off the rock.

(2) He can tag another player only when that player is out of goal and has touched or picked up his own duck since throwing it from the goal line. It is usual for every player after making a throw to go and stand by his duck, waiting until the duck is knocked off the rock or for a good chance to pick up and run in. On a chill November day boys can get a good deal of fun, warmth, and exercise out of this old-fashioned game.

DUCKS, TREATMENT OF:

Ducks do not really require a pond or stream of water; give them, especially the well-advanced young ones, a shallow box, sunk into the ground, of water, which should be constantly supplied, and they will thrive well. Very young ducklings should be kept away from the water, merely giving them plenty of drink, fresh and pure. When they have attained a fair size, have feathered up considerably, and are 3 or 4 weeks old, introduce them to the puddle made for them and they will be all right. Where it can be done, let the water-box be in a good-sized inclosure, so that they cannot wander away and fall an easy prey to hawks, snakes, turtles, etc.

About the same food that is given turkeys is suitable for young ducks, although they like plenty of green food as well as soft food while young. Worms, flies, bugs, etc., are eagerly shoveled in by them, and relished accordingly, in the absence of which occasional feeds of shreds of well-cooked beef—the cheap of all parts will do—come in very nicely to supply the deficiency. Like other young poultry they require care during the earlier stages of growth and development.

DUSTING:

For dusting tufted furniture a house-painter's brush is the best implement. It goes into nooks and crevices, removing fluff and lint. Such brushes may be bought at almost any hardware store or house-furnishing establishment. The bristles are so much softer than those of the ordinary whisk-broom that they are less likely to fray the fabric with which the furniture is covered. For wood-work, marble, etc., the invaluable cheesecloth duster surpasses every other, unless, perhaps, an old silk handkerchief. Feather dusters take off the superficial deposit, but do not clean thoroughly. They are indispensable, however, when attached to long poles, for brushing curtain-rods, cornices, and picture-frames that cannot be reached by the arm alone. Spider-webs must also be watched for especially in warm or damp weather. They appear with incredible rapidity, and give a look of shiftlessness not equaled even by finger-marked paint or dingy windows.

DUST-PAN, PROPER SHAPE:

When you want a dust-pan have it made to order, with the handle turned down instead of up, so as to rest on the floor and tip the dust-pan at a proper angle for receiving the dust. It is a great convenience, as you do not have to stoop and hold it while you are sweeping.

DWELLINGS AND HEALTH:

Importance of a Healthful Location: The healthiness of dwellings depends upon their faultless situation, construction, and management. It is, therefore, of primary importance that the foundation of houses be on dry ground free from decaying matters. Houses built upon a soil saturated with putrid moisture or upon old swamps or cess-pools, or similar filthy ground, are notoriously unhealthy, because such a soil, especially in the warm season, evolves deleterious exhalations, and vitiates the water of the ground and the air.

In the construction of buildings it is also necessary to protect their foundations against dampness from underground by means either of drainage or of a damp-proof ground floor. A construction conducive to a free and ample supply of light and air is then the main condition for a healthy habitation; however large or small, elegant or plain, the house may be, its salubrious condition may be maintained and regulated by these two simple and cheap correctors, light and air.

Location of Dwellings in Cities: Dwellings which face on free and open streets are to be preferred to those which open into courts, because the motion of the air is freer in the former. In a closely built city the corner house, having the sweep of two streets, is, in this respect better located than others in the block. It is not well that high blocks of dwellings should so surround the rear court as to shut out the wind, nor that streets should terminate against the middle of a block at right angles to it. In the country any open, dry portion of land will make a good building spot.

Shade-trees Around our Dwellings: Farm-houses or other dwellings, whether for man or beast, should not be closely shaded, as such shade obstructs both sunlight and air-currents. The aim should be to so arrange the trees in the lawn as to permit the ingress of the sun's rays and of the free and healthful air.

High Ceilings and Health: Lofty ceilings are regarded by some as a principal means of insuring a sufficient measure in cubic feet for each person. Unless ventilation is secured for the upper portion of a room, a lofty ceiling only makes that portion of space above the tops of the windows a receptacle for foul air, which accumulates and remains to vitiate the stratum below.

How to Dry Damp Walls: The most effective method is by letting them evaporate the water into the air. This is best accomplished by heating all the chimneys and stoves, and the constant ventilation of all the rooms until the necessary degree of dryness is obtained. Ventilation is also constantly necessary to maintain the proper degree of dryness to counteract their tendency to re-absorb the various gases, and the emanations resulting from inhabitation, and the vapors arising from the culinary department.

Caution against Damp Floors: Floors of cellars and basements should not be made of brick or similar soft and porous material; apparently these can be easily kept clean, but they absorb and retain moisture, and not only remain cold and damp, but by their porosity expose the impurities of the absorbed moisture to evaporation, and thus pollute the air and render otherwise healthy cellars and basements damp and unwholesome. Floors of water-tight cement of or wood, well ventilated underneath, are therefore preferable.

How to Make Dry Cellar Floors: For making floors the following method is said to produce very desirable results: 4 parts course gravel or broken stone and sand, and 1 part each of lime and cement, are mixed in a shallow box and well shoveled over from end to end. The sand, gravel, and cement are mixed together dry. The lime is slaked separately and mixed with just water enough to cement it well together. Six or 8 in. of the mixture is then put on the bottom, and when well set another coating is put on, consisting of 1 part cement and 2 of sand. This will also answer for making the bottom of a cistern that is to be cemented up directly upon the ground without a lining of bricks.

Danger from Wetting Coal in Cellars: The habit of wetting coal in bulk in the cellar, which is sometimes practiced, causes it to emit poisonous gases deleterious to health, and it should be carefully avoided.

Kitchen Sink and Health: A little sink near a kitchen door-step, inadvertently formed, has been known, although not exceeding in its dimensions a single square foot, to spread sickness through a whole household. Hence every thing of the kind should be studiously obviated, so that there should be no spot about a farm-house which can receive and hold standing water, whether it be for pure rain from the sky, the contents of a wash-basin, the slop-bowl, or the water-pail.

Death in the Dish-cloth: A lady correspondent of the *Rural World*, having been startled by typhoid fever in her neighborhood some time ago, gives the following good advice about dish-cloths: "If they are black and stiff, and smell like a barn-yard, it is enough; throw them in the fire, and henceforth and forever wash your dishes with cloths that are white, cloths that you can see through, and see if you ever have that disease again. There are sometimes other causes, but I have smelled a whole houseful of typhoid fever in one 'dish-rag.' I had some neighbors once—clever, good sort of folks; one fall four of them were sick at one time with typhoid fever.

The doctor ordered the vinegar barrels whitewashed, and threw about 40 cents' worth of carbolic acid in the swill-pail and departed. I went into the kitchen and made gruel; I needed a dish-cloth, and looked around and found several, and such 'rags!' I burned them all, and called the daughter of the house to get me a dish-cloth, and looked around on the table. 'Why,' she said, 'there were about a dozen here this morning,' and she looked in the wood-box and on the mantel-piece, and felt in the cup-board. 'Well,' I said, 'I saw some old black rotten rags lying around, and I burned them, for there is death in such dish-cloths as those, and you must never use such again.'

I took turns at nursing that family for weeks, and I believe those dirty dish-cloths were the cause of all that hard work. You may only brush and comb your head on Sundays, you need not wear a collar unless you go from home—but you must wash your dish-cloths."

DYSENTERY:

A disease arising from inflammation of the mucous membrane of the large intestines, and characterized by stools consisting chiefly of blood and mucus, or other morbid matter, accompanied with griping of the bowels, followed by straining at stool. There is generally more or less fever, and the natural feces are either retained or discharged in small hard balls. The common causes are marsh miasms, improper diet, excessive exhaustion and fatigue, and, above all, exposure to the cold and damp air of night after a hot day.

Treatment: Give gentle aperients, $^1/_2$ ounce of castor oil or the same quantity of Epsom salts to cleanse the bowels; then dilute the muriatic acid 2 fluid drams; sulphate of morphia, 2 grains; water, 3 fluid ounces; mix, take 1 tea-spoonful 3 times a day. The symptoms, which frequently hang about for some time, are best combated by mild tonics and vegetable bitters; compound tincture of cinchona(1), compound tincture of gentian(2), of each 1 ounce; mix, take 1 teaspoonful 3 times a day, before meals.

Homeopathic: Mercurius corrosivus should be given for the acute symptoms, a drop dose in a dessert-spoonful of water every 2 or 3 hours; an occasional dose of aconite will reduce any feverish symptoms and moisten skin; arsenicum is of value in the chronic form, a drop dose 3 times a day.

DYSPEPSIA(3), CAUSES AND TREATMENT OF:

The majority of people know far less than they ought of the rules of diet which one must observe to maintain good health. Very little intelligence is, as a rule, shown in the selection of the different dishes which make up a meal, and as a consequence some of the most indigestible mixtures are indulged in; whereas were any one or perhaps two or more eaten and the others excluded, they would be quickly and easily digested. To make our meaning clear we will consider the principal dishes we find on the breakfast-table in many American families.

There is broiled steak, on which butter has been melted, fried bacon, boiled or fried eggs, and hot dry toast. Now, any one of these foods alone is easy of digestion, but when eaten together they are no little burden to the stomach, by reason of the admixture of the different kinds of fats. There is one kind in the butter, another in the bacon, another in the steak, and another in the eggs. Again, while these fats are in an unchanged state easily digestible, they are no longer so after being exposed to heat. Many must know from experience that when they eat toast which has been allowed to cool before being buttered in "sets well" on the weakest stomach, and yet toast buttered while hot is likely to distress them.

Fried sausages are very palatable, and hence appear often on the breakfast-table. In almost all families they are served while hot, and in the majority of people they cause some disturbance. They say they can "taste them" for several hours afterward. Let those who complain eat sausages only when cold, and but few will find them difficult of digestion. And so it is with hot roast lamb. To many persons that proves burdensome to the stomach, and for several hours after eating it they feel dull and heavy. Yet, when cold, that meat so cooked is one of the most easy of digestion. The same difference in digestibility is noted in nearly all fats or fatty foods;

(1) From the bark of the cinchona tree.
(2) From the dried root of the Gentiana Lutea, a bitter stomachic tonic.
(3) Indigestion.

when hot they are much less quickly disposed of by the digestive organs. We might go on and cover pages with such illustrations of the common errors in diet, but we have given sufficient for purpose.

If people would only learn what and how to eat, the last case of dyspepsia would soon be recovered from. Among the direct causes of the disease under consideration must be included the excessive use of alcoholic liquors, particularly the concentrated forms. The English people are much heavier drinkers than us, and yet they are far less frequent sufferers from the habit. One potent reason is that we take our liquors but slightly diluted, while they add much water, and instead of swallowing without stopping to take breath, they slowly sip them. Raw spirits are very irritating to the stomach, and also cause disturbance to the associated organs.

In a large proportion of cases dyspepsia is due to mental disturbances. The sympathy which exists between the mind and body is of the closest character. If the former becomes disturbed, the functions of the latter are more or less deranged. Persons of certain mental constitution are especially prone to dyspepsia; viz., those so constituted as to be constantly anxious about something, such as acquiring success in life, getting out of debt, securing an independent position, or about imaginary troubles.

We come now to the treatment of dyspepsia. If a person suffering from it has fortitude, and can practice self-denial, he may, in nearly all instances, cure himself, if he properly selects and restricts his diet. But few care to make the effort, or at least persist in it long enough. It is easier and far more agreeable for them to take medicine, and so they go on eating and dosing until the disease becomes chronic, for rarely can it be cured by drugs alone.

A person with dyspepsia, treating himself, should first ascertain what foods are easy of digestion, and confine himself to them, reducing the quantity taken to the smallest amount upon which he can live and still retain his strength and full vigor. He must religiously deny himself those articles of food which he has found by experience to be burdensome to his stomach. If the dyspepsia is recent and not an aggravated form, this simple method, if persisted in for a few weeks, will very often be sufficient to effect a cure.

We will give a list of foods which dyspeptics are likely to find the least tax upon digestion. It is, of course, impossible to make a diet table which will be suited to all cases. "What is one man's meat is another's poison" is a trite yet true saying. The testimony of the stomach should prevail against the inclinations of the palate, and each should eat the food which he has found to be easiest of digestion.

The dyspeptic may, as a rule, eat of the following:

Clear soup made from meat, raw oysters, raw beefsteak, mutton chop, stale bread baked twice, cold roast beef and cold roast mutton, cream, butter but no other fat, rice and milk, sago, tapioca, etc., boiled with milk. The drinks should be plain soda-water, milk and the same or lime-water; tea and coffee made weak by the addition of much milk. Pepper may be used on the food, but vinegar, mustard, horse-radish, and the like are prohibited.

We urge a careful avoidance of the following common foods:

Fried potatoes, fried fish, fritters, fried cakes, veal cutlets breaded, pork, liver, crabs, lobsters, chicken salad, cheese, boiled cabbage, lettuce and salads generally. Mixed dishes, "made dishes," hot bread, corned beef, sausage, plumb-pudding, suet-pudding, pies, and pastry.

KITCHEN, DRESS FOR THE:

"The uniform insisted upon for women by those who direct gymnastic exercises is the only one appropriate for housework, so far as the under-garments are concerned..................."

"The accessories of a working toilet are as important as those of a ball attire. A white collar is indispensable...................."

"Kitchen aprons, gloves, and caps to be worn when sweeping, dusting, and attending to fires are essential to cleanliness and soft hands..................... Consider, too, how much more soothing the touch of soft hands to the little ones and invalids than that of hard palms and rough cracked fingers."

E

EAR-ACHE, REMEDIES FOR:

(1) Put some live coals in an iron pan, sprinkle with brown sugar, invert a funnel over it, and put the tube in the ear. The smoke gives almost instant relief.

(2) Carbolic acid(1) diluted with warm water and poured into the ear is a sovereign cure for the ear-ache.

(3) Take equal parts chloroform and laudanum, dip a piece of cotton into the mixture and introduce into the ear, and cover up and go to sleep as soon as possible.

(4) Four drops of oil of amber and 2 drams of oil of sweet almonds. Four drops of this mixture to be applied to the part affected.

(5) For ear-ache dissolve asafetida in water; warm a few drops and drop in the ear, then cork the ear with wool.

(6) Cotton wool wet with sweet-oil and laudanum often relieves ear-ache, it is said.

EARS, CARE OF THE:

(1) Never put any thing into the ear for relief of toothache.

(2) Never wear cotton in the ears if they are discharging pus.

(3) Never attempt to apply a poultice to the inside of the canal of the ear.

(4) Never drop any thing into the ear unless it has been previously warmed.

(5) Never use any thing but a syringe and warm water for cleaning the ears from pus.

(6) Never strike or box a child's ears; this has been known to rupture the drum and cause incurable deafness.

(7) Never wet the hair if you have any tendency to deafness; wear an oiled silk cap when bathing, and refrain from diving.

(8) Never scratch the ears with any thing but the finger if they itch. Do not use the head of a pin, hair-pin, pencil tips, or any thing of that nature.

(1) Phenol alcohol, coal-tar creasote.

(9) Never let the feet become cold and damp, or sit with the back toward the window, as these things tend to aggravate any existing hardness of hearing.

(10) Never put milk, fat, or any oily substance into the ear for the relief of pain, for they soon become rancid and tend to incite the inflammation. Simple warm water will answer the purpose better than any thing else.

(11) Never be alarmed if a living insect enters the ear. Pouring warm water into the canal will drown it when it will generally come to the surface and can be easily removed by the fingers. A few puffs of smoke blown into the ear will stupefy the insect.

(12) Never meddle with the ear if a foreign body, such as a bead, button, or seed, enters it; leave it absolutely alone, but have a physician attend to it. More damage has been done by injudicious attempts at the extraction of a foreign body than could ever have been done from its presence in the ear.

EARTHENWARE, TO PREVENT CRACKING:

Before using new earthenware place in a boiler with cold water and heat gradually till it boils; then let it remain in the water till it is cold. It will not be liable to crack if treated in this manner.

EASTER-EGGS, TO DYE:

In Paris, where more than 1,000,000 of these eggs are sold during the season, the red ones, which are the favorites, are dyed by boiling, (not violently, however), about 500 at a time, packed in a basket in a decoction of logwood(1), and then adding some alum to convert the violet color to red. Various aniline dyes are used for a similar purpose.

EATING, HEALTHFUL:

Appetite not an Infallible Guide: The opinion prevailing among many, that if people like a thing they may eat it without harm, is a great mistake. If sweetened drinks, candies, or things containing poison be given children, they will eat them readily without detecting the danger. Brute animals are guided in the selection of food by their instinct and their wonderfully developed organs of smell. Human individuals do not show such instinct, but are, or should be, governed by their superior intelligence.

Evil of Rapid Eating: Eat slowly, thoroughly masticating your food. Rapid eating is one of our national evils, and is the chief cause of dyspepsia. The saliva does not flow too rapidly to mix with the food to promote digestion, and the

(1) Dye from the logwood tree.

coarse pieces swallowed resist the action of the digestive fluid. The food washed down with drinks which dilute the gastric juice, and hinder its work will not supply the place of the saliva. Failing to get the taste of the food by rapid mastication, we think it insipid, and hence use condiments which over-stimulate the digestive organs. In these ways the system is over-worked, and the tone of the stomach being affected, a foundation is laid for dyspepsia.

How to Regulate the Quantity of Food: If the food be swallowed no faster than the gastric fluid is prepared to be mixed with it hunger or the desire for food will cease when just enough has been taken; but if the food is crowded down rapidly, after the manner of thousands of American eaters, the appetite will continue until more than enough is eaten, and often until 2 or 3 times too much is eaten. Remember that the appetite will only cease with the secretion and flow of the gastric fluid; hence we should eat slowly, or we shall eat too much. The slow eater should stop with the cessation of his appetite; the rapid eater before. Rapid eating frequently begets irritability, dyspepsia, or disease of the stomach.

Eating Too Much: Eating too fast generally involves eating too much—more than is needed for the support and nutrition of the body—and the reason for this is that the organs of taste, which are our guide in this matter, are not allowed sufficient voice; they are not allowed time to take cognizance of the presence of food ere it is pushed past them into the recesses of the stomach. They do not, therefore, have opportunity to represent the real need of the system, and hence allow the crowding of the stomach.

Food should be Thoroughly Chewed: There is one simple rule, the observance of which will go a great way toward securing full benefit of what we eat, and so will be conducive to good health; it is that all food should be thoroughly chewed before being swallowed. The effects, both mechanical and chemical, of thorough mastication are the preliminary conditions for healthy digestion and nutrition. Aside from the grinding, the service which the saliva is capable of performing if we give it time is similar to, if not identical with, that of the juice of the stomach. And in a general way it may be said that the more nearly the food is reduced to a fine pulp in the mouth the less remains for the rest of the digestive apparatus to do, the more completely their task is performed, and the more perfect is the preparation of the food for its purpose—the formation of blood and the nutrition of the whole body.

Loss of Appetite, and How to Recover It: The appetite is often lost through excessive use of stimulants, food taken too hot, sedentary occupation, liver disorder, and want of change of air. To ascertain and remove the cause is the first duty. Exercise, change of air, and diet will generally prove sufficient to recover the appetite. Children, if they have plenty of outdoor exercise, are regular in their habits, and eat only plain nourishing food, will seldom, if ever, complain of a lack of appetite.

Eating between Meals: This is another of the causes of dyspepsia, for which the foundations are laid in childhood. When the ordinary meals of the day are sufficiently near each other nothing should be taken into the stomach between meals. Even fruit, which so many consider healthy at all times, robs the stomach of its needed rest.

Dangers in Eating: The close alliance between food and poison is one of the most remarkable combinations known to man. For instance, if the juice of a sweetbread, which makes such a delicious morsel, were injected into a vein of one's body it would be as fatal as prussic acid.

- Of food that rapidly begins to decompose mackerel is perhaps one of the most common. Being both cheap and usually plentiful when in season, it is largely consumed. Putrefaction sets in very rapidly, especially about the gills of this fish, sometimes almost as soon as it is taken out of the water. The poisonous principle that has been extracted from mackerel is called hydrocollidine, a very violent poison, so powerful that the seven-thousandth part of a grain will cause death in a bird.
- From beef and other flesh meat when bad a poisonous body known as neuridine has been extracted. Bullock's sweetbread when decomposed yields a principle named collidine. Putriscine is another poisonous substance that has been extracted from meat flesh and fish when putrid.
- Muscles are a common article of diet largely eaten by some classes, and they frequently occasion fatal cases of poisoning. This is attributed to a principle which has been extracted from the muscle called mytilotoxine, also a powerful poison, about $1^1/2$ grains being a fatal dose.
- Cheese that has become moldy coated causes serious illness, doubtless due to the formation of trimethylamine or tyrotoxicon, which are its putrefactive products.
- Milk, that universal diet of daily use, may also produce in hot weather the same poison. Its symptoms are nausea, vomiting, and fever, followed by great prostration, and it often causes diarrhea among infants.
- Sausages, another common food, often give rise to hurtful effects due to an animal poison. Being frequently composed of imperfectly cooked and old pork and beef in which putrefaction has already begun, they sometimes produce very alarming symptoms after eating.

- High game and grouse have occasionally the same result, with more or less severity; and even roast goose that had become decomposed has caused death to those who have partaken of it. Tinned lobster and other meats have been known to generate poisonous bodies which will produce vomiting and other symptoms.

We might enumerate many other foods which give similar results. With some shell fish it is possible they may have the power of naturally secreting a venomous substance when alive which might cause like results.

- Mackerel and other fish should be as fresh as possible, and kept on ice or very cool. A little of the boracic acid solution should be sprinkled over it directly when bought in warm weather.
- Muscles should always be boiled before eaten, and a table-spoonful of bicarbonate of soda added to the water in which they are boiled will prevent the formation of any poisonous principle.
- Milk in hot weather should be boiled before being used. Great care should be exercised that all vessels in which it is kept are made perfectly clean, especially when intended for children.
- Saüsages and game should be thoroughly well cooked throughout before being eaten.

In cases of poisoning from decomposed food the symptoms soon show themselves, usually commencing with headache and vomiting, and all the symptoms of an irritant poison. Medical assistance should be promptly obtained.

Notions about Eating: It has been an old-wives' notion from way back that certain kinds of food must be avoided because they tend to produce certain kinds of disease. This notion has been fostered by alleged physicians who publish health journals, and are always laying down rules about living, which, if any one undertook to follow literally and scrupulously, would make life a burden from the cradle to the grave.

- Some years ago Dr. Dio Lewis, who was regarded as somewhat of a health expert, announced that tomatoes were unhealthy, were the cause of cancer, loosened and destroyed the teeth, etc.
- For generations boys and girls had been warned not to eat so much butter or their faces would break out with "butter sores." It is an old-time tradition that buckwheat cakes are productive of skin diseases, and the Scotch are said to be cursed with the itch because they eat so much oatmeal.

- Dr. James C. White, Professor of Dermatology in Harvard University, in a recent article on cutaneous diseases, pricks some of those annoying traditional bubbles. He says that uncooked butter is perfectly harmless food so far as the skin is concerned, and it is difficult to conceive how any one would have thought otherwise unless, possibly, the use of bad butter in food otherwise indigestible may have disturbed the stomach and produced impure blood.

Buckwheat cakes do not produce cutaneous diseases unless improperly cooked and eaten hot with too much syrup, they upset the digestion. Oatmeal is perfectly harmless food, and the idea that tomatoes cause cancer is ridiculous. Mr. White says that the eating of fruits, nuts, and fish may lead to irritation of the skin in certain individuals, but this arises from some cause peculiar to the individual.

Choice in Eating: In regard to eating many traditions have come down from the past which must be got rid of. One of the most erroneous is that attaching to farinaceous food. That has been usually regarded as the rock of hope for weak stomachs, the natural nourishment of the young, and the backbone of strength generally. This is a total mistake in some respects. For some men it may be good, and for others bad, not so much on account of the difference of stomachs as from the difference in the sort of labor they are engaged in.

Eating at Bedtime: As to the general principle whether eating before going to bed is advisable or not, the sensible advice of New York doctors is that those who do not work at night, and who retire early, are better off without a late bite; so also are those who take no exercise in the evening and who dine heartily. But if a person is up and works long enough after dinner for the stomach to be empty and to crave food, the natural and necessary thing to do is to eat a little. The stomach is better full than empty to sleep on.

One great English doctor is quoted as recommending that an apple be eaten every night before going to bed. He is said to assert that if this is habitually done it will prolong the life of a man 10 yrs.

A New York doctor who was asked what he thought of that prescription replied that there was no harm in it, but that he thought the good claimed for it was too extravagant, and showed it to be that particular doctor's fad. It is to be classed with the familiar recommendation of a glass of water on retiring, and that other one of a few crackers or milk and crackers at that time.

All these recommendations proceed from the known fact that many persons sleep best upon a full stomach. Of all prescriptions, that of the glass of water is perhaps most sensible, because water dilutes whatever the stomach contains, so that the kidneys perform their function more easily.

Either an apple or a glass of water at night will be found efficacious where there is a tendency toward constipation. For those who need the merest trifle of food at bedtime it is wiser to resort to hot milk diluted with apollinaris or soda-water. The reason for diluting the milk in this way is that it is thus rendered less hearty and less apt to curdle, and thus produce biliousness.

ECONOMICAL HINTS:

- Look carefully to your expenditures. No matter what comes in, if more goes out you will always be poor.
- The art is not in making money but in keeping it; little expenses, like mice in a barn, when they are many make great waste.
- Hair by hair heads get bald; straw by straw the thatch goes off the cottage; and drop by drop the rain comes in the chamber.
- A barrel is soon empty if the tap leaks but a drop a minute.
- When you mean to save begin with your mouth; many thieves pass down the red lane.
- The ale-jug is a great waste. In all other things keep within compass.
- Never stretch your legs farther than the blanket will reach, or you will soon take cold.
- In clothes, choose suitable and lasting stuff and not tawdry fineries.
- To be warm is the main thing; never mind looks.
- A fool may make money, but it takes a wise man to spend it.
- Remember it is easier to build two chimneys than to keep one going.
- If you give all to back and board there is nothing left for the savings-bank.
- Fare hard and work hard when you are young, and you will have a chance to rest when you are old.

ECZEMA:

This is an eruption of minute vesicles, closely crowded, often running into each other so as to form, on being ruptured, a moist sore, which becomes more or less covered with scabs, attended, usually, with feverishness and restlessness.

Treatment: Light, nutritious diet, cooling drinks, and saline laxatives, as Rochelle salts, cream of tartar, etc., and warm or tepid baths of bran-water, elm-bark or flax-weed infusions, with 20 grains of bicarbonate of soda to 4 ounces of the wash. If there is inflammation and burning, limewater and linseed oil in equal parts, with the addition of 2 or 3 grains of carbolic acid to 1 ounce of the mixture, is an excellent application; later, use benzoated oxide of zinc ointment.

In chronic cases cover the inflamed surface with oiled silk or rubber cloth, these being removed several times daily and the surface washed with a lotion of equal parts of glycerine and water. If the system is debilitated use tonics in some form. Another good application is citrine ointment, 2 drams; olive-oil, 1 ounce; sulphate of morphia, 2 grains; mix, and make an ointment; rub this ointment faithfully into the part affected with eczema 2 or 3 times a day.

EGGS:

Eggs, like milk, are a perfect food, yet they contain absolute poison to some people. But these are very few. As a rule eggs must be regarded as one of the most valuable articles of food for business men. They are of highly concentrated nutritive elements, and for the stomach of a man engaged in intellectual pursuits they should form a staple article.

EGGS, HOW TO INCREASE PRODUCTION:

In the winter and early spring, to keep up egg production, the fowls must have something to work on. The best way to supply them, if there is not enough of waste meat scraps from the breeder's table to meet the required demand, is to get scraps from the butcher or slaughter-house. The waste meat, offal, and the bloody pieces which are unsalable can be bought for a cent or two a pound. The best way to utilize these scraps and to render them more digestible and nutritious is to cut them into fine pieces, put them into a boiler with plenty of water, and boil them until the bones separate from the flesh. Then stir cornmeal into it until it makes a thick mush, season with salt and pepper, and cook till done. Feed this when cold to the poultry, and they will eat it with evident relish, and you have a most excellent food which will keep during cold weather.

EGGS, PRESERVING:

The several modes recommended for preserving eggs any length of time are not always successful. The egg, to be preserved well, should be kept at a temperature so low that the air and fluids within its shell shall not be brought into a decomposing condition, and at the same time the air outside of its shell should be excluded in order to prevent its action in any way upon the egg.

The following mixture was patented several years ago by a Mr. Jayne. He alleged that by means of it he could keep eggs 2 yrs. A part of his composition is often made use of; perhaps the whole of it would be better. Put into a tub or vessel 1 bushel of quicklime, 2 lbs. of salt, 1/2 lb. of cream of tartar, and mix the same together with as much water as will reduce the composition or mixture to that consistence that will cause an egg put into it to swim with its top just above the liquid, then put and keep the eggs therein.

EGGS, TO LIME:

To 3 gallons of water add 1 pint of lime and $1^1/_2$ pints of salt; put this brine in an earthen crock and place in the cellar. Put in the eggs; they will keep a year.

EGGS, TO TEST:

A good egg will sink in a body of water; if stale, a body of air inside the shell will frequently cause it to float. When boiled a fresh egg will adhere to the shell, which will have a rough exterior; if stale, the outside will be smooth and glassy. Looking through a paper tube directed toward the light, an egg held to the end of the tube will appear translucent if fresh; but if stale it will be dark—almost opaque.

EGGS FOR THE NEST:

Use only good-sized eggs with strong shells. Make in the small end a hole about one-eighth in. across, and in the other end a $^1/_2$ in hole. By blowing through the smaller hole the contents of the shell will be driven out. Plaster of Paris is mixed with water thin enough to pour. The shells are to be filled with this, using a spoon to fill them if necessary. When the shells, are full they are set aside for 24 hours. Trim off any superfluous plaster with a knife. These eggs are in appearance exactly like real eggs, and, being heavy, are not thrown out of the nest.

EGGS IN WINTER:

If hens have been carefully fed during the moulting season their owner may fairly expect a crop of eggs when the price is highest, usually about or a little after the holidays. One of the most stimulating foods is bran liberally dosed with pepper and mixed with skim-milk. In cold weather corn or other grain should be added. The best method is to mix with their food every other day about a tea-spoonful of ground Cayenne pepper to each dozen fowls. While upon this subject it would be well to say that if your hens lay soft eggs, or eggs without shells, you should put plenty of old plaster, egg-shells, or even oyster-shells broken up where they can eat at it.

ELECTRO-PLATING, GOLD SOLUTION FOR:

Dissolve 5 pennyweights(1) gold coin, 5 grains pure copper, and 4 grains pure silver in 3 ounces nitro-muriatic acid, which is simply 2 parts

(1) 24 grains or 1/20 of an ounce.

muriatic acid and 1 part nitric acid. The silver will not be taken into solution as are the other two metals, but will gather at the bottom of the vessel. Add 1 ounce pulverized sulphate of iron, $^{1}/_{2}$ ounce pulverized borax, 25 grains pure tale-salt, and 1 quart hot rain-water. Upon this the gold and copper will be thrown to the bottom of the vessel with the silver. Let it stand till fully settled, then pour off the liquor very carefully and refill with boiling rain-water as before. Continue to repeat this operation until the precipitate is thoroughly washed; or, in other words, fill up, let settle, and pour off so long as the accumulation at the bottom of the vessel is acid to the taste.

You now have about an 18 carat chloride of gold. Add to it $1^{1}/_{2}$ ounces of cyanuret potassa and 1 quart of rain-water—the latter heated to the boiling point. Shake up well, then let it stand about 24 hours, and it will be ready for use. Some use platina as an alloy instead of silver, under the impression that plating done with it is harder. I have used both, but never could see much difference.

Solution for a dark-colored plate to imitate Guinea gold may be made by adding to the above 1 ounce dragon's blood(1) and 5 grains iodide of iron. If you desire an alloyed plate proceed as first directed without the silver or copper, and with $1^{1}/_{2}$ ounces of sulphuret potassa in place of the iron, borax, and salt.

ELEMENTS, THE GAME OF:

Seated around the room, one of the company holds in his hand a ball, round, which should be fastened to a string, so that it may be easily drawn back again. Sometimes a ball of worsted is used, when 1 or 2 yds. is left unwound. The possessor of the ball then throws it first to one person, then to another, naming at the time one of the elements, and each player as the ball touches him must, before 10 can be counted, mention an inhabitant of that element. Should anyone speak when fire is mentioned he must pay a forfeit.

EMERGENCIES, HOW TO MEET THEM:

Bleeding:

(1) Ordinary bleeding from small cuts or injuries may be stopped by cold water or ice, or pressure until a clot has had time to form. The wisdom of our Maker has made this wonderful provision, that as soon as blood ceases to circulate in its proper channels, or comes in contact with air, it will coagulate. By this means a plug is formed at the mouth of an open vessel to stop the flow of blood. Cold water and various styptics, like sulphate of iron, tannin, alum, and matico, hasten this result.

(1) Red resin from tropical palms native to the Malayan islands.

(2) It is said that bleeding from a wound on man or beast may be stopped by a mixture of wheat flour and common salt, in equal parts, bound down with a cloth. If the bleeding be profuse use a large quantity, say from 1 to 3 pints. It may be left on for hours, or even days, if necessary.

(3) Bleeding from a larger artery is indicated at once by coming in jets at each beat of the heart, and being of bright scarlet color instead of purple. If the wound be such a character that the end of the artery can be seen, it can be readily taken up with a hook or sharp-pointed fork by any one who keeps his wits about him in spite of the sudden alarm, and tied with a strong thread. Otherwise tie the limb between the wound and the heart, the simplest device being to bind the handkerchief around, and running a stick beneath the knot, twisting it up until the requisite pressure be attained to stop the bleeding.

Bleeding from the Teeth: The following is an excellent remedy for hemorrhage arising from the extraction of teeth: Cut a piece of clean dry sponge into cone shape. This should be compressed tightly and introduced into the cavity left by the tooth. As soon as the sponge is dampened it begins to swell, and this will in most cases effectually close the cavity and prevent bleeding.

Rupture of a Large Blood-vessel: In case a large artery or vein is cut, especially in a limb, make a knot in a handkerchief and tie it loosely about the limb, placing the knot on the wound. Then with a stick twist the handkerchief until the flow of blood ceases. A pad can be used instead of a knot. If the artery is ruptured apply the pressure between the wound and the heart. If a vein, beyond the wound.

Fracture of the Skull: Send for the physician. If there be a collapse, hot bottles and blankets should be applied to the extremities, and the circulation stimulated by friction with the hands. Diluted injections may be given. These efforts must cease when reaction is secured.

Fainting, and its Relief: In mild cases of fainting, where partial consciousness remains, stimulating substances, as vapor of ammonia or cologne-water, may be inhaled, and cold water sprinkled in the face, and fresh air introduced into the apartment.

Insensibility: No violent measures should be used to arouse a patient who may or may not be insensible. Lay him in bed, loosen his clothes, and let him have a free access of air; notice whether the breathing is quiet or noisy, regular or irregular; whether there are any convulsive movements of the limbs;

whether the urine or feces are passed involuntarily; whether the pupils of both eyes are alike, or larger or smaller than usual, or whether the patient will bear to have his eyes touched; and whether he can be aroused at all. In all cases of apparent insensibility the attendant should be careful to say nothing to the patient within his hearing, for while he can neither speak nor move he may yet be perfectly conscious of all that is passing around him and the effort to speak may do him great injury.

Dislocation: This is the displacement of two or more bones where articular surfaces have lost wholly or in part their natural connection, either owing to external violence or to disease of some of the parts about the joint. Dislocation is complete when the bones have entirely lost their connection, incomplete when they partly preserve it, and compound when a wound communicates with the dislocated joint. The first thing to be done is to reduce the protruded bone to its original place, then to retain it in that position by means of splints, ligatured as tightly as the circulation will allow. The circulation must by no means be impeded, otherwise mortification(1) will ensue.

Sprains: A sprain is often more painful and dangerous that a dislocation. It requires immediate attention. The injured part should be wrapped in flannels wrung out of hot water, and covered with a dry bandage, or, what is better, oiled silk. The limb should not be allowed to hang down, but kept in a quiet, easy position, until after all pain has ceased.

Fracture of the Collar-bone: If the collar-bone is fractured the attendants must keep the patient in bed without a pillow, with the arm on the injured side folded across the chest. Keep the part moist with water until the doctor comes.

Fracture of the Ribs: If the ribs are fractured the patient should remain in bed; have a spittoon within reach, so that the expectorations may be duly noted by the physician when he arrives.

Lock-jaw: Take a small quantity of turpentine, warm it, and pour it on the wound, no matter where or of what nature it is, and relief will follow in less than a minute. Lobelia(2) has been successfully used in several cases of lock-jaw.

Choking:

(1) To relieve choking break an egg into a cup and give it to the patient to swallow. The white of the egg seems to catch around the obstacle and remove it. If 1 egg does not answer the purpose try another. The white is all that is necessary.

(1) The complete death of parts of the body.
(2) A medicine made from a plant of the lobelia family, used as an expectorant, an emetic and as a diuretic.

(2) Often a smart blow between the shoulders, causing a compression of the chest and a sudden expulsion of air from the lungs, will throw out the substance.

(3) If the person can swallow, give plenty of bread and potatoes, and water to wash them down.

(4) Press upon the tongue with a spoon, when, perhaps, the substance may be seen and drawn out with a pair of dull scissors.

(5) If these fail, give an emetic of ipecac, or mustard and water.

Cut-wounds: Protect the wounded parts from the air and dust instantly if possible. Press the parts together and keep them so by adhesive plaster or bandage, and give them instant and permanent rest till healed, which in most cases will be rapidly accomplished. It is the inherent property of all wounds (on the surface or deep) to heal up by "first intention."

How to Relieve Pain: A correspondent of the Country Gentleman gives the following remedy for painful wounds: "Take a pan or shovel with burning coals, and sprinkle upon them common brown sugar and hold the wounded part in the smoke. In a few minutes the pain will be allayed, and recovery proceed rapidly."

Delirious Patients: Avoid any roughness in dealing with such cases, but be firm, and not permit them to know you are afraid of them or inclined to let them have their own way. Do not attempt to argue with them or contradict any of their assertions, but at the same time it is well to appear interested in their conversation. See that all escape is prevented and that there are no knives or dangerous weapons within reach. Immediate aid should be within call.

Convulsions, and How to Stop Them: Some children are liable to convulsions from derangement of the digestive organs. They sometimes occur when a child is teething. The attack is often preceded by involuntary movements of the mouth or eyelids; then the eyes become fixed and the body rigid, the breathing is irregular, often suspended for a few moments, and the face and surface of the body becomes dark red or livid. This is followed by twitching or jerking of the limbs, and often of the arms and legs and the muscles of the face. The attendant should at once prepare a warm bath, and the child be immersed in the water up to the head, which should have cold water applied to it. It should be kept in the bath until the convulsions cease, keeping up the temperature to about 98 degrees. After the bath wrap the child in a warm blanket.

EMETIC, PROMPT-ACTING:

The ingredients are tartar emetic, 1 grain; powdered ipecac, 20 grains. Take the above in a wine-glassful of sweetened water.

ENEMAS:

Enemas are a peculiar kind of medicines, administered by injecting into the rectum or outlet of the body. The intention is either to empty the bowels, kill worms, protect the lining membrane of the intestines from injury, restrain copious discharges, allay spasms in the bowels, or nourish the body. These clysters or glysters are administered by means of bladders and pipes, or a proper apparatus.

ENGRAVINGS, TO CLEAN:

It frequently happens that fine engravings, despite the care taken of them, will in some unaccountable manner become stained and dirty to such an extent as to seriously impair their beauty. To those who own engravings that have been injured in this way a simple recipe for cleaning them will prove of value. Put the engraving on a smooth board and cover it with a thin layer of common salt, finely pulverized; then squeeze lemon-juice upon the salt until a considerable portion of it is dissolved. After every part of the picture has been subjected to this treatment elevate one end of the board so that it will form an angle of about 45 degrees with the horizon. From a tea-kettle or other suitable vessel pour on the engraving boiling water until the salt and lemon-juice be all washed off. The engraving will then be perfectly clean and free from stain. It must be dried on the board, or on some smooth surface, gradually. If dried by the fire or sun it will be tinged with a dingy, yellowish color.

ENGRAVINGS, TO MOUNT:

Look up all your engravings and nice wood-cuts and trim them off evenly. At the stationer's you can get a cheap kind of Bristol board. Cut it up into two sizes, one large and the other smaller. Make a smooth paste of starch, cover the back of the picture with it, taking care that the edges are all wet, but do not put on so much that it will squeeze out. Place it on the Bristol board, taking care to get it in the middle. Have a sheet folded and lay the picture face downward on it. Lay a soft, thin cloth over it and press it a few minutes with a hot iron, then turn it over and spread on the cloth as before, and press till dry.

EPILEPSY, TREATMENT OF:

Prof. W. H. Gobrecht employed in the treatment of this disease the following:

Sodie bromide, 2 ounces; zinc bromide, 32 grains; glycerine, 1 ounce; aqua cinnamonia, 7 ounces. Dose, 1 table-spoonful 3 times a day in half a wine-glassful of water. This is an excellent prescription, not only useful in epilepsy, but in many diseases of the nervous system, especially when persons are sleepless and restless at night. One or two doses of this medicine will quiet the most excited lunatic.

EPIZOOTIC(1), REMEDY FOR:

One of the simplest remedies for the epizootic, it is said, is a mixture of tar and assafetida, 10 drops of which are given twice a day in the feed. Besides this a warm bran mash once a day is recommended.

ERUPTIVE FEVERS:

For the early stages, when the skin is hot, a warm bath or tepid sponging will be useful. Cleanse the eyes and nostrils with water and a piece of lint as often as necessary. If small-pox, and the pustules have burst, this is all that is practicable. Light poultices to the face will prevent pitting. To allay itching oil the pustules on the face and neck with olive-oil and cold cream. The same will apply in scarlet fever. In small-pox the nurse must examine the body, and if she finds any signs of abscesses forming should report to the physician; she should also use every precaution against bed-sores.

ESSENCE FROM FLOWERS:

(1) Procure a quantity of the petals of any flower which have an agreeable fragrance; card thin layers of cotton, which dip into the finest Florence or Lucca oil; sprinkle a small quantity of fine salt on the flowers alternately until an earthen vessel or wide-mouthed glass bottle is full. Tie the top close with a bladder, then lay the vessel in a south aspect to the heat of the sun, and in 15 days, when uncovered, a fragrant oil may be squeezed away, leaving a whole mass quite equal to the high-priced essences.

(2) Take any flowers you choose; place a layer in a clean earthen pot, and cover over them a layer of fine salt. Repeat the process until the pot is filled; cover closely and place in the cellar. Forty days afterward strain the essence from the whole through a crape(2) by pressure. Put the essence thus expressed in a clear bottle, and expose it for 6 weeks in the rays of the sun and evening dew to purify. One drop of this essence will communicate its odor to a pint of water.

ESSENCE OF ROSES:

Take 4 parts of clean fresh leaves of rose flowers—damask roses are best—put them into a still with 12 parts of water; distill off one half; repeat

(1) Epidemic diseases among animals.
(2) A gauzy fabric made of raw silk.

the process, and when a sufficient quantity of this liquid has been obtained it must be used as water upon fresh rose-leaves, and the same process must be continued 4 or 5 times until the quantity desired is obtained. If carefully done this essence will be very powerful.

ESSENCES, TO MAKE:

Essences are made with 1 ounce of any given oil added to 1 pint of alcohol. Peppermints are colored with tincture turmeric; cinnamon with tincture red sanders; wintergreen with tincture kino(1).

ESSENTIAL OIL(2) FROM WOOD, BARKS, ROOTS, HERBS, ETC.:

Take balm, mint, sage, or any other herb, etc., put it into a bottle, and pour upon it a spoonful of ether; keep in a cool place a few hours, and then fill the bottle with cold water; the essential oil will swim upon the surface and may be easily separated.

ETCHING ON GLASS:

Druggists' bottles, bar tumblers, signs, and glassware of every description can be lettered in a beautiful style of art by simply giving the article to be engraved or etched a thin coat of engraver's varnish, and the application of fluoric acid. Before doing so the glass must be thoroughly cleaned and heated, so that it can hardly be held. The varnish is then to be applied lightly over and made smooth by dabbing it with a small ball of silk filled with cotton. When dry and even the lines may be traced on it by a sharp steel, cutting clear through the varnish to the glass. The varnish must be removed clean from each letter, otherwise it will be an imperfect job. When all is ready pour on or apply the fluoric acid with a feather, filling each letter. Let it remain until it etches to the required depth, then wash off with water and remove the varnish.

ETCHING VARNISH:

Take of virgin wax and asphaltum, each 2 ounces; of black pitch and Burgundy, each 1/2 ounce; melt the wax and pitch in a new earthenware glazed pot, and add to them by degrees the asphaltum, finely powdered. Let the whole boil, simmering gradually, till such time as, taking a drop upon a plate, it will break when it is cold, or bending it double 2 or 3 times between the fingers. The varnish being then boiled enough, must be taken off the fire, and, after it cools a little, must be poured into warm water, that it may work the more easily with the hands, so as to be formed into balls, which must be kneaded and put into a piece of taffeta for use. The sandblast is not in extensive use for ornamenting on glass.

(1) Powerful astringents made from the gum of various trees, used as a gargle and for pyrosis and diarrhea.
(2) A volatile oil which gives a distinctive odor.

ETHER, DANGERS IN THE USE OF:

The false cry that ether anesthesia is entirely free from danger has led to another grave condition of things observed among the young men who seek and gain hospital positions. Nowhere else did the reader of this paper see an amount of recklessness exhibited in the administration of anesthetics equal to that in the cities where chloroform is tabooed; especially in cases that take ether badly, and in whom relaxation is not easily accomplished, matters are formed in such a way that must excite the gravest apprehensions for the safety of the patient. Usually these are the cases of those addicted to the immoderate consumption of alcohol, persons of enfeebled circulation and impaired respiratory organs.

More and more ether is turned on, until the cyanosed patient relaxes, his stertorous breathing indicating that an ever-increasing mass of viscid mucus and saliva is flooding his trachea and bronchi. The sensitiveness of the larynx and trachea is abolished, and if vomiting occurs, especially where the inexperienced anesthetizer neglects to conduct the vomited matter out of the mouth, gastric contents find their way into the bronchi, and a catarrhal or even septic pneumonia follows resulting in death, which, however, is never charged to the account of ether.

EXERCISE:

Exercise invigorates the brain, expands the lungs, quickens the circulation, and braces the nerves. All exercise should, as far as possible, be in the open air. It facilitates the full and thorough oxygenation of the blood, the development of the muscles and the nervous system, and promotes sound digestion. Children especially should have the benefit of outdoor exercises in all seasons, except in inclement weather, and when confined within doors should have all the benefits of through ventilation.

Many of the diseases of women are attributable to too close confinement to the household drudgery and neglect of proper outdoor exercise. Every person should take a daily walk in the open air. Horse-back riding calls into activity and develops many of the muscles. Gardening is one of the most healthful exercises; the use of the various tools employed brings into play every muscle in the body, and with the ennobling pleasure to the mind it affords it imparts a vigor and freshness to the entire system. Of all modes of exercise of children, that of jumping the rope is the most dangerous. It produces continuous concussion of the joints which impinge upon the bone, often causing periostitis, and finally resulting in the death of the bone. Children should be encouraged in all their games to take exercise, but rope-jumping should be forbidden.

It was wisely deemed that man should earn his bread by the sweat of his brow. Without exertion scarcely any of the gifts of Providence are available; observation of external nature indicates this necessity, and that he was designed for a life of action. To fit man for existence, and with ability to maintain it, he is furnished with a system of muscles complete in number and arrangement. This system is dominated by another, the mental system, exercise being essential to both, and suffering alike from injudicious use. To maintain the natural force of the muscular system exercise should be regular.

Disuse from any cause for a length of time tends to diminish the strength of the muscles, soften their texture, and render them weak and sluggish. While regular exercise is essential to the welfare of the body, it is important that an error be not committed in the exertion incident to daily labor, as well as in amusements, so often attended by over-exertion and excess. The exercise of any particular limb does little more than increase the size and strength of that member; in order to increase the general strength, the whole system must be engaged.

How and When to Exercise: The time for exercising is in the morning; that is to say, the thorough exercising of the day should be performed at that time. Morning exercise fits a man for the day that lies ahead of him; it drives the cobwebs from his brain and sends new blood up there. In olden times, when boxing was either unknown or in disrepute, fencing was considered the *ne plus ultra* of all forms of exercise, because the rule always must be that the best form of exercise is that which exercises the most muscles, and succeeds best in shaking up the internal organs. But today, with the facilities for practicing boxing that modern demand has provided in all large cities, the noble art of self-defense, as it is called, is generally regarded as by far the most advantageous form exercise can take. It requires more activity and force, and the more constant play of all muscles, than fencing. It brings about profuse perspiration also, which is very desirable. In modern houses or boxing halls the necessary adjuncts of a bath and rough towels, and even of a lounge to rest on after the exercise, are always at hand.

Those machines which provide the means of lifting weights, or of imitating the exercise of an oarsman, are only to be recommended to those who cannot indulge in the actual and legitimate forms of exercise of which they are designed to take the place.

Daily Exercise: The importance of sufficient daily exercise to the health of intellectual men cannot be exaggerated. The same may be said also of adequate and regular repose, as few causes are more potent in shattering the nervous energies, weakening the constitution, and hastening on the infirmities of old age than deficient or irregular sleep. For those devoted to intellectual employment frequent relaxation and amusing recreation are imperative. The natural tendency of the student is to avoid society and its innocent frivolities. Such a course is deplorable, as it tends to pervert nature and make one gloomy, irritable, and misanthropic.

Few can profitably devote to study more than 7 hours a day, and the intellectual effort should cease when the brain grows weary, as its capabilities diminish, and productions, in consequence, are labored and feeble. It has been truly said that "there is scarcely any book which does not savor of painful composition in some part of it, because the author has written when he should have rested."

EYE, HOW TO REMOVE A MOTE FROM:

To remove a mote from the eye take a horsehair and double it, leaving a loop. If the mote can be seen lay the loop over it, close the eye, and it will come out as the hair is withdrawn. If the irritating object cannot be seen raise the lid of the eye and roll the ball around a few times; draw out the hair; the substance which caused so much pain will be sure to come with it. This method is practiced by ax-makers and other workers in steel.

EYELASHES:

The mode adapted by the beauties of the East to increase the length and strength of their eyelashes is simply to clip the split ends with a pair of scissors about once a month. Mothers perform the operation on their children, both male and female, when they are mere infants, watching the opportunity while they sleep; the practice never fails to produce the desired effect. We recommend it to the attention of our fair readers as a safe and innocent means of enhancing the charms which so many of them, no doubt, already possess.

EYELIDS, INFLAMMATION OF:

The following ointment has been found very beneficial in inflammation of the eyeball and edges of the eyelids:

Take of prepared calomel, 1 scruple; spermaceti ointment, 1/2 ounce; mix them well together in a glass mortar; apply a small quantity to each corner of the eye every night and morning, and also to the edges of the lids if they are affected. If this should not eventually remove the inflammation, elder-flower water may be applied 3 or 4 times a day, by means of an eye-cup. The bowels should be kept in a laxative state by taking occasionally 1/4 ounce of Epsom salts.

EYES, CARE OF THE:

There are some simple rules for preserving the health and vigor of the eyes. Sit up straight when you read; you gorge the eyes with blood if you lean forward with the head down when reading. Let the light fall on your back over your shoulders or across one shoulder. Don't read by fire-light or a dim light, or in the cars. Reading in bed is hurtful; if you find it puts you to sleep, remember that is at the cost of good eyesight. Bedroom window-shades should be red or gray, and the head of your bed should be toward the window. When you come to spectacles do not put off the resort to them a day longer than it takes you to discover the need of them. It is false pride that shuns spectacles. Get two pair instead of one, a pair adjusted to long sight for out of doors and a pair for reading. And remember that spectacles often cure chronic headache in those whose eyes have been the unsuspected cause of it.

EYES, WEAK, REMEDIES FOR:

(1) When the eyes are weakened or distressed by over-exertion few remedies will be found more effectual than bathing them every morning with clean spring water in which has been placed just sufficient brandy to make the mixture cause a slight stinging sensation when applied to the eyes. This weak brandy-and-water lotion may be kept ready mixed in a bottle. Another useful eye-water is made by mixing 40 drops of laudanum with 2 table-spoonfuls of milk and the same quantity of water.

(2) There is no better recipe for curing weak eyes, it is said, than cold water. Sluice plentifully not only the eyes, but the ears, especially the orifice.

EYESIGHT, HOW TO PRESERVE:

For the cure of the eyes the following rules are laid down by a noted oculist:

- Keep a shade on your lamp or gas burner. Avoid all sudden changes from light to darkness.
- Never begin to read, write, or sew for several minutes after coming from darkness to light.
- Never read by twilight, moonlight, or on cloudy days.
- Never read or sew directly in front of the light, window or door. It is best to let the light fall from above obliquely over the left shoulder.
- Never sleep so that on first awakening the eyes shall open on the light of a window.
- Do not use the eyesight by light so scant that it requires an effort to discriminate.
- The moment you are instinctively prompted to rub your eyes, that moment stop using them.
- If the eyelids are glued together on waking up do not forcibly open them, but apply saliva with the finger; it is the speediest dilutant in the world; then wash your eyes and face in warm water.

EYESIGHT, TO PROLONG THE USE OF:

Sooner or later our eyesight must become impaired. When beginning to use glasses use them as short a time as possible, only on deficient light, or on minute objects. By a judicious attention to these two points the ageing of the sight will be retarded years. And as reading is one of the luxuries of the age, and one of the most delightful pastimes, we cannot be too careful of the eyesight, and should study how to husband its powers.

EYESIGHT, TO STRENGTHEN:

Let there be an occasional pressure of the finger on the ball of the eye. Let the pressure always be from the nose and toward the temples, and wash the eyes 3 times a day in cold water. If this simple advice is followed the day is not far distant when partial blindness will disappear from the world.

EYE-WASHES:

Alum: Dissolve 1/2 dram of alum in 8 ounces of water. Use as an astringent. When the strength of the alum is doubled, and only half of the quantity of water used, it acts as a discutient(1).

Common: Add 1 ounce of diluted acetic acid to 3 ounces of decoction of poppy-heads. Use as an anodyne wash.

Zinc and Camphor: Dissolve a scruple of white vitriol in 8 ounces of water, then add 1 dram of spirit of camphor, and strain. Use as a stimulant.

Compound Zinc: Dissolve 10 grains of white vitriol in 8 ounces of camphor water, *(Mistura camphoroe),* and the same quantity of decoction of poppy-heads. Use as an anodyne and detergent; useful for weak eyes.

EYE-WATER FOR HORSES AND CATTLE:

Alcohol, 1 table-spoonful; extract of lead, 1 tea-spoonful; rain-water, 1/2 pint.

(1) Having the power of dissipating morbid matter.

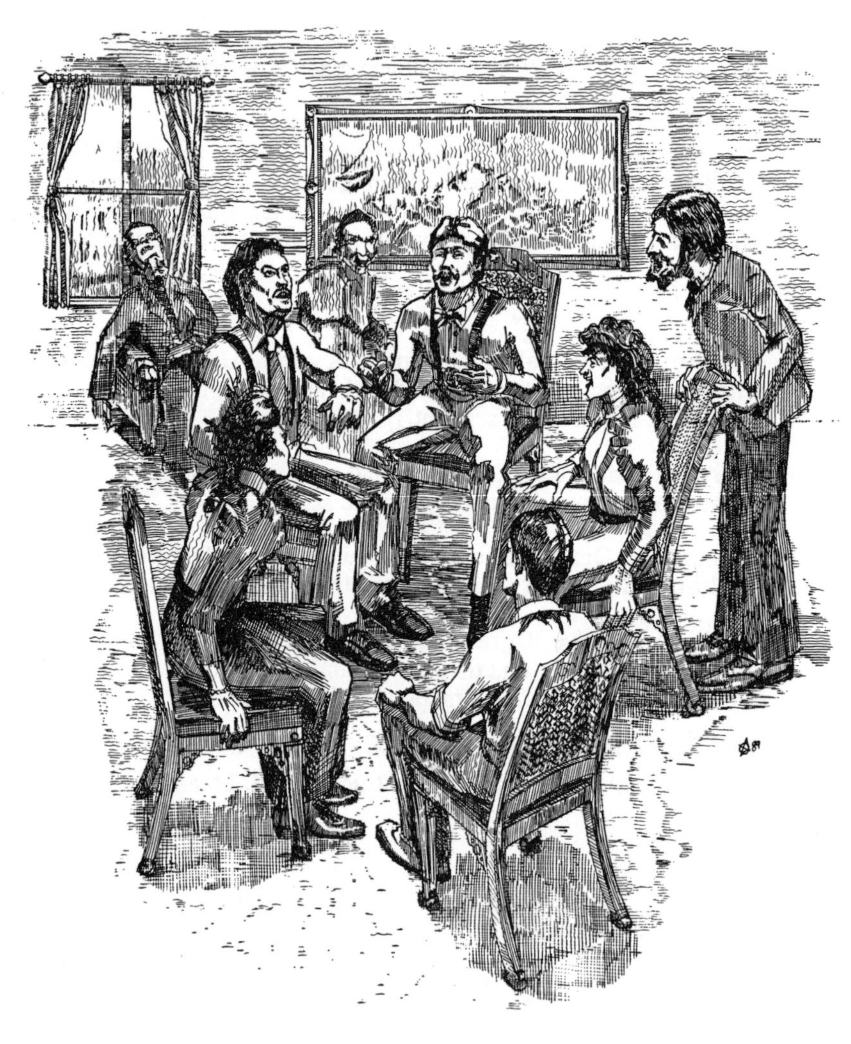

• *Game of Feather* •

F

FACADES, STONE, TO CLEAN:

It has been ascertained that the jet of water thrown from a steam fire-engine has the power of removing the discoloration produced by smoke without injuring the face of the stone. The work is done from the ground, the force of the stream thrown by the steam fire-engine being quite sufficient to effect the necessary cleansing.

FARM IMPLEMENTS, TO PREVENT DECAY OF:

When not in use have them sheltered from the sun, wind, rain, and snow. By this means sleighs, wagons, carts, plows, threshing-machines, harrows, and the like would last twice as long as they would if left in the open air, swelling from moisture one week and shrinking the next from the influence of the sun and wind.

FAT, HOW TO GROW:

"Every woman who is thin would like to be stouter," says a witty and observant Frenchman, and the observation is undoubtedly correct. While there may be considerable difference of opinion as to the aesthetic merits of embonpoint(1), every one will agree that a scrawny neck, pinched features, a gaunt figure, or spare shanks are not elements of beauty. Like excessive plumpness, meagerness is in some cases a family trait, and is only in a measure amenable to treatment, but unless there is some pernicious cause constantly in action, reducing nutrition or preventing assimilation, more or less improvement can generally be secured by proper management.

Among the more prominent causes of leanness must be classed an irritable, worrying, or overworked condition of the nervous system. Any thing which interferes with the proper digestion or assimilation of food may be the cause of a spare frame. This is particularly liable to influence the body during the period of growth. For this reason children should not be stinted in proper food. Any conditions which depress the general vitality, such as deprivation of sleep, loss of blood, painful and long-continued diseases, or acute diseases accompanied by high fever, violent passions, consumption, and other wasting maladies, may all be determining causes of leanness.

Girls not unfrequently bring about a meager habit of body during school-life. The inordinate consumption of pickles, lemons, and other acid

(1) Plumpness.

condiments, or later in life the almost entire dependence upon tea as a nervous stimulant, with a minimum of nutritious food, are frequently causes of this undesirable condition. According to my observations teachers are as blamable in this regard as are the pupils, and they suffer probably to no less extent than the latter from their ignorance or carelessness in matters of personal hygiene.

The prevention of leanness should be a care with parents while their children are growing up. Any marked decrease in weight or want of the normal fullness of body and limbs should attract attention to the cause, and any pernicious influences removed or bad habits corrected. If the individual is the subject of chronic, wasting disease, this will naturally first claim attention; but even in such a case medicine is of less value than abundance of appropriate food, for here "in food there is medicine," as one of the old writers quaintly expresses it.

Saccharine and starch foods are of special value in making fat, and hence should receive preference if they can be digested. Even in disorders of the digestive organs certain artifically prepared ailments and digesive principals will be assimilated. Thus modern physiological and chemical researches have taught us how to aid or even supplant natural digestion with pepsine, pancreatine, and other peptic preparations, until we are almost able to dispense with salivas, gastric juice, bile, and the secretions of the pancreas in converting the food taken into the mouth into assimilable aliment.

A dietary for a lean person might include the following articles: Coffee with cream, chocolate, milk, good, well-baked wheaten bread, rice, hominy and grits well cooked, rich purees and pastes, the old-fashioned "mush and milk," with which the Orientals are said to fatten their women as the Strassburgers grow geese; eggs, oysters, fat fish, such as shad and salmon; brains, fats of all kinds, pates, pastry and sweet cakes, confectionery, avoiding of course the poisoned kinds; heavy-bodied wines, as port or Burgundy; beer, ale, porter, or malt extract. As a table beverage the arsenical water of La Bourboule is often useful, but should not be drunk to excess.

Oatmeal, Graham bread, tea, light acid wines, and acid foods and condiments, like pickles and lemons, should be avoided. Although the first 2 contain much nutriment, they are so irritant to the mucous membrane of the digestive organs that they are not only imperfectly digested themselves, but they interfere with the assimilation of other foods by causing the contents of the intestinal canal to be swept onward before all the nutriment has been absorbed. Aside from eating such foods as are easiest converted into fat, the individual of meager habit should avoid excessive exertion, sleep much, shun worry and nervous excitement, and surround himself with as many comforts as circumstances will permit.

FAT, TO REDUCE:

There are 3 modes by which fat can be reduced, diet, exercise, and specific medicines. The patient may eat lean mutton, beef, veal, lamb, tongue, sweetbread, soups not thickened, beef-tea and broths, poultry, game, fish, cheese, eggs, bread, in moderation; also greens, spinach, watercress, mustard and cress, lettuce, asparagus, celery, radishes, French beans, green peas, Brussels sprouts, cabbage, cauliflower, onions, broccoli, sea-kale, jellies, flavored but not sweetened; fresh fruit in moderation, without sugar or cream, and pickles. He may not eat fat bacon and ham, fat of meat, butter, cream, sugar, potatoes, carrots, parsnips, beet-root, rice, arrowroot, sago, tapioca, macaroni, vermicelli, semolina, custard, pastry and pudding of all kinds, and sweet cakes.

He may drink tea, coffee, cocoa from nibs, with milk, but without cream or sugar; dry wines of any kind in moderation brandy, whisky, or gin in moderation, without sugar; light bitter beer, Apollinaris water, soda water, and seltzer water. He may not drink milk, except sparingly, porter and stout, sweet ales, sweet wines; as a rule alcoholic liquors should be taken very sparingly, and never without food.

Among specific medicines certain natural mineral waters are the best. Sea-water is the best of all, as taken internally it acts as a diuretic and purgative, particularly the latter. A small glassful of it should be taken 3 times a day in a little fresh water or milk. Sea-water baths are also to be resorted to; free exercise should be practiced. Five drops of Flower's solution 3 times a day will sometimes restore the patient to health in 2 months. Turkish baths have a reputation for reducing obesity.

FEATHER, GAME OF THE:

A small flossy feather with very little stem must be procured. The players then draw their chairs in a circle as closely together as possible. One of the party begins the game by throwing the feather into the air as high as possible above the center of the ring formed. The object of the game is to keep it from touching one, as the player whom it touches must pay a forfeit; and it is impossible to imagine the excitement that can be produced by each player preventing the feather from alighting upon him. The game must be heartily played to be fully appreciated, not only by the real actors of the performance, but by the spectators of the scene. Indeed, so absurd generally is the picture presented, that it is difficult to say whether the players or the watchers have the most fun.

FEATHER FLOWERS:

The art of making feather flowers, though a very easy and inexpensive accomplishment, and yielding pretty ornaments for the mantel-piece or the chiffonier, is but little pursued. Many persons are under the impression that they can only be made from the feathers of exotic birds, and that these are expensive. But following instructions will dispel this misconception, and remove the difficulty. Procure the best white geese or swans' feathers, have them plucked off the fowl with care not to break the web, and free them from down, except a small quantity on the shaft of the feather. Having procured two good specimens of the flower you wish to imitate, carefully pull off the petals of one, and with a piece of tissue-paper cut out the shape of each size, taking care to leave the shaft of the feather at least 1/2 in. longer than the petal of the flower. Carefully bend the feather with the thumb and finger to the proper shape, taking care not to break the web.

To Make the Stem and Heart: Take a piece of wire 6 in. long; across the top lay a small piece of cotton wool, turn the wire over it, and wind it round until it is the size of the heart or center of the flower you are going to imitate. If a single flower cover it with paste or velvet of the proper color, and round it must be arranged the stamens; these are made of fine India silk, or feathers may be used for this purpose. After the petals have been attached the silk or feather is dipped into gum and then into the farina. Place the petals round, 1 at a time, and wind them on with Moravian cotton, No.4; arrange them as nearly like the flower you have for a copy as possible. Cut the stems of the feathers even, and they make the calyx of feathers, cut like the pattern of natural flower. For the small flowers the calyx is made with paste. Cover the stems with paper or silk the same as the flowers; the paper must be cut in narrow strips, about 1/4 in. wide.

To Make the Calyx, Hearts, and Buds: Take common white starch and mix it with gum-water until it is the substance of thick treacle; color it with the dyes used for the feathers, and keep it from the air.

To Make the Farina: Use common rice, mixed into a stiff paste with any dye; dry it before the fire, and when quite hard pound it to a fine powder. The buds, berries, and hearts of some double flowers are made with cotton wool, wound around wire, molded to the shape with thumb and finger. Smooth it over with gum-water, and when dry cover the buds, berries, or calyx with the proper colored pastes; they will require 1 or 2 coats, and may be shaded with a little paint and then gummed and left to dry. Flowers of 2 or more shades or colors are variegated with water-colors, mixed with lemon-juice, ultra-marine and chrome for blue, and gold may also be used in powder, mixed with lemon-juice and gum-water(1).

To Dye Feathers Blue: Into 2 pennyworths(2) of oil of vitriol mix 2 pennyworths of the best indigo in powder; let it stand 1 or 2 days; when wanted shake it well, and into a quart of boiling water put 1 table-spoonful of the liquid. Stir it well, put the feathers in, and let them simmer a few minutes.

(1) A distillation from gum.
(2) A small quantity.

Yellow: Put a table-spoonful of the best turmeric(1) into a quart of boiling water; when well mixed put in the feathers. More or less of the turmeric will give them different shades, and a very small quantity of soda will give them an orange hue.

Green: Mix the indigo liquid with turmeric, and pour boiling water over it; let the feathers simmer in the dye until they have acquired the shade you want them.

Pink: Three good pink saucers in a quart of boiling water, with a small quantity of cream of tartar. If a deep color is required use 4 saucers. Let the feathers remain in the dye several hours.

Red: Into a quart of boiling water dissolve a tea-spoonful of cream of tartar, put in 1 table-spoonful of prepared cochineal, and then a few drops of muriate of tin. This dye is expensiuve, and scarlet flowers are best made with the plumage of the red Ibis, which can generally be had of a bird-fancier or bird-stuffer, who will give directions how it may be applied.

Lilac: About 2 tea-spoonfuls of cudbear(2) into about a quart ofboiling water; let it simmer a few minutes before you put in the feathers. A small quantity of cream of tartar turns the color from lilac to amethyst.

Before the Feathers are Dyed: They must be put into hot water, and let them drain before they are put into the dyes. After they are taken out of the dye rinse them 2 or 3 times in clear cold water, except the red, which must only be done once. Then lay them on a tray, over which a cloth has been spread, before a good fire; when they begin to dry and unfold draw each feather gently between your thumb and finger until it regains its proper shape.

The Leaves: Are made of green feathers, cut like those of the natural flower, and serrated at the edges with a very small pair of scissors. For the calyx of a moss-rose the down is left on the feather and is a very good representation of the moss on the natural flower.

FEATHERS, TO CLEAN:

Cut some white curd soap in small pieces, pour boiling water on them, and add a little pearlash(3) when the soap is quite dissolved, and the mixture cool enough for the hand to bear, plunge the feathers into it and draw them through the hand till the dirt appears to be squeezed out of them; pass them through a clean lather with some blue in it, then rinse them in cold water with blue to give them a good color; beat them against the hand to

(1) A plant of the ginger family whose powdered form is used as a yellow dye.
(2) A crimson die manufactured in Scotland by heating certain lichens.
(3) Crude carbonate of potash, made from the ashes of plants.

shake off the water, and dry by shaking them near a fire. Black feathers may be cleaned with water and some gall, proceeding as above.

FEATHERS, TO WASH AND CURL:

Wash in warm soap-suds and rinse in water a very little blued, if the feather is white; then let the wind dry it. When the curl has come out by washing the feather or getting it damp place a hot flat-iron so that you can hold the feather just above it while curling. Take a bone or silver knife and draw the fibers of the feather between the thumb and the dull edge of the knife, taking not more than 3 fibers at a time, beginning at the point of the feather and curling one half the other way. The hot iron makes the curl more durable. After a little practice one can make them look as well as new feathers. When swan's-down becomes soiled it can be washed and made to look as well as new. Tack strips on a piece of muslin and wash in warm water with white soap, then rinse and hang in the wind to dry. Rip from the muslin and rub carefully between the fingers to soften the leather.

FEET, BLISTERED, REMEDY FOR:

A good remedy for feet blistered from long walking: Rub the feet at going-to-bed with spirits mixed with tallow dropped from a lighted candle into the palm of the hand.

FEET CARE OF THE:

Warm Feet Essential to Health: Unless the feet be kept warm the circulation of the blood to the extremities is prevented, the whole system becomes deranged, and fever or any kind becomes aggravated as a result. A distinguished medical man declares that as a result of many years' careful observation in a large practice in his profession he believes a large part of the sickness prevalent in any community is "nearly or remotely the result of cold feet."

How to Cure the Habit of Cold Feet: The feet should be placed in a basin of cold water every morning for a few seconds, just deep enough to cover the toes; wipe dry, dress, and walk off. Once or twice a week the feet should be held in water made comfortably warm for some 10 minutes, adding hot water from time to time, using a little soap; if at the end of this bathing at night the feet were placed in a pan of cold water, toe-deep, for less than a 1/4 minute, it would greatly aid in giving tone and softness to the skin, and vigor to the circulation, and thus do much toward keeping them warm.

Foot Odor: A table-spoonful of chloride of lime in a basin of warm water is an excellent wash for removing foot odor.

How to Sleep with Warm Feet: Before retiring to bed, especially in winter, hold both feet before a blazing fire, stockings removed, for 10 minutes at least, rubbing them with the hands all the time until they feel perfectly dry and warm; such a process will warm the feet more effectually in 5 minutes than can be done in 1 hour by holding them to the fire with the stockings and shoes on.

Waking up with Cold Feet: Sometimes without apparent cause a person will suddenly wake up to the knowledge that his feet are cold, and a disagreeable sensation is caused which pervades the whole body, and the mind and temper become fretful and morose. This is often the case in the very midst of summer. When this is observed you are taking cold, and you should instantly treat the feet to a blazing fire as named above. If this is not practicable, give them a hot foot-bath as just directed. In either case you will not only avert the cold, but you will also experience a feeling of comfortableness which is delightful. This same kind of bath is the speediest and most comfortable means of warming the feet when they are found to be uncomfortably cold after coming in from a walk or a long day's work.

Bunions: These may be checked when they first appear by binding the joint with adhesive plaster and keeping it on until all indications of an enlargement disappear. An inflamed bunion demands large shoes and a poultice. An ointment to be rubbed on gently 2 or 3 times a day may be made of iodine, 12 grains; lard or spermaceti(1) ointment, 1/2 ounce.

To Cure Frosted Feet: Warm some pine tar, and apply with a feather to the affected part; heat it by the fire before going to bed. In very bad cases it may need the second or third application. It is a sure cure, and the tar can easily be removed with lard and soap.

Treatment of Scalded Feet: When the legs and feet are scalded they should be plunged as soon as possible into cold water, and kept immersed in it a considerable length of time before the stockings are removed. By this means blisters are often prevented.

FEETACHE, PANACEA FOR:

When your work is finished sit down with your feet in as hot water as can be borne, adding water if convenient for as long a time as possible. Three or 4 times will effect a cure, and you will not be troubled again in a good while.

FELONS(2), TESTED CURES:

(1) Take a pint of common soft-soap, and stir in air-slaked lime till it is of

(1) Waxlike substance from the head of a sperm whale or dolphin.
(2) Painful pus infection of the finger or toe.

the consistency glazier's putty(1). Make a leather thimble, fill it with this composition, and insert the fingers therein, and a cure is certain.

(2) As soon as the parts begin to swell get tincture of lobelia(2), and wrap the part affected with a cloth saturated thoroughly with the tincture, and the felon is dead. An old physician says he has known it to cure in scores of cases, and it never fails if applied in season.

(3) As soon as the disease is felt put directly over the spot a fly blister about the size of your thumb-nail, and let it remain for 6 hours, at the expiration of which time, directly under the surface of the blister, may be seen the felon, which can be instantly taken out with the point of a needle or a lancet.

(4) When the felon first appears procure some poke root, and roast a piece sufficient to cover your finger. When it is roasted tender cut it open and bind it on the felon as hot as can be borne; repeat this when the root becomes dry until the pain subsides. If the felon is too far advanced to "put back," this same remedy will hasten it on and cure it in a few days, as it softens the skin.

(5) Probe the swelling of the finger, making a small incision where the pain appears greatest. The pain of the operation may be lessened by the local application of ether or inhalation of chloroform. The after-treatment is equally simple. The small wound is to be covered with lint and carbolic acid, and bathed morning and evening in tepid water. In a few days it is perfectly healed.

(6) Take an earthen crock, put in a quantity of live coals, throw on a handful each of hops, rye flour, and brown sugar; then steam the affected part for about 15 minutes, repeating 2 or 3 times, by holding it over the vessel. The better way is to bore a hole through the board, thus having the affected part only coming in contact with the steam. This is guaranteed as a certain cure.

FENCE-POSTS, TO MAKE DURABLE:

It was discovered many years ago that wood could be made to last longer than iron in the ground.

The following is the recipe: Take boiled linseed oil and stir in it pulverized charcoal to the consistency of paint; put a coat of this over the timber, and there is not a man that will live to see it rotten.

FERN-CASE, TO MAKE:

This fern-case consists of 3 bars crossed at the top and fastened into

(1) Window sealing putty.
(2) Medicine from the lobelia plant used as an expectorant, and emetic and as a diuretic.

a triangular base. A basket is suspended from the center of the case and the base is decorated with shells, acorns, or corals. The best method of making this case is to have the base first made of wood, then lined with zinc. The sides should hold glass neatly filled into the bars, thus inclosing the plants from the outer air. The height should be about 3 ft., and width of base 2 ft. on each side. Any florist can supply ferns for such a structure. Choose only the smaller growing sorts, and avoid those which branch widely.

FERN-WORK:

The handsome articles that come under this head are made simply by pinning ferns or leaves in any form desired upon white cloth, and drawing a comb through a small brush of indelible ink, so that minute particles will be scattered over the cloth. Upon removing the ferns their impression, uncolored, is distinct. Doylies made in this way are charming. Paper-hanging and other wall ornaments are made of white paper and spotted with common ink. Gilt paper can be used with fine effect.

FETID BREATH:

Scarcely any thing is more disgusting.

Treatment: Various means depend principally on aromatics, which by their odor smother it for a time; but these require continual repetition, and are liable to interfere with digestion. The real cause of ill-smelling breath may generally be traced to a diseased stomach, or to decayed teeth. When the former is the case mild aperients should be administered; if these do not succeed, an emetic may be given. When decayed teeth are the cause they should at once be thoroughly cleaned and then filled, or, if this is impracticable, they should be removed.

FETTERED BUFF, GAME OF:

In fettered buff the hands are tied behind, and the player has to move quickly and turn suddenly in order to seize a captive. This game can be played indoors or out-of-doors, and must be limited to a certain space.

FEVER, SYMPTOMS AND PREVENTIVES OF:

Fevers and many acute diseases are often preceded by a loss of appetite, headache, shivering, "pains in the bones," indisposition to work, etc. In such cases sponge with tepid water, and rub the body till all aglow. Go to bed, place hot bricks to the feet, take nothing but a little gruel or beef-tea, and drink moderately of warm cream-of-tartar water. If you do not feel better the next morning, call a physician. If that be impossible, take a dose of castor-oil or Epsom salts.

FEVER AND AGUE:

There are several varieties, differing from each other in the length of time that elapses between the attacks. There is one called quotidian(1), occurring every 24 hours; another named tertian, every 48 hours; and the third, quartan, the interval lasting 72 hours. There is a very severe form of it called congestive, which is quite fatal and requires energetic treatment. The symptoms commence with yawning, stretching, and uneasiness; this is succeeded by slight shiverings that end in a violent shaking of the whole body; this is the cold fit, and is immediately followed by the fever; the pulse rises, skin becomes hot with pain in the head, tongue white, and all the marks of fever, terminating in a produce sweat which leaves the patient in his natural state, though somewhat weakened.

Treatment: In the cold stage give hot stimulating drinks; use the hot foot-bath, and put the patient to bed with hot bricks or bottles of hot water to the feet, sides, and back; administer a tea-spoonful of chloroform or 1/2 tea-spoonful of laudanum to cut short the paroxysm(2).

In the hot stage give 20 or 30 drops of spirits of niter, or a table-spoonful of the spirits mindererus(3) every hour until the fever subsides; bathe the head and hands occasionally, and even the whole body, if agreeable to the patient, with water; when the sweating sets in rub the patient with dry towels; in the outset of the paroxysm, if the bowels are constipated, give an active cathartic, as the infusion of senna and salts, or 3 or 4 cathartic pills; as soon as the fever has subsided give quinine in 3-grain doses every 4 hours, until some ringing in the ears is produced or the time for the next paroxysm is past; the quinine may be taken in pills or in powder packed in capsules, 4 to 6 grains twice a day. Iodine may be substituted for quinine in doses of 12 to 15 minims for adults, 3 times a day; for children 5 to 10 min-ims, 3 times a day. The best form in which to take it is as follows: Compound tincture of iodine, 6 drams; syrup of acacia, 18 drams.

FIGS, TO DRY:

When ripe the figs are picked and spread out in the sun to dry; those of the better quality being much pulled and extended by hand during the process. Thus prepared, the fruit is packed closely in barrels, rush baskets, or wooden boxes.

FILES, TO RE-SHARPEN:

Remove the grease and dirt from your files by washing them in warm potash water, then wash them in warm water and dry with artificial heat; next, place 1 pint warm water in a wooden vessel and put in your files; add 2 ounces of blue vitriol, finely pulverized, 2 ounces borax, well-mixed, taking care to turn the files over, so that each one may come in contact with the mixture. Now add 7 ounces sulphuric acid and 1/4 ounce cider vinegar to

(1) Daily
(2) A sudden outburst or convulsion.
(3) Acetate of ammonia solution.

the above mixture. Remove the files after a short time, dry, sponge them with olive-oil, wrap them up in porous paper, and put aside for use. Coarse files require to be immersed longer than fine.

FILES AND RASPS, TO RE-CUT:

The worn files are first cleaned with potash and hot water, after which they are left for 5 minutes in a solution composed of 1 part of sulphuric acid and 7 parts of water; a quantity of nitric acid equal to the sulphuric is then added to the solution and as much water also, and the files are left in it for about 40 minutes longer. They are now ready for use, but if to be stored, they must be brushed over with a little oil or grease to prevent rusting. The files must not be allowed to touch each other in the solution, being supported by their tangs only. In order to obtain the most complete results possible the proportions of acid are varied according to the size of the files; e.g., for large files, one sixth acid; for bastard files, one eighth, one ninth, to one eleventh; and for the fines, one twelfth to one thirteenth.

FILIGREE WORK(1) ON SILVER, TO CLEAN:

A tooth-brush is just the thing for cleaning the filigree of jewelry, and will answer as well for silverware.

FINGERS, WHAT MAY BE EATEN WITH THE:

There are a number of things that the most fashionable and well-bred people now eat at the dinner-table with their fingers. They are: Olives, to which a fork should never be applied. Asparagus, whether hot or cold, when served whole, as it should be. Lettuce, which should be dipped in the dressing or in a little salt. Celery, which may properly be placed on the table-cloth beside the plate. Strawberries, when served with the stem on, as they usually are in most elegant houses. Bread, toast, and all tarts and small cakes. Fruit of all kinds, except melons and preserves, which are eaten with a spoon. Cheese, which is almost invariably eaten with the fingers by the most particular people. Even the leg or other small piece of a bird is taken in the fingers at fashionable dinners, and at most of the luncheons ladies pack small pieces of chicken without using a fork.

FIRE IN A CHIMNEY, TO EXTINGUISH:

So many serious fires have been caused by chimneys catching fire and not being quickly extinguished that the following method of doing this should be made generally known:

Throw some powdered brimstone on the fire in the grate, or ignite some on the hob(2), and then put a board or something in the front of the fire-place to prevent the fumes descending into the room. The vapor of the

(1) A lace-like ornament made of gold or silver wire.
(2) A flat iron shelf next to a grate to keep things warm.

brimstone ascending the chimney, will then effectually extinguish the soot on fire.

FIRE-KINDLERS:

To make very nice fire-kindlers take resin any quantity and melt it, putting in for each pound being used from 2 to 3 ounces of tallow, and when all is hot spread it out about 1 in. thick upon boards which have fine sawdust sprinkled upon them, to prevent it from sticking. When cold break up into lumps about 1 in. square. But if for sale take a thin board and press upon it while yet warm to lay it off into inch squares; this makes it break regularly, if you press the crease sufficiently deep; grease the marking board to prevent it from sticking.

FITS, FAINTING:

Fainting is caused by the blood leaving the brain. Place the patient flat and allow the head to be lower than the body. Sprinkle cold water on the face. Hartshorn(1) may be held near the nose, not to it. A half tea-spoonful of aromatic spirits of ammonia in a wine-glassful of water will tend to revive the patient. If the symptoms recur, send for a physician.

FITS, OR SPASMS:

During the period of childhood the nervous system is so easily excited or irritated that these are of frequent occurrence. During the first 4 yrs. of its life the child is especially liable.

Treatment: When a child is attacked place the lower extremities up to the knees in water, hot as can be borne, for 10 or 15 minutes; when taken out, rub them thoroughly dry and wrap in a warm flannel, at the same time enveloping the whole head in a cold cloth and changing it often. If the spasm is caused by indigestion or constipation, give an injection of warm slippery-elm or flaxseed tea. An emetic, a tea-spoonful of mustard in a tumbler of warm water, may be given. Mustard poultices or chloroform liniment to the spine may also be used if necessary. If the gums are swollen and tender, lance them.

FIVE-DOT GAME:

Any number can play, but each player must be provided with a sheet of white paper and a pencil. All must then mark 5 dots in any arrangement on the piece of paper before him, and pass it to his next neighbor at the left hand. He then takes the dotted paper which has been handed to him, and tries to draw on it some human figure in such a posture as to bring one of the dots at the middle top of the forehead, one at the point of each foot, and one at each hand. But no one must take longer than a certain time, say

(1) An odorous liquid extracted from the horn of a deer.

5 or 10 minutes, in making his picture. The results sometimes are very laughable, and the game calls for a good deal of invention and skill.

FIVE O'CLOCK TEA:

Five o'clock tea now exists in half a dozen different forms. There is, first, the original English afternoon tea, imported and adhered to by some 3 or 4 women who understand thoroughly how to entertain. Tea, as served by them is a needed simplification of our forms of social intercourse. It makes their houses a daily rendezvous where young men, after business hours and while it is yet too early to assume the formalities and responsibilities of the dress coat, can count on finding one or more of the ladies of the house, surrounded by a home atmosphere and the center of attraction for a group of pleasant women and girls. At such a daily tea there are no floral decorations beyond a vase or two of roses, no music, and no menu more elaborate than thin bread and butter, wafers, tea, and cake.

At the other end of the scale, and coming but once or twice a season, is the tea as it has been elaborated by the competition of society matrons with *débutante* daughters to introduce. Combined with a reception to some hundreds of people, costing more for flowers than a ball and more for viands than a state dinner, tea and the *débutante* have fallen foul of each other with results satisfactory to the *débutante*, but causing the tea to doubt its identity. Between these two extremes come weekly teas, monthly teas, occasional teas, all sorts of teas, but all, in spite of their diversity, amenable to much the same general social laws.

Decoration: Flowers for afternoon teas have assumed of late years an importance they never aspired to before. It was the original tradition that you should offer your guests comparatively little to eat or drink and so, however much you depart from the traditions, it still influences you mentally to feast their eyes right royally in addition, if not instead. The flower of all flowers for afternoon tea is the orchid. Next the orchid comes the rose, and next the rose the violet, but the orchid by all means if you can. The orchid is a weirdly delicate and luxurious flower, and it wants luxurious surroundings. No orchids unless you have a silken cloth for the table, and unless your silver and your glass is of quality graceful in shape and curiously wrought.

The splendidly decorative blossoms of the *lycaste skinneri*, *catteya maxima*, *oncidium varicosum*, and *odonto-glossum cordatum* are the tea-table queens, if you can give them royal welcoming. Mass them in low open baskets of delicate porcelain or white enamel. Roses for the tea-table are wholesome flowers that suit a robust taste better than the unearthly orchids. Use a single variety of one of the larger hybrids and cut them with long stems, filling a couple of dozen slender silver vases.

Small Tables: When the number of guests is large enough and the menu elaborate enough to set small separate tables, it is a pretty trick of flower decoration to put a dish of fine posies divided into nose gays in the middle of each table, so that every lady may take with her when she goes a bunch of violets or valley lilies or white Roman hyacinths. The waxy camellia, which your mother wore in her hair when she was married, is a long ago favorite lately revived, and the fragrant *daphne ordora* is liked everywhere. Ferns and mignonette, if you like. But don't mix flowers. All roses, all violets, or no flowers at all.

The Cloth: The cloth for 5 o'clock tea-drinkings is a delicate thing to spread. The acme of elegance for orchid people is a set of hand-woven silk cloths, in delicate colors, adapted to the tiny tea-tables in vogue. There are women who have put $2,000 or $3,000 into embroidered silk spreads. Next these, for rose or violet tables, are tea-cloths and sets of tea-cloths in momie. These are a novelty and come with inserted borders of hand-made lace costing $100 or $150. Fine linen cambric is occasionally used for tea-spreads. Heavy damask, when used for tea-spreads is lace-trimmed or embroidered or edged with drawn work. Tea-cloths are the only variety of table linen on which a fringe is now allowable, and even here it is not commonly used.

Menu Cards: Menu cards are essential at the more elaborate teas only. When used it is the latest thing to have them of tinted fine gauze, lined with soft silk, of an oblong shape, with a painted conventional design on the gauze, fringed at one end and having a tiny card for the name attached by a narrow ribbon. Each tea-table should seat not over 4 guests, preferably intimates or congenial spirits; and a card should lie by each plate; favors of small dainty baskets of a delicate straws in pale shades of pink and blue heaped with flowers being added if desired.

Tea-service: Porcelain, silver, and glass for the tea-service should be delicate in shape and dainty in design. Porcelains from the English factories are preferred, as superior in design and wearing better as to metallic decoration than the French. Sevres ware(1) especially has degenerated, the makers being hampered by the conventionalities that always surround a factory under government supervision. English crystal is the preferred glass, though Venetian is used by some people.

Costumes: Frocks for afternoon teas assume a character distinctively their own. The contrast between hostess and guests is less marked than last season, visitors now assuming bonnets and gowns ceremonious enough as well as pretty enough to do honor to the occasion. Tea-drinkers wear fancy combinations of silk, velvet, and lace, or fine embroidered cloth frocks, altogether too dressy for the promenade, but invariably short, and

(1) Porcelain of fine quality.

distinguished from evening gowns by being cut high in the neck and by the artistic simplicity of drapery appropriate to day wear.

Jewels are not out of place, but too many are not desirable. Gloves may be in mousquetaire(1) or button style. Suede gloves are the first choice in tan colors, lavender, pale silver gray, and other tints. The corsage bouquet, which is tabooed for evening dress, is in favor for teas. It consists of 3 or 4 roses, long stemmed, all of a color and kind; a spray of valley lilies, heliotrope, or something not too large and harmonizing with the gown.

The Tea-gown: The tea-gown par excellence, the privilege of the hostess, is responsible for much of the popularity of the tea. It is not only the prettiest, it is the only comfortable gown made. It exhibits no striking novelties but the best designers are putting some of their best work into it. Tea-aprons are in delicate shades of china silk, hand embroidered, and edged with real lace.

FIVES, GAME OF:(2)

There is a very old game at ball, called "Fives," which was known in the days of Queen Elizabeth, and declared by her to be "the best sport she had ever seen." For this game a garden wall with a piece of smooth ground before it is necessary. A line is drawn with chalk on the wall at the distance of about a yard from the bottom. On the ground a long line is marked out, with 2 other lines at right angles with it reaching to the wall, forming an oblong square. This space marks the "bounds."

The players stand in a row outside the boundary-line, a player on each side standing alternately; for, of course, as it is a trial of skill, the players divide as at croquet. The first begins the game by bouncing the ball on the ground, in the Chinese manner of playing ball. On its rebounding, she strikes it with the palm of her hand against the wall in such a manner that at its descent it shall fall outside bounds. This is done only for the first stroke; after it the ball must be struck so as to fall within bounds, otherwise the opposite party count "one." The players strike the ball in turn, first one then the other. If any player misses the ball at the rebound, or strikes it beneath the line on the wall, or hits it out of bounds, the opposite side count "one." "Fifteen" is the game, and the side which counts it first wins.

FLANNELS, CARE OF:

Soap should never be rubbed on flannels, but they should be washed in warm suds, and rinsed in water of the same temperature as that in which they were washed. A little blueing in the second water will improve their color. They should be hung out at once, dried in the shade, and, if possible, ironed while still damp. Flannels thus treated will never become stiff and yellow, but will retain the color and texture of new goods. Where there are

(1) Musketeer.
(2) Handball.

fine baby flannels it is well to have a special time for washing them, so that they may be ironed before they are quite dry without interrupting the general wash.

FLANNELS, TO BLEACH:

(1) Hang the flannels loosely in a tight barrel over the fumes of burning sulfur.

(2) A solution of $1^1/4$ lbs. of white soap and three eights ounce spirits of ammonia, dissolved in 12 gallons soft water, will impart a beautiful and lasting whiteness to any flannels dipped in it, no matter how yellow they have been previous to their immersion. After being well stirred round for a short time the articles should be taken out and well washed in clean, cold water.

FLANNELS, TO SHRINK:

New flannel should always be shrunk or washed before it is made up, that it may cut out more accurately and that the grease which is used in manufacturing it may be extracted. Cut off the list along the selvage edge of the whole piece; then put it into warm water without soap; begin at one end of the piece and rub it with both hands till you come to the other end; this is to get out the grease and blue with which new white flannel is always tinged; then do the same through another water; rinse it through a clean lukewarm water; wring it length-wise, and stretch it well. In hanging it out spread it along the line straight and lengthwise. If dried in festoons(1) the edges will be in great scallops, making it very difficult to cut out. It must be dried in the sun. When dry, let it be stretched even, clapped with the hands, and rolled up tightly and smoothly till wanted.

FLAXSEED TEA, WAYS TO MAKE:

(1) Put 2 table-spoonfuls whole flaxseed in a pint of boiling water and boil 15 minutes; cut up 1 lemon and put in a pitcher with 2 table-spoonfuls of sugar. Strain the tea boiling hot through a wire strainer into the pitcher and stir together. Good for cough and sore throat.

(2) Take 3 table-spoonfuls of linseed, about 1 pint of water, and boil for 10 minutes. Strain off the water, put in a mug with 2 lemons, 1 cut in thin slices; put in also some brown sugar. A wine-glassful of wine is an improvement. This has been found most nourishing for invalids.

(3) Macerate 1 once flaxseed and $^1/2$ ounce of bruised liquorice-root in 1 pint of boiling water for 2 hours in a tightly closed vessel; filter, and add 1 fluid ounce of lemon-juice. This is a good drink in cases of catarrh.

(1) Suspended from two points.

FLESH-WORMS ON THE SKIN:

When black spots—"flesh-worms," as they are called—become troublesome, it would be advisable to adapt the following remedy, which, though simple, is very efficacious:

Mix some flour of sulfur in a little milk, let it stand for a couple of hours, and then, without disturbing the sulfur, use the milk as a lotion to be well rubbed into the skin with a towel. Almost immediately afterward the skin may be washed with soap and cold water. Cold cream should be rubbed in at bed-time. The spots will shortly disappear.

FLIES, TO DESTROY:

To destroy flies in a room take 1/2 tea-spoonful of black pepper in powder, 1 tea-spoonful of brown sugar, and 1 table-spoonful of cream, mix them well together, and place on a plate in the room where the flies are troublesome, and they will soon disappear.

FLOORS, CARE OF:

To prepare floors for coloring or hard polish proceed as follows: If the floor is already painted or spotted with paint, cover with caustic potash; leaving this on till the paint is dissolved. It will take perhaps 36 hours if the paint is old and hard; then scour the floor, not letting the mixture deface the wash-boards. In case of wide cracks between the flooring have them puttied, or the dust will gather in them, allowing ugly stripes between the shining boards. If the planks are narrow and of equal width, color alternately oak and walnut, by first staining the entire floor oak and then the alternate stripes dark. It would be safe to dilute the mixture with an equal quantity of turpentine, as it is too thick when bought. In staining in stripes lay a board on each side of the stripe to be stained, and then draw the brush between. This guards the plank from a false stroke of the brush and saves time. But if the dark staining should run over on the light plank, wipe it off with a bit of flannel dipped in turpentine before it dries.

If the floor is to be all walnut, stain without a brush. Buy at a grocer's, for a medium sized room, a 1 lb. can of burnt umber ground in oil; mix a sufficient amount of this with boiled linseed oil to color without perceptibly thickening the oil; by trying the mixture upon a bit of wood till the desired color is attained, the quantity may be easily determined. It should be rich walnut brown. Rub this thoroughly into the wood with a woolen cloth till the stain ceases to come off. Never use boiled oil on the floor. Like a varnish it attracts and holds the dust, which can only be removed by caustic potash, sand-paper, or the plane. If the coloring matter is not dark enough when dry, rub on another coat. The floors may look dull, but in a few weeks, with proper care, will be satisfactory.

When the staining is done prepare for the next day's waxing. Mix 1 gallon of turpentine with 1 lb. of beeswax shaved thin. Soak the wax all night in the turpentine before using; rub it on with a woolen cloth. When the wood finally becomes well polished the wax need not be applied once a week for fortnight. When the floor is polished lay rugs on it. Floors are frequently made of oak, disposed in patterns, grooved and tongued together. The wood is usually 1 in. thick, and great care is taken in laying it, the wood being keyed at the back for further security.

Different colored woods are frequently employed with great effect, small pieces being so disposed as to produce geometrical patterns. All angular figures can be used as bases for the patterns. Large rooms may be finished by a border of parquetry, and sometimes a large center ornament is introduced. Floors of this kind are extremely durable, but necessarily expensive from the careful workmanship needed. A thin parquetry, something like stout veneer, is also used. This is affixed to the original flooring-boards of the room by means of glue, or glued on a backing of cloth, then called "wood carpet."

FLOORS, STAIN FOR:

To strong lye of wood ashes add enough copperas for the required oak shade. Put this on with a mop and varnish afterward.

FLOORS, TO STAIN AND POLISH:

An authority who thinks that carpets are too expensive for daily use, and that something that is cheaper and at the same time more easily kept clean is needed, says that a friend's hall and kitchen were floored as he supposed with black walnut and pine; but he was informed that the owner had caused the floors to be smoothly laid, and with his own hands had stained each alternate board a dark color, and then with shellac had finished the whole with a fine polish.

He says: "I shall have my hall and living-room floors planed smoothly and evenly by a carpenter, and then myself rub carefully with a sponge or brush, avoiding any daubs over the seam, into each alternate board a stain prepared as follows:

1/4 lb. of asphaltum and 1/2 lb. of beeswax; if too light in color, add asphaltum, though that must be done with caution, as very little will graduate the shade, and black walnut is not what its name indicates, but a rich dark brown; or burnt umber in alcohol to the proper consistency of easy application may be used without the beeswax; and, after a thin coat of shellac has been laid over the whole and the surface smoothed over with sandpaper, a coat of common varnish will give it a splendid finish. A breadth of carpet or matting or a piece of oilcloth laid down will protect it where the greatest wear comes. The narrower the floor the finer will be the effect, but in any case it will excite your own and your friends' admiration and prove a joy forever."

FLORIDA WATER:

Half pint proof spirits, 2 drams oil lemon, 1/2 dram oil rosemary; mix.

FLOUNDERS, HOW TO SELECT:

Flounders and all white flat fish are rigid and firm when fresh; the under side should be of a rich cream color. When out of season or too long kept this becomes a bluish white and the flesh soft and flaccid. A clear, bright eye in fish is also a mark of being fresh and good.

FLOUR, HOW TO SELECT:

Look at its color; if it is white, with a slightly yellowish or straw-colored tint, it is a good sign. If it is very white, with a bluish cast with white specks in it, the flour is not good. Examine its adhesiveness; wet and knead a little of it between the fingers; if it works dry and elastic, it is good; if it works soft and sticky, it is poor. Flour made from spring wheat is likely to be sticky. Throw a little lump of dry flour against a dry, smooth, perpendicular surface; if it adheres in a lump the flour has a life in it; if it falls like powder, it is bad. Squeeze some of the flour in your hands; if it retains the shape given by the pressure, that, too, is a good sign. Flour that will stand all of these tests it is safe to buy.

FLOWERS, ARRANGEMENT OF:

Flowers may be arranged either according to the harmony or contrast of colors. Red harmonizes with orange, orange with yellow, violet with red, indigo with violet, blue with indigo, and green with blue. Green is the contrast of red, sky-blue to orange, yellow to violet, blue to orange-red, indigo to orange-yellow, and violet to bluish-green. To find the contrast to any flower cut a small, circular piece out of its petals, place it upon white paper, look at it steadily with one eye for a few seconds without letting the eyelids close, then look from the colored circle to another part of the white paper, when the circle of another color will be apparent. This color is the true contrast or complimentary color. Tastes differ as to whether the effect of arranging the flowers according to contrast or complimentary color is more pleasing to the eye than according to harmonies. The former, however, is the most in favor. To carry it out a blue flower should be placed next to an orange flower, a yellow near a violet, and a red or a white should have plenty of foliage around it. White contrasts with blue or orange, or, still better, with red or pink, but not with yellow or violet.

FLOWERS, FOR EXHIBITION:

To place flowers on exhibition and keep fresh and to show off to good advantage, get large flakes of moss from logs, and after putting an inch or so of sand in the bottom of a shallow box, lay on this the moss, and thrust into this the flower stems; then, by watering occasionally, they keep perfectly fresh for a number of days. Crosses, rings, etc., can be formed in these boxes, and having sprigs of evergreens tacked on the sides of the boxes, the effect is beautiful. Moss placed in fancy-shaped baskets, and in these the flowers, make a pretty show.

FLOWERS, TO PACK FOR SHIPMENT:

Cut flowers should be packed in a perfectly dry condition, and whatever packing materials are used should also be dry. Considerable quantities are sent in boxes by rail to distances varying from 50 to 300 miles in the following manner with perfect success:

The bottom and sides of the box are lined with spray and fern fronds; upon that at the bottom is placed a compact layer of buds and such flowers as will not suffer from a little pressure; then comes another layer with more delicate flowers enveloped singly in a thin piece of wadding, all packed closely. This is followed by a sheet of silver paper, upon which a third and last layer of padded flowers is placed. A thin sheet of soft wadding is placed upon the top; and the lid fastened in the same manner as the fruit boxes.

FLOWERS, TO PRESERVE:

By the following process flowers may be preserved without losing their beauty of tint or form:

Get a quantity of fine sand, wash it until the last water that runs off is quite clear; then put wet sand on a board placed aslant over a pan to drain the water off. Dry the sand perfectly by the fire or in the sun. Sift it twice—once through a fine sieve, next through a coarse one; thus the sand will become nearly all of the same-sized particles, and be very fine.

Cut the flowers when full blown and in dry weather, not moist with dew or rain. Get a box of sufficient size, fill it with dry sand so high that the flowers may stand erect in it by their imbedded stems. Then put some sand in the sieve and tenderly sift it over the flowers so as not to break them; do not crumple or displace a petal. Keep the box in a warm, dry place, but not too hot. The temperature should never exceed 100 degrees. The sand absorbs the moisture of the flowers. As soon as you think the flowers are thoroughly dry open the box and slant it so as to let the upper sand run out gently; then lift them out by their stems. The flowers will be perfect, but a little brittle. In time the atmosphere will make them less so.

FLOWERS, TO PRESERVE IN WATER:

Mix a little carbonate of soda with the water in which flowers are immersed, and it will preserve them for a fortnight. Common saltpeter(1) is also a very good preservative.

(1) Potassium nitrate.

FLOWERS, TO REVIVE WHEN WITHERED:

Plunge the stems into boiling water and keep them there till the water is cold. They will quite revive. The stems may then be cut and the flowers put to stand in cold water.

FLOWER SEEDS, AUTUMN SOWING OF:

Persons say that the finest flowers they ever had of certain annuals were from "volunteer" plants from self-grown seeds. The real reason for their superiority is not due to the manner, but to the time of sowing. Seeds are "self-grown" soon after they are ripe, and the superiority of the plants from these suggests autumn sowing. The annual flowers classed as "hardy" should as a general thing, if practicable, be sown in autumn. Larkspurs and pansies are incomparably finer when thus sown. Clarkia, whitlavia, gilia, and nearly all the rest of the California annuals, to give the best results, should be sown in autumn.

FLOWER-STAND, TO MAKE:

A very pretty flower-stand can be made out of a table, a bucket, and half a dozen old tin cans. Place the bucket in the center of the table. Punch several holes in the bottom of each can and screw them firmly to the table by screws in the holes. Arches of stout wire may be made across the top of the cans. For ferns planted in the cans, which require a great deal of water, cover the top of the table with a shallow pan to catch the drip. Other plants should only have the soil kept damp. Geraniums are fine for winter blooming, as also coleus, fuchsias, and petunias. Some kind of vine should be planted in each of the corner cans. Trailing plants produce a good effect.

FLY IN TURNIPS, TO PREVENT:

From experiments lately made it has been ascertained that lime sown by hand or distributed by a machine is an infallible protection to turnips against the ravages of this destructive insect. It should be applied as soon as the turnips come up, and in the same daily rotation in which they were sown. The lime should be slaked immediately before it is used if the air be not sufficiently moist to render that operation unnecessary.

FLY-PAPER:

Coat paper with turpentine varnish, and oil it to keep the varnish from drying.

FOOD, HOW TO CHOOSE GOOD:

Nothing is more important in the affairs of housekeeping than the choice of wholesome food.

Mackerel: Must be perfectly fresh, or it is a very indifferent fish; it will neither bear carriage nor being kept many hours out of the water. The firmness of the flesh and the clearness of the eyes must be the criterion of fresh mackerel, as they are of all other fish.

Flounders: Flounders and all flat white fish are rigid and firm when fresh; the under side should be of a rich cream color. When out of season or too long kept this becomes a bluish white, and the flesh soft and flaccid. A clear, bright eye in the fish is also a mark of the being fresh and good.

Cod: Is known to be fresh by the rigidity of the muscles, (or flesh), redness of the gills, and a clearness of the eyes. Crimping much improves this fish.

Salmon: The flavor and excellence of this fish depends upon its freshness and the shortness of time since it was caught; for no method can completely preserve the delicate flavor it has when just taken out of the water.

Lobsters: Lobsters recently caught have always some remains of muscular action in the claws, which may be excited by pressing the eyes with the finger; when this cannot be produced, the lobster must have been too long kept. When boiled, the tail preserves its elasticity if fresh, but loses it as soon as it becomes stale. The heaviest lobsters are the best; when light they are watery and poor. Hen lobsters may generally be known by the spawn or by the breadth of the "flap."

Crabs: Crabs must be chosen by observations similar to those given above in the choice of lobsters. Crabs have an agreeable smell when fresh.

Prawns and Shrimps: When fresh, are firm and crisp.

Oysters: If fresh, the shell is firmly closed; when the shells of oysters are opened they are dead and unfit for food. The small-shelled oysters are the finest in flavor. Larger kinds, called rock oysters, are generally considered only fit for stewing and sauces, though some persons prefer them.

Beef: The grain of ox beef when good is loose, the meat red, and the fat inclining to yellow. Cow beef, on the contrary, has a closer grain, a whiter fat, but meat scarcely as red as that of ox beef. Inferior beef, which is meat obtained from ill-fed animals, or from those which had become too old for food, may be known by a hard, skinny fat, a dark red lean, and, in old animals, a line of horny texture running through the meat of the ribs. When meat pressed by the finger rises up quickly it may be considered as that of an animal which was in its prime; when the dent made by pressure fills slowly, or remains visible, the animal had probably passed its prime, and the meat consequently must be of inferior quality.

Veal: Should be delicately white, though it is often juicy and well-flavored when rather dark in color. Butchers, it is said, bleed calves purposely before killing them, with a view to making the flesh white, but this also makes it dry and flavorless. On examining the loin, if the fat enveloping the kidney be white and firm-looking, the meat will probably be prime and recently killed. Veal will not keep so long as an older meat, especially in hot or damp weather; when going, the fat becomes soft and moist, the meat flabby and spotted and somewhat porous, like sponge. Large, over-grown veal is inferior to small, delicate, yet fat, veal. The fillet of a cow calf is known by the udder attached to it, and by the softness of the skin; it is preferable to the veal of a bull calf.

Mutton: The meat should be firm and close in grain and red in color, the fat white and firm. Mutton is in its prime when the sheep is about 5 yrs. old, though it is often killed much younger. If too young the flesh feels tender when pinched; if too old, on being pinched it wrinkles up and so remains. In young mutton the fat readily separates; in old, it is held together by strings of skin. In sheep diseased of the rot the flesh is very pale-colored, the fat inclining to yellow, the meat appears loose from the bone, and, if squeezed, drops of water ooze out from the grains; after cooking the meat drops clean away from the bones. Whether mutton is preferred to that of the ewe; it may be known by the lump of fat on the inside of the thigh.

Lamb: This meat will not keep long after it is killed. The large vein in the neck is bluish in color when the fore-quarter is fresh, green when becoming stale. In the hind-quarter, if not recently killed, the fat of the kidney will have a slight smell, and knuckle will have lost its firmness.

Pork: When good, the rind is thin, smooth, and cool to the touch; when changing from being too long killed, it becomes flaccid and clammy. Enlarged glands, called kernels, in the fat are marks of an ill-fed or diseased pig.

Bacon: Bacon should have a thin rind and the fat should be firm and tinged red by the curing; the flesh should be of clear red, without intermixture of yellow, and it should adhere firmly to the bone. To judge the state of a ham, plunge a knife into it to the bone; on drawing it back, if particles of meat adhere to it, or if the smell is disagreeable, the curing has not been effectual, and the ham is not good; it should in such a state be immediately cooked. In buying a ham, a short, thick one is to be preferred to one long and thin.

Venison: When good the fat is clear, bright, and of considerable thickness. To know when it is necessary to cook it a knife must be plunged into the haunch, and from the smell the cook must determine on dressing or keeping it.

Turkey: In choosing poultry the age of the bird is the chief point to be attended to. An old turkey has rough and reddish legs, a young one smooth and black. Fresh killed, the eyes are full and clear and the feet moist. When it has been kept too long the parts about the vent begin to wear a greenish, discolored appearance.

Domestic Fowls: When young, have the legs and combs smooth; when old, they are rough, and on the breast long hairs are found instead of feathers. Fowls and chickens should be plump on the breast, fat on the back, and white-legged.

Geese: The bills and feet are red when old, yellow when young. Fresh killed, the feet are pliable, stiff when too long kept. Geese are called green when they are only 2 or 3 months old.

Ducks: Choose them with supple feet and hard, plump breasts. Tame ducks have yellow feet, wild ones red.

Pigeons: Pigeons are very indifferent food when too long kept. Suppleness of the feet show them to be young; the state of the flesh is flaccid when they are getting bad from keeping. Tame pigeons are larger than the wild.

Partridges: When young, have yellow legs and dark-colored bills. Old partridges are very indifferent eating.

Woodcocks and Snipes: When old, have the feet thick and hard; when these are soft and tender they are both young and fresh killed. When their bills become moist and their throats muddy they have been too long killed.

FOOD AND HEALTH:

Amount of Food Daily Needed: To replace the daily outgo we need about 2 lbs. of food and 3 lbs. of drink. With the 800 lbs. of oxygen taken from the air, a man uses in a year about 1½ tons of material. Our bodies are but molds in which a certain quantity of matter receives a definite form. They may be likened to an eddy in a river which retains its shape for a while, yet every instant each particle of water is changing.

Our strength comes from the food we eat. The food contains within it a latent force, which it gives up when it is decomposed. Putting food into our bodies is like placing a spring within a watch; every motion of the body is only a new direction given to this spring-force, as every movement of the hand on a dial is but the manipulation of the power of the bent spring in the watch. We use the pent-up energies of meat, bread, and vegetables which are placed at our service, and transfer them to a higher sphere of action.

Kinds of Food Needed: *In order to produce heat and force we require something that is combustible, something with which oxygen can combine. Three kinds of food are needed:*

(1) *Nitrogen:* That which contains a considerable proportion of nitrogen. This is a prominent constituent of the tissues of the body, and is necessary to their growth and repair. The most common forms are whites of eggs, which are nearly pure albumen; caseine, the chief constituent of cheese; lean meat, and gluten, the viscid substance that gives tenacity to dough. Bodies that have much nitrogen readily oxidize.

(2) *Carbon:* The next is carbonaceous food, or that which contains much car-bon. This consists of two kinds; first, the sugars. These contain hydrogen and oxygen in proportion to form water, and about the same amount of carbon. They may, therefore, be considered as water with carbon diffused through them. In digestion starch and gum are changed into sugar. All these are burned to produce heat. The second are the fats, which are like sugars in composition, but contain less oxygen, and not in the proportion to form water. They combine with more oxygen in burning, and thus give off more heat.

(3) *Mineral Matters and Water Needed for Food:* Food should contain mineral matter in addition to water—such as iron, sulphur, magnesia, phosphorus, salt, and potash. About 3 pints of water are needed daily to dissolve the food and carry it through the circulation, to float off waste matter, to lubricate the tissues, and by evaporation cool the system. A man weighing 154 lbs. contains 100 lbs. of water; enough if collected in a body to drown him. Iron goes to the blood-disks; lime combines with phosphorus and carbonic acid to give solidity to the bones and teeth; phosphorus is essential to the activity of the brain; salt is necessary to the secretions of some of the digestive fluids, and also to aid in working off the waste products.

Nutritious and Healthy Articles of Food: There are some articles of food of the greatest nutritive value. We mention the following: beef, mutton, fish, milk, cheese, eggs, bread, potatoes, corn, oatmeal, rice, ripe fruits, tomatoes, peas, beans etc., all of which articles of food are more or less nutritive.

- Beef and Mutton possess the greatest nutritive value of any of the meats.
- Lamb is less strengthening, but more delicate. Like the young of all animals, it should be thoroughly cooked, and at a high temperature, to properly develop its flavor.

- Pork has much carbon, and hence is very heating; the delicate and sedentary have no need of such food. It sometimes contains a parasite called trichina, which may be transferred to the human system, and produce disease and death. If eaten it should be cooked thoroughly.
- Fish is rich in phosphorus and is commended as food for the brain. It loses its mineral constituents and juices when salted.
- Oysters are highly nutritious, and are more easily assimilated when eaten raw.
- Milk is a model food, containing albumen, starch, fat, and mineral matter.
- Cheese is very nourishing, 1 lb. being equal in value to 2 lbs. of meat.
- Eggs are most easily digested when cooked soft.

Fresh or Stale Bread, Which? Fresh bread and warm biscuits are less digestible and less nutritious than old bread. In Germany bakers are prohibited from selling bread until 24 hours old. Nothing is more common in Germany than to hear the buyers at bake-shops ask for "*Alt gebackenes Brod.*"

Oatmeal: Oatmeal is a food of great strength and nutrition. It is especially serviceable as a brain food. It contains phosphorous enough to keep a man doing an ordinary amount of brain-work in good health and vigor. All medical authorities unite in the opinion that, for the proper development of the system, it is a pre-eminently useful food for growing children and the young generally. Oatmeal requires much cooking to effectually burst its starch-cells, but when it is well cooked it will thicken liquid much more than equal its weight in wheaten flour.

The oats of this country are superior to those grown on the Continent and the southern parts of England, but certainly inferior to the Scotch, where considerable pain is taken to cultivate them; and it is needless to point out that the Scotch are an example of a strong robust nation, which result is justly set down as being derived from the plentiful use of oatmeal. Dr. Guthrie has asserted that his countrymen have the largest heads of any nation in the world—not even the English have such large heads—which he attributes to the universal use of oatmeal.

Healthfulness of Fruits: The liberal use of various fruits as food is conducive to good health. Fruit is not a solid and lasting element like beef and bread, and does not give strength to any great extent. But fruits contain those acids which refresh and give tone to the system during the season when it is most needed. They should never be eaten unless thoroughly ripe or cooked. Stale fruits or those which have been plucked some time are unhealthy in the extreme. The proper time to eat fruit is in the morning

TO PREVENT HARM FROM DRINKING COLD WATER:

"It is a very safe rule to wet your wrists before drinking cold water if at all heated. The effect is immediate and grateful, and the danger of fatal results may be warded off by this simple precaution."

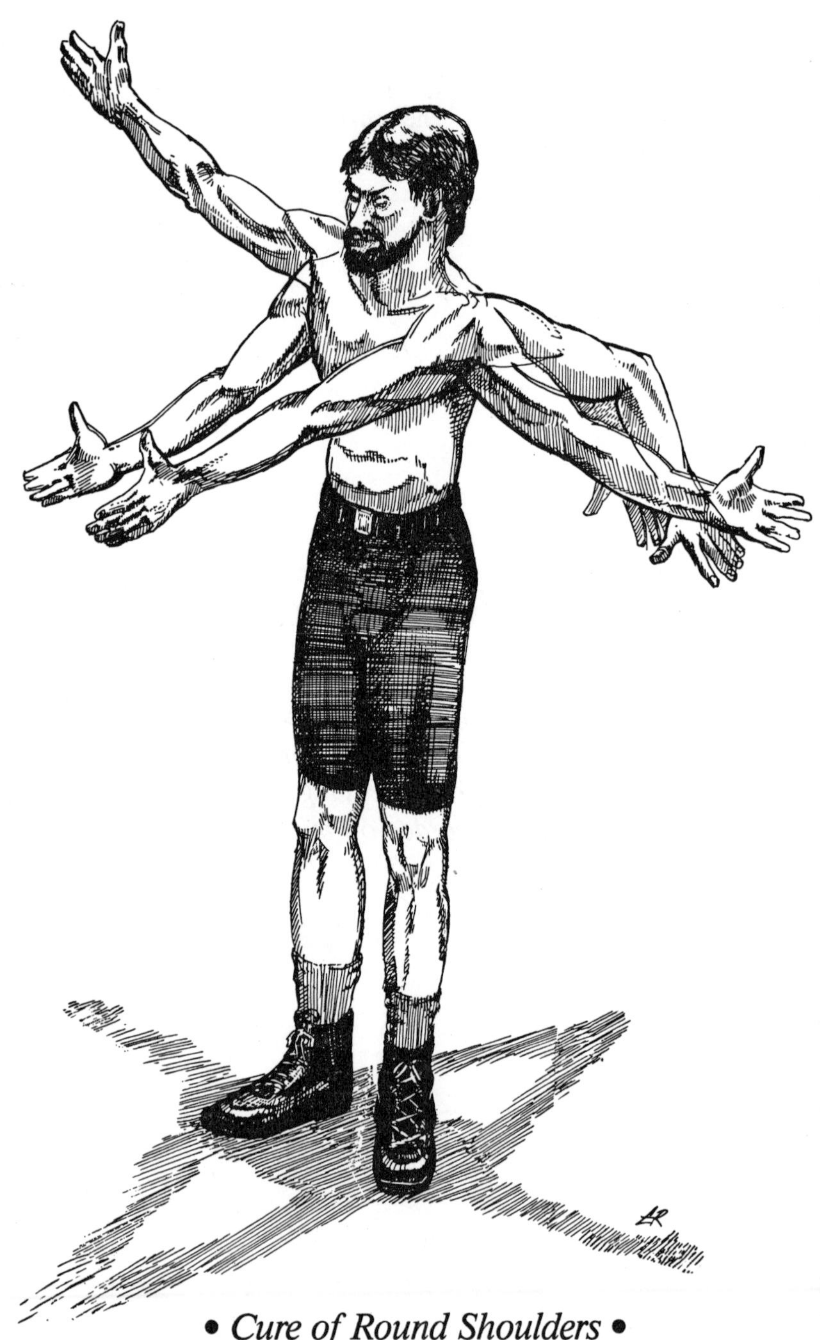

• *Cure of Round Shoulders* •

G

GALL-STONES:

Generally found in the gall bladder, but occasionally in the larger biliary ducts. They vary in size from a grain of wheat to a large hazel-nut, and some have been found as large as an hen's eggs, roundish or angular in form, and having the feel and consistence of soapstone. The pain is felt about 3 in. to the right and a little below the point of the breast-bone, is of a continuous, dull, aching character, at times becoming most excruciating. The paroxysms cause nausea and vomiting, cold sweat, small, frequent pulse, pallid face, and great exhaustion. The attacks usually come on without warning, continue from 1 to 3 hours, and stop suddenly as the stone escapes through the duct. Attacks having once occurred, are liable to be repeated.

Treatment:

(1) Sulphate of morphia, 1/4 to 1/2 grain; dissolve in 1/4 dram of water and inject under the skin of the arm with hypodermic syringe; keep the patient under the influence of this narcotic by repeating the injections 2 or 3 times in 24 hours until the obstruction has passed the gall-duct.

(2) The prolonged hot bath is often of signal benefit.

(3) To promote the solution of the gall-stone, give muriate of ammonia and extract of dandelion, of each 1/2 ounce; water, 6 fluid ounces; mix; a dessert-spoonful 3 times a day.

(4) Oil of turpentine, 3 fluid drams; sulphuric ether, 2 fluid drams, mix; 1/2 tea-spoonful night and morning.

GAPES IN FOWLS:

The parasite that causes gapes in fowl is of a red color and about three-fourths in. long. The remedies are numerous, but chiefly consist in removing the worms. One way is to moisten a feather from which all but the tip of the web has been stripped with oil, salt water, or a weak solution of carbolic acid, introduce it into the windpipe, twist it around once or twice, and then withdraw it. A tea-spoonful of sulphur mixed with a quart of corn-meal and water, and fed to the fowls morning and evening, is also a good remedy. Camphor pills will cure a chicken of the gapes. No medicine can reach them unless it does so by vapor. An hour after the chicken has swallowed the pill it smells of camphor. Camphor is a very strong vermifuge(1), and the worms die.

GARDEN PARTIES:

June, the loveliest month in the year, suggests the most charming form of outdoor entertainment—the garden party, with all its provisional beauties. The first thing to consider in respect to a festivity of this kind is the weather.

Invitations: It is considered good form to send the invitations from 2 to 4 weeks in advance, and if the party takes place some distance from town, to inclose a card stating the departure and arrival of trains, etc. The invitation should be engrossed on the note-paper bearing the family crest, (if the family are so fortunate as to have a crest).

The following is the most approved style:

Mr. and Mrs. John Brown request the pleasure of Mr. and Mrs. Tomkin's company on Wednesday, the twenty-fifth of July, at four o'clock

GARDEN PARTY. TARRYTOWN.

Locality: The garden party should be entirely in the open air; even the refreshments served under a tent, as they do in England, or, on one of our splendid dry summer days, under a wide-spreading tree or on a broad plazza, covered with rugs, and where there is an abundance of chairs and sofas. No festive scene is quite so pretty as a banquet served in the lingering twilight, or in the light made by hundreds of Chinese lanterns effectively disposed. The lawn tennis ground should be in order, the croquet ground as well, and all the adjuncts of Punch and Judy which delight grown-up children. Orchestral music of the best should be at such distance from the guests as to charm them if they choose to listen, but not to interfere with the conversation and the games. A servant should be in attendance at the gate to direct the visitors to the hostess, who stands in a conspicuous part of the grounds and receives them with her round hat or bonnet on, showing that it is an outdoor party. At Newport the hostess and her visitors remain outdoors until weary, and they adjourn to the house; but at Newport they are intensely English, following every caprice of the great court ladies to the extreme. For a private garden party it is allowable to request an invitation for a friend. If it is refused no offense should be taken.

Dress: Bonnets and short dresses are the rule for an affair of this kind; i.e., the head should be covered and the costume of a length suitable for walking, tennis, and dancing.

(1) A drug for expelling intestinal parasites.

Games: Ours is essentially a country for garden parties. Even England is famed for entertainments of the kind, where a shower may at any moment destroy Worth costumes and loves of bonnets. Queen Victoria is said to be passionately fond of garden parties, and attends several each season, either freezing her attendants by her haughty ways or making sunshine by her smiles and good cheer. It is a pretty fashion for the young girls who are to play tennis to dress in harmonizing colors—say half in blue and half in white, their partners adapting their colors as nearly as possible. A pretty woman once said: "I will not attend a garden party. I look blousy at such an affair, my face gets red, my hair gets out of curl, my dress is torn, spiders crawl over me, angle worms cross in the paths, and all sorts of abominations get into my lemonade; in fact, it destroys my temper for days to attend an affair of this kind." This, however, is a woman who has greater consideration for her personal appearance than for the beauties of nature or the charm of outdoor companionship.

Duties of Servants: Servants should be taught the proprieties of an outdoor festival, and attend to the removal of plates, knives and forks, and the fragments from the table, and constantly replenish all that is needed.

Refreshments: Fruit is now served on such occasions; strawberries, pines, melons, peaches, grapes; tea, coffee, soda-water, and apollinaris water are served at a separate table. Gentlemen help themselves and serve the ladies. If fruit is served, a small napkin should be placed between the plate and the saucer holding it. Ices and creams are served in lint paper cups. Camp-stools and small tables scattered over the grounds are indispensable as centers for gatherings of guests and for refreshments. As much destruction of glass and china takes place, a hostess generally hires the dishes and the glass, and has an abundance of the cheap and pretty Chinese paper napkins ready for use.

Etiquette: A garden party is a very troublesome and costly affair, but it is very pretty, often picturesque. There is no prescribed etiquette about them, an inventive hostess making her own rules and routines, and, after receiving her guests, letting them amuse themselves. There are people who are at ease anywhere. A garden party is a good place to test one's capabilities in this direction. The garden party is first cousin to the picnic. It is more exclusive, more elegant. The English borrowing the idea from the French, and the Americans from the English. The first parties of the kind were given at Newport, and are now popular summer entertainments throughout the country.

GARGET(1) IN COWS:

It is said that 8 drops of tincture of aconite dropped on a piece of bread and mixed with the food at night, and next morning 4 drops more given in the same manner, will generally complete the cure of garget in cows.

GARGLES:

Gargles are used to stimulate chronic sore throats or relaxed state of the swallow or uvula.

- *Acidulated:* Mix 1 part of white vinegar with 3 parts of honey of roses and 24 of barley-water. Use in chronic inflammations of the throat, malignant sore throat, etc.
- *Astringent:* Take 2 drams of roses and mix with 8 ounces of boiling water, infuse for 1 hour, strain, and add 1 dram of alum and 1 ounce of honey of roses. Use in severe sore throat, relaxed uvula, etc.
- *For Slight Inflammation of the Throat:* Add 1 dram of sulphuric ether to $^1/_2$ ounce of syrup of marsh-mallows and 6 ounces of barley-water. This may be used frequently.

GAS-METER, TO PREVENT FROM FREEZING:

Half a pint of good glycerine is said to prevent the freezing of 1 gallon of water, though at least double the proportion is preferable in the country, whatever the temperature in the winter may happen to be.

GEESE, HOW TO SELECT:

In old birds the bills and feet are red, in young ones they are yellow. When fresh killed the feet are pliable, when long kept they become quite stiff. It is said that geese will thrive better and their flesh be more delicately flavored if fed upon raw potatoes than upon any other substance.

GERANIUMS, HOW TO PRESERVE OLD PLANTS THROUGH THE WINTER:

Take them out of the borders in autumn, before they have received any injury from frost, and let this be done on a dry day. Shake off all the earth from their roots, and suspend them with their heads downward in a cellar or dark room where they will be free from frost. The leaves and shoots will become yellow and sickly, but when potted about the end of May, and exposed to a gentle heat, they will recover and vegetate luxuriantly. The old plants, stripped of their leaves, may also be packed closely in sand, and in this way, if kept free from frost, they will shoot out from the roots, and may be re-potted in the spring.

(1) Distemper in cattle, accompanied by a swelling of the throat and neighboring parts.

GERMAN PASTE, FOOD FOR SINGING-BIRDS:

Take 1 pint of pea-flour, in which rub a new laid egg; then add 2 ounces of fresh lard and 3 ounces of honey or treacle; continue to rub this well, so as to prevent its being in a large lumps; when reduced to a fine powder, put it into a clean earthen pipkin(1), and place it over a slow and clear fire until warmed through, stirring it all the while to prevent its burning. When sufficiently hot take it off and pass it through a fine wire sieve; then add about 2 ounces of maw-seed, and if hemp-seed is thought essential, give the small Russian whole, in preference to the common sort bruised, as it only tends to bring on the husk or dry cough.

Birds will eat it whole, and it will do them equal good, and prevent nasty and troublesome complaints, which oftentimes stop them when in full song, until they bring up the small particles of the hulls of the bruised hempseed.

GIANTESS, GAME OF THE:

This is a very amusing deception. A tall young lad is dressed in a petticoat. Then a large umbrella is covered over its silk ribs with a gown and cloak; a ball, and a bonnet and thick veil put on it. The umbrella is partially opened, so that its ribs set out the dress and cloak as a crinoline does.

The player gets under it, and holding the handle up as high as the hall-door to pretend that there is an arrival, and a minute or two afterward the footman is to open the drawing-room door and announce, "Miss Tiny Littlegirl." The giantess then walks into the drawing-room, to the amazement of the company, bows, etc. It has a good effect to enter holding the umbrella-handle naturally, and then to raise it by degrees, which will give a comical appearance of growth. We have seen the giantess thus appear to rise till she peered over the tops of the highest pictures in the room. The effect is exceedingly funny. She may talk to the company also, bending her head down toward them, and speaking in a shrill tone of voice. In clever hands the giantess causes a great deal of fun.

GILDING, TO CLEAN:

Remove all dust with a soft brush; then wash the gilding lightly and rapidly with warm water in which an onion has been boiled. Dry it by rubbing with soft cloths.

GILDING CHINA AND GLASS:

Powdered gold is mixed with borax and gum-water, and the solution applied with a camel's-hair pencil. Heat is then applied by a stove until the borax fuses, when the gold is fixed and afterward burnished.

(1) A small earthen boiler.

GILDING LIQUID:

Take of fine gold, 5 ounces, (troy); nitromuriatic acid, 52 ounces; dissolve by heat, and continue the heat until red or yellow vapors are evolved; decant the liquid into a proper vessel; add of distilled water 4 gallons; pure bicarbonate of potash, 20 lbs.; boil for 2 hours.

GILDING ON WOOD:

To gild in oil the wood, after being properly prepared, is covered with a coat of gold size, made of drying linseed oil mixed with yellow ocher; when this has become so dry as to adhere to the fingers without soiling them, the gold-leaf is laid on with great care and dexterity and pressed down with cotton wool; places that have been missed are covered with small pieces of gold-leaf, and when the whole is dry the ragged bits are rubbed off with the cotton. This is by far the easiest mode of gilding; any other metallic leaves may be applied in a similar manner.

Pale leaf gold has a greenish yellow color, and is an alloy of gold and silver. Dutch gold-leaf is only copper-leaf colored with the fumes of zinc; quantities of gilding are required in places where it can be defended from the weather, as it changes color if exposed to moisture, and it should be covered with varnish. Silver-leaf is prepared every way the same as gold-leaf, but when applied should be kept well covered with varnish, otherwise it is liable to tarnish; a transparent yellow varnish will give it the appearance of gold. Whenever gold is fixed by means of linseed oil it will bear washing off, which burnished gold will not.

GILT CORNICES, TO CLEAN:

Wash them well with warm milk, and polish them with a soft wash-leather.

GILT FRAMES, TO CLEAN:

(1) White of eggs, 2 ounces; chloride of potash or soda, 1 ounce; mix well, blow off the dust from the frames; then go over them with a soft brush dipped in the mixture, and they will appear equal to new.

(2) Take sufficient flour of sulphur to give a golden tinge to about $1^1/_2$ pints of water, and in this boil 4 or 5 bruised onions, or garlic, which will answer the same purpose. Strain off the liquid, and with it, when cold, wash with a soft brush any gilding which requires restoring, and when dry it will come out as bright as new work.

(3) When the gilt frames of pictures or looking-glasses, or the moldings of rooms, have specks of dirt upon them from flies or other causes, they may be cleaned with white of egg laid on with a camel's-hair pencil.

GIRAFFE, GAME OF THE:

Provided with an artificial head as nearly like that of a giraffe as possible, no difficulty need be feared. First of all, the head must be fastened to the end of a long stick. One of two performers must then hold the stick aloft, while his companion, standing close behind, must place himself in a stooping position, so as to make the outline of his own person like that of the lower part of the giraffe's body. The long stick will, of course, form part of the body. A cloth is then pinned round the stick and round the bodies of the two performers, leaving the legs, of course, to represent the legs of the giraffe. A rope tail must be stuck in by some means of other, and, if cleverly managed, it is astonishing what an excellent imitation of the real animal can thus be manufactured.

GIRDLING:

This is usually done to fruit-trees to promote early and full bearing by preventing the sap from returning into the roots, and forcing it to expand itself among the fruits and flowers. It is done by taking out a rim of bark entirely around the tree, limb, or vine not over 1/4 inch wide. Sometimes this space is healed up the first year, but certainly the second year, if the tree be not too feeble and sickly. Another method is to take coarse twine or fine wire and wind it several times around the tree above the lower limbs and tie it as tight as possible. Girdling is also performed in clearing new ground of timber when there is not time to remove it entirely. A portion of the bark 1 or 2 ft. in length is cut out all around the butt in spring. This kills the tree.

GLASS, HOW TO CUT:

It is not generally known that glass may be cut under water with a strong pair of scissors. If a round or oval be required, take a piece of common window glass, draw the shape upon it in a black line; sink it with your left hand under water as deep as you can without interfering with the view of the line, and with your right use the scissors to cut away what is not required.

Another way is to dip a worsted thread in spirits of turpentine, and tie it close round the glass where it is intended to be cut; then set fire to the thread, and while it is burning, plunge the glass into cold water, or well wet the thread with it. The glass will break easily in the direction of the thread.

GLASS, TO PREVENT CRACKING:

(1) While pouring very hot water into a tumbler or other glass vessel never hold the tumbler in your hand, but leave it on a tray or table. It is advisable also to warm the glass before using it, and to keep a spoon in it during the time of pouring. These are the best methods to prevent the cracking of the glass.

(2) Place your tumblers, chimneys, or vessels which you desire to keep

from cracking in a pot filled with cold water and a little cooking salt; allow the mixture to boil well over a fire, and then cool slowly. Glass treated in this way is said not to crack, even if exposed to very sudden changes of temperature. Chimneys become very durable by this process, which may also be extended to crockery, stoneware, porcelain, etc. The process is simply one of annealing, and the slower the process, especially the cooling portion of it, the more effective will be the work.

GLASS AND CHINA, TO DRILL:

To drill china use a copper drill and emery, moistened with spirits of turpentine. To drill glass use a steel drill tempered as hard as possible and camphor and water as a lubricant. Moisten the tool with dilute sulphuric acid. This last is better than turpentine.

GLASS AND CHINA, TO SEASON:

To season glass and china ware to sudden changes of temperature, so that it will remain sound after exposure to sudden heat and cold, is best done by placing the articles in cold water, which must gradually be brought to the boiling point and then allowed to cool very slowly, taking several hours to do it. The commoner the material the more care in this respect is required.

GLASSES, HINTS UPON USING:

Persons finding their eyes becoming dry and itching on reading, as well as those who find it necessary to place an object nearer than 14 in. from their face to read, need spectacles. Persons under 40 yrs. of age should not wear glasses until the accommodating power of the eyes has been suspended and the exact state of refraction determined by a competent ophthalmic surgeon.

The spectacle in glasses sold by peddlers and by jewelers generally are hurtful to the eyes of those who read much, as the lenses are made of inferior sheet glass and are not symmetrically ground. No matter how perfectly the lenses may be made, unless they are mounted in a suitable frame and properly placed before the eye discomfort will arise from their prolonged use.

There are three systems of grading spectacle lenses, the English, the metric, and the Prussian. Those made to supply the demands of the trade in this country are carelessly made, and are poor imitations of either the English or the metrical system. The metrical scale has no English equivalent, is not graded by any uniform rule of dividing the inter-focal spaces, and is therefore unsuited to the exacting demands of science.

Persons holding objects too near the face endanger the safety of their eyes, and incur the risk of becoming near-sighted. The near-sighted eye is an unsound eye, and should be fully corrected with a glass, notwithstanding the fact that it may need no aid for reading. The proper time to begin wearing glasses is just as soon as the eyes tire on being subjected to prolonged use.

GLASS STOPPERS, TO LOOSEN:

(1) Put 1 or 2 drops of sweet-oil round the stopper, close to the mouth of the bottle; then put a little distance for the fire. When the decanter gets warm, have a wooden instrument with a cloth wrapped tightly round it; then strike the stopper, first on one side, then on the other; by persevering a little while you will most likely get it out.

(2) Lay the bottle in warm water, so that the neck of the stopper may be under water. Let it soak for a time, then knock it with a wooden instrument as before.

(3) Drop some glycerine in the surrounding crevice and after an hour or two it will loosen.

GLASS TUBES, TO BEND:

Hold the tube in the upper part of the flame of a spirit-lamp, revolving it slowly between the fingers; when red hot it may be easily bent into any desired shape. To soften large tubes a lamp with a double current of air should be used, as it gives a much stronger heat than the simple lamp.

GLOSS ON LINEN, TO PRODUCE:

Put boiling water in a vessel, and add pieces of white wax and spermaceti about the size of a half dollar, boil well together, then remove from the fire and add starch mixed with cold water. Stir well while mixing, and put it back on the fire; boil 2 or 3 minutes, stirring well. Rub well into the clothes, and when ironing use a common iron, and then take a damp cloth, wrung out well in hot water, and rub over the shirt and collar, and use the polisher right away, and I can really say you will have as nice a polish as any one could wish for.

GLOVES, HOW TO PUT ON:

A great deal depends on the first putting on of gloves. Have the hands perfectly clean, dry, and cool, and never put on new gloves while the hands are warm or damp. Where a person is troubled with moist hands it is well to powder them before trying on the gloves; but in most cases, if the hands are dry and cool, this is not needed. First work on the fingers, keeping the thumb outside of the glove and the wrist of the glove turned back. When the fingers are in smoothly, put in the thumb and work the glove on very carefully; then, placing the elbow on the knee, work on the hand. When this is done smooth down the wrist and button the second button first, then the third, and so on to the end; then smooth down the whole glove and fasten the first button.

Fastening the first button last when putting on a glove for the first time makes a good deal of difference in the fit, although it may seem but a very little thing. It does not strain the part of the glove that is the easiest to strain at first, and prevents the enlarging of the button-hole, either of which is sure to take place if you begin at the first button to fasten the glove.

When removing gloves never begin at the tips of the fingers to pull them off, but turn back the wrist and pull off carefully, which will, of course, necessitate their being wrong side out. Turn them right side out, turn the thumb in, smooth them out lengthwise as near as possible the shape they would be if on the hands, and place away with a strip of white canton flannel between if the gloves are light, but if dark colored the flannel may be omitted. Never roll gloves into each other in a wad, for they will never look as well after. There is always some moisture in them from the hands; consequently, when rolled up this moisture has no chance of drying, and must work into the gloves, making them hard and stiff, and of very little use after, as far as looks or fit are concerned.

GLOVES, KID, TO CLEAN:

(1) Pour 1 tea-cupful of benzine into a pint bowl and put a pair of gloves into it, soaking them completely and rubbing them together just as if you were washing cotton rags; then rinse them in fresh, clean benzine; squeeze them as dry as you can; beat them against each other and hang them out in the air. In an hour or less the odor will be gone and they will be found to be clean and soft.

(2) Go over them with a clean towel dipped in skim-milk, wearing them during the process and until they are quite dry.

(3) Procure some gasoline, put on one glove, pour some of the fluid into a saucer, and cork the bottle to prevent evaporation; then rub the glove all over quite hard with a sponge wet with the contents of the saucer; keep the glove on your hand until nearly dry, but avoid stoves and lamps; then repeat the operation with the other. The odor of gasoline is disagreeable. Hang the gloves out of the window for a while. Then put away with a sachet.

GLOVES, LANGUAGE OF:

For "yes," drop one glove from the right into the left hand. "No" is said by rolling both gloves in the right hand. If you want to express that you are indifferent to a partner, take the right-hand glove partly off. If you wish a male friend to follow you into the next room, strike your left arm with both gloves. "I love you still" is expressed by slowly and carefully smoothing both gloves. If the fair she desires to know whether her affection is reciprocated, she is to put on half the left-hand glove, one finger at a time.

"Be on your guard against the governor," or "my mother-in-law" as the case may be, is a message often sent, and is given by delicately twisting the glove fingers round the thumb. If the damsel is in a quarrelsome mood, she simply makes a cross with both her gloves and proceeds to lay them on her lap in this position. These are the principal and most simple rules.

GOLD, TO CLEAN:

Dissolve a little sal-ammoniac in urine; boil your soiled gold therein, and it will become clean and brilliant.

GOLD ARTICLES, TO RESTORE COLOR:

Tarnished gold colored articles may be restored by the following method: Dissolve 1 ounce of bicarbonate of soda, 1/2 ounce of chloride of lime, and 1/2 ounce of common salt in about 4 ounces of boiling water. Take a clean brush, and wash the article with the hot solution for a few seconds and rinse immediately in 2 clean waters. Dry in warm sawdust, and finally rub over with tissue-paper.

GOLD-FISH:

Where gold-fish are kept in vessels in rooms they should be in spring water. The water will require to be changed, according to the size of the vessel or the number of fish kept therein; but it is not well to change the water too often. In a vessel that will hold a common sized pail of water 2 fish may be kept by changing the water once a fortnight; and so on in proportion. If any food is supplied them, it should be few crumbs of bread dropped into the water once or twice a week.

GOLD LACQUER:

Gold lacquer, closely resembling the real Chinese article, is made by first melting to a perfectly fluid mixture 2 parts copal and 1 part shellac. Top this add 2 parts good boiled oil. Remove the vessel from the fire, and gradually mix in 10 parts of turpentine. To give color, add a solution of gum guttæ in turpentine for yellow, or of dragon's blood(1) for red; a sufficient quantity of coloring material being used to give the desired shade.

GOUT REMEDY:

Half an ounce of niter (saltpeter), 1/2 ounce of sulphur, 1/2 ounce of flour of mustard, 1/2 ounce of Turkey rhubarb, 1/4 ounce of powdered guaiacum. Mix, and take a table-spoonful every other night for 3 nights, and omit 3 nights, in a wine-glassful of cold water—water which has been previously well boiled.

(1) A red resin from the ripe fruit and leaves of several palms.

GOOD MANNERS:

At Home:

- Wake up good-natured.
- The first cross word spoils the day.
- Wash, arrange your hair, clean your nails and teeth, clean out your throat and head in the privacy of your own room. Personal cleanliness is one of the first conditions of good health and good manners. What seems inoffensive to you may be disgusting to others.
- Say "Good morning" to the different members of the family.
- Notice the servants pleasantly. Show your appreciation of their desire to please, yet avoid being too familiar with them. "Fair words don't butter the cabbage," but they have a tendency to improve the cook.
- Don't monopolize the morning paper.
- Don't take possession of the only easy-chair.
- Don't take up more room than you are entitled to. Remember that other people have their rights and privileges.
- Don't snuffle.
- Avoid picking your teeth. Avoid picking your face. Avoid picking your nose. Avoid biting your nails. Avoid scratching your head. Avoid drumming with hands or feet. Avoid shaking your foot continually. Avoid making grimaces. Avoid staring at people. Avoid speaking sharply, or scolding. Avoid slang expressions. Avoid fault-finding.
- Don't laugh at your own jokes. Don't run out the tongue when speaking. Don't make fun of people behind their backs.
- Observe what refined people do, and do likewise. If you imitate the vulgar, you will soon be as vulgar as they.
- Have a place for every thing, and see that every thing is in its place.
- Brush your clothes carefully, and clean off unsightly spots. For this purpose keep liquid ammonia and alcohol among your toilet articles.
- Do not go about the house in untidy dress. Ladies and gentlemen should never be seen in soiled or ragged wrappers, or in garments minus the buttons and strings that are essential to their proper appearance.
- Don't go whistling, singing, or shouting through the house. If

you want to find people, go where you think they are, and don't call out to them.

- Be as civil to your own folks as you would be to strangers.
- Knock at a closed door before entering.
- Do not listen to private conversations.
- Do not repeat what you hear.
- Do not make trouble by being too particular.
- Learn to take care of your own room. Practice making the bed; it is an art to make one nicely.
- Study how to make home attractive.
- Devise games for the children.
- Read only good literature. Talk about what you have read; it is a good way to impress it upon your mind.
- Be ready to help where ever help is needed. Be sympathetic and kind. Do not turn a deaf ear to the complaints of the afflicted; sympathy heals many wounds.
- Seek the society of those older than yourself, that you may learn something from them.
- Cultivate the society of young people, that you may impart what you have learned, and keep your heart from growing old.
- Be busy. There is plenty of work to do in the world. See to it that you are doing your share. Find your place and strive to fill it acceptably.
- Form a habit of prayer.
- Quiet manners are everywhere a mark of good breeding. It is ill-bred to walk heavily or to slam doors.
- Profane and indecent words degrade you. If you respect yourself you will not use them, nor listen to them.
- Civilities, even from members of our own household, should always be received with some kind of an acknowledgment. The atmosphere of a house is what makes it home-like. Every living creature has an atmosphere of his own. He can be as chilly and damp and disagreeable as a March wind; he can be as bright, cheerful, and charming as a June morning; he can be as dark and impenetrable as a November fog, or as crisp and electric as a day in December. It depends entirely on ourselves whether we are ugly, cross, tyrannical, fretful, nagging, sulky, and unbearable, or kind, considerate, tender, thoughtful, cheery, sweet, and wholesome. The atmosphere of

one person can destroy the comfort of a roomful; in fact, upset the whole house.

- Learn to accommodate yourself to the unavoidable circumstances.
- Be companionable. Bring into the house all the sunshine you possibly can, that your presence may be its chief attraction.

At Table:

- Parents should train their children by example as well as by precept to be attentive and polite to each other at every meal.
- Be thankful for what is set before you.
- Do not unpleasantly criticise the food.
- Do not sit either crowded against the table or at an inconvenient distance.
- Unfold your napkin, which should be at the left side of the plate. Spread it over your lap.
- It is rude and awkward to place your hands or elbows on the table, or to move them so as to incommode those on either side of you.
- Eat without noise. Part the lips widely enough to admit the spoon, so that when you take soup or other liquids you will not make a sound suggestive of a pig at a trough.
- Do not put large pieces of food into the mouth.
- Test your tea or coffee with a spoon, so that when you drink it from the cup you will not run the risk of scalding your mouth. Never blow it to cool it.
- Never drink from the saucer, not even at home, for if you make a practice of doing it there you will involuntary perform the same trick elsewhere, to your great mortification.
- Never tip your chair back at table—or anywhere else.
- Eat slowly. Chew your food well.
- Don't talk with your mouth full.
- Drink as little as possible with your meals.
- Be cheerful. Avoid talking about diseases, accidents, medicines, bad dreams, sores, wounds, or any thing that would be likely to offend.
- Spitting, sneezing, or hard blowing of the nose at table are all alike objectionable. If obliged to use your handkerchief do it quietly, and turn your head from the table.

- Never spit out upon your plate bones, cherry-stones, grape-skins, etc., but either carry them to it with the hand or upon the spoon or fork.
- Do not gormandize upon one or two articles that are especially to your taste. It is extremely vulgar.
- Avoid stiffness or formality. We may be decorous without being ceremonious.
- When there are waiters, ask one of them quietly for what you want, not loudly nor rudely.
- Always lift and pass food to others courteously, and never shove it across the table.
- Avoid putting your knife in your mouth. The knife should never come near the lips. Use your fork.
- Avoid putting your own knife, spoon, or fork into any dish but your own.
- If it is necessary to remove any obstruction from between the teeth let it be done in an unobtrusive manner, holding the napkin before the mouth with the left hand. Even this is to be avoided if possible.
- Do not blow your breath in any one's face. Turn your head aside when you cough. Breathe gently.
- If you enjoy picking bones, gratify your taste at your own table, or among intimate friends.
- If you prefer corn from the cob, break the cob in two in your napkin, and you will find it thus very easily managed.
- Don't gnaw like a brute creature.
- Do not grasp the fork, but handle it gracefully in carrying food to the mouth. In olden times, when the steel or iron fork with two formidable prongs was in use, there was some excuse for bringing the knife into play.

On The Street:

- In the first place, dress within your means.
- Too glaring colors, "loud" costumes, and a profusion of showy jewelry are not in good taste.
- Neatness in a lady's dress is one of the first requisites.
- Do not accustom yourself to loud talking on the street, in stores, or public conveyances, or anywhere else. Emerson says, "A gentleman makes no noise; a lady is serene."

- A gentleman offers his right arm to a lady on the street or in the house, that she may have her right hand free for holding her parasol or guiding her train.
- A gentleman precedes a lady in passing through a crowd; ladies precede gentlemen under ordinary circumstances.
- One should never stare at another.
- Ladies should not talk or call across the street.
- In public conveyances all should endeavor to make room for passengers entering, and no gentleman will retain his seat when there are ladies standing.
- No lady will accept a seat vacated by a gentleman for her convenience without a smile, a bow, or thanks.
- Violent swinging of the arms when walking in the street is an ill-bred habit.
- Never obtrude talk on politics or religion in a public conveyance.
- In the cars one has no right to keep a window open if the current of air thus produced annoys or endangers the health of another.
- In shaking hands always present the whole hand, and never one or two fingers.
- To eat any thing, even confectionery, in the street, is decidedly ill-bred.
- Never put on your gloves in the street.
- Avoid humming or rocking continually in company.
- Do not drum on the back of the car seat, or on the window or floor, or keep up a tapping on the toe of your boot or shoe when traveling, as these sounds are very disturbing to many persons. A loud noise is far less irritating than these little scratches or scrapes, or that which has been appropriately designated as "the devil's tattoo."
- Study the comfort of others more than your own.
- Always endeavor to conceal a yawn.
- A gentleman should always return the bow of a lady.
- Turn out your toes when walking, and allow the weight of the body to rest upon the hip joints, unless you wish to appear as ungraceful as the ostrich.
- Avoid hawking and spitting.

- Do not sit cross-legged in company, especially in a public conveyance.
- Make no display of your feet or your hands. Do not call attention to them on account of their size.
- Self-consciousness is the trade-mark of vanity and the scourge of modesty. "Handsome is that handsome does," is an old proverb that can never be worn out by oft repeating. Johnson's uncouth manners gave him marked individuality, but added not to his list of personal friends. Had Carlyle cultivated the graces of the heart he would have been a wiser and lovelier man, and would not have known the pangs of remorse which tormented him at the last.

In Church:

- Cultivate reverence, and manifest it by respectful manners.
- If a habit has been formed of being invariably behind time, it ought to be broken up as soon as possible, because it is offensive and, to say the least, impolite.
- Be attentive to strangers.
- The house of God is not the proper place for the display of gaudy apparel. Dress neatly, and richly if you can afford it, but not showily. Be clothed upon with humility.
- Don't fidget about uneasily or stare at the congregation.
- Do not form the habit of offensively criticising the minister.
- Pay diligent attention to the sermon. The pulpit receives its inspiration from the pews, and the more sympathetic the hearers the better the preaching.
- Be not cold and exclusive. Rich and poor, strangers and friends, should meet as in a common home in a place dedicated to the Father of all.
- Take part in the singing. Every one can sing praise in his heart, if he does not know one note of music from another.
- Make no unnecessary noises with fan, book, cane, umbrella, throat, or pew-door, and attract as little attention to yourself as possible.
- Do not criticise your neighbors.
- "Remember the Sabbath day to keep it holy." Let its influence be felt in your looks, your speech your manners, and your mind. A devotional attitude may be as impressive as a sermon to young children who cannot understand the minister, but are

very observing of those who sit in sacred places. Be careful not to offend these little ones.

Golden Rules for Boys and Girls:

(1) Shut every door after you, and without slamming it.

(2) Never shout, jump, or run in the house.

(3) Never call to persons up stairs, or in the next room; if you wish to speak to them, go quietly where they are.

(4) Always speak kindly and politely to the servants, if you would have them do the same to you.

(5) When told to do, or not to do, a thing by either parent, never ask why you should or should not do it.

(6) Tell of your own faults and misdoings, not those of your brothers and sisters.

(7) Carefully clean the mud or snow off your boots before entering the house.

(8) Be prompt at every meal hour.

(9) Never sit down at the table or in the parlor with dirty hands or tumbled hair.

(10) Never interrupt any conversation, but wait patiently your turn to speak.

(11) Never reserve your good manners for company, but be equally polite at home and abroad.

(12) Let your first, last, and best friend be your mother.

GOOSEBERRIES, RED, TO KEEP.

Pick gooseberries when fully ripe, and for each quart take 1/4 lb. of sugar and 1 gill of water; boil together until quite a syrup; then put in the fruit, and continue to boil gently for 15 minutes; then put them into small stone jars; when cold, cover them close; keep them for making tarts and pies.

GOOSEBERRIES, TO DRY:

To 7 lbs. of red gooseberries add 1 1/2 lbs. of powdered sugar, which must be strewed over them in the preserving pan; let them remain at good heat over a slow fire till they begin to break; then remove them. Repeat this process for 2 or 3 days; then take the gooseberries from the syrup, and spread them out on sieves near the fire to dry. This syrup may be used for other preserves. When the gooseberries are quite dry, store them in tin boxes or layers of paper.

GRACES, GAME OF:

Two players are each provided with 2 small hoops and 2 sticks, and the game is to throw the hoops from the sticks and to catch them again on the sticks in the same succession as the bags are thrown and caught in the game of that name. The hoops are also sometimes thrown from both sticks, and caught on one or both, according to the wish or the ability of the players; the object being not to allow the hoops to fall to the ground. This game is sometimes called by its French name, *Les Graces*.

GRAFTING WAX, TO MAKE:

Common grafting wax is made by taking 1 part of tallow, 3 of beeswax, and 4 of resin, and melting them together over a slow fire. Melt the resin first, and put in the other ingredients after, stirring well together.

GRAMMAR IN RHYME:

Of course the whole science of grammar cannot be comprised in 20 lines of verse, but the 10 couplets which are here given have started many young learners upon the difficult road which leads to the mastery of language. The lines are worth remembering.

Three little words you often see
Are articles a, an, and the.

A noun's the name of any thing.
As school or garden, hoop or swing.

Adjectives tell the kind of noun,
As great, small, pretty, white, or brown.

Instead of nouns the pronouns stand—
Her head, his face your arm, my hand.

Verbs tell of something to be done—
To read count, laugh, sing, jump, or run.

How things are done the adverbs tell
As slowly, quickly, ill, or well.

Conjunctions join the words together,
As men and women, wind or weather.

The preposition stands before A noun,
As in or through the door.

The interjection shows surprise.
As O! how pretty, Ah! how wise.

The whole are called nine parts of speech,
Which reading, writing, speaking teach.

GRANITE, TO IMITATE:

For the ground color stain your white-lead to a light lead color with lamp-black and a little rose pink. Throw on black spots, with a graniting machine, a pale red, and fill up with white before the ground is dry.

GRAPES, TO DRY:

The grapes are allowed to remain on the vine until of a golden color and translucent; they are then picked and put on wooden trays, 2 by 3 ft. in size, placed between the rows, sloping to the sun. When half dried they are turned by putting a tray on the top, and by inverting them both are transferred to the new tray. When the grapes lose their ashy appearance, and after removing the green ones, the rest are put into large sweat boxes, left there for 2 weeks, when the stems are tough and the raisins soft. The packing follows, in which iron or steel packing frames are used, the raisins being assorted, weighed, inspected, and made presentable.

GRAPES, TO PRESERVE:

Pick off all unsound or unripe ones and lay the clusters in an empty room on papers until dry, for in all packages some will be crushed and dampen others. Any empty crate will do to pack them in. First a layer of grapes, then a layer of paper, so as to exclude the air and keep them separate, then grapes and then paper, until you have 3 or 4 layers, not more than 4. If the box is to hold more put in a partition to support the others that are to be packed. Thus put up in the fall, grapes will keep perfectly until past the middle of March.

GRAPEVINES, WINTER CARE OF:

All varieties of grapevines not thoroughly hardy should receive some winter protection to secure best results, and it is claimed by many that it pays to give protection to the hardiest kinds even. Some growers attribute their success with Delaware, Duchess, Roger's Hybrids, etc., simply to covering, while their neighbors signally fail with the same varieties. As the treatment in both cases is exactly alike, the different results can only be attributed to the protection given in one case and its omission in the other. The process is simple, and depends on the extent of the operation.

After the vines have shed their leaves and matured their wood they should be pruned, and on the approach of cold weather loosened from the trellis, bent down on the ground, and held there with stakes, rails, or something similar. This is sometimes found sufficient, especially when snow lies till late in the spring. If not satisfied with this dependence, a slight covering with leaves, straw, cornstalks, or limbs of evergreens will prove effectual.

If danger is to be apprehended from the depredations of mice, which in some sections are very troublesome, a slight covering of earth on top is all that is necessary. It should be remembered that it is the young wood of the present season's growth that is to be protected; this contains the buds in which are the embryo fruit cluster for next year's crop. Of course, similar protection would not hurt in the old wood, but it is not always feasible to provide it. But the main question necessary preceding all this, on which depends the success or entire failure of the whole operation, is the maturity and thorough ripening of the wood.

GRASSES, TO CRYSTALLIZE:

Ladies who admire beautiful bouquets of grass will appreciate the following recipe: Take 1½ lbs. of rock alum, pour on 3 pints of boiling water; when quite cool put in a wide-mouthed vessel, hang in your grasses, a few at a time. Do not let them get too heavy, or the stems will not support them. You may again heat alum and add more grasses. By adding a little coloring matter it will give a pleasing variety.

GRAVEL:

Steep ½ lb. of hops in a quart of water and give it as hot as the horse can stand it.

GREYNESS, PREMATURE:

There is a premature grayness which sometimes occurs in the young, chiefly in those of light complexions and light-colored hair, which is the consequence of weakness of the nervous power. This, as well as the loosening and falling out of the hair, which come often from the same cause, may be checked by increase of the general vigor and the use of proper local remedies. A useful practice, when the hair is sufficiently short to admit of it, is to plunge the head in cold water morning and night, and, after thoroughly drying, to brush it briskly until the scalp is warmed to a glow. A simple lotion composed of ½ ounce of vinegar of cantharides, and an ounce each of cologne and rose waters, rubbed on the scalp, will probably be found beneficial.

GREASE-SPOTS, TO REMOVE:

(1) Cover the spots with French chalk, buckwheat, potter's clay, or magnesia; over this place a piece of brown paper; set a moderately warm iron on this, and let it remain till it gets cold. Be careful not to have the iron so hot as to scorch or change the color of the cloth.

(2) Gasoline or benzine is excellent for cleaning coat-collars, etc. The stained portion should be laid between 2 sheets of blotting-paper, and the upper sheet well soaked with benzine. In this way, if sufficient time be given, the whole of the fatty matter becomes dissolved and absorbed by the paper.

(3) Turpentine, chloroform, and ammonia in water are all good for removing grease-spots.

(4) Oil of turpentine and oil of lemons, equal parts; both of the ingredients should have been recently distilled or rectified.

To Eradicate Grease-spots from Silk: Upon a deal table(1) lay a piece of woolen cloth or baize, upon which lay smoothly the part stained, with the right side downward. Having spread a piece of brown paper on top, apply a flat-iron just hot enough to scorch the paper. About 5 or 8 seconds is usually sufficient. Then rub the stained part briskly with a piece of cap-paper.

GREEN FLY:

These are not always green, but vary from yellow to green, according to what they eat. They are very common and easy to get rid of.

(1) They may be destroyed by tobacco smoke or tobacco-water.

(2) The stems and leaves of the tomato plant are well boiled in water, and this decoction, when strained and cold, is syringed over plants which are infested by the green fly and other insects. The liquor, when once applied, leaves behind a peculiar odor which prevents insects from coming again for a long time.

(3) Take a 2-gallon water-pot full of water, put into it 2 wine-glasses of paraffine; then mix well with the syringe; afterward syringe the roses with the mixture. It will kill every fly, and will not injure the tenderest shoot or the rose blooms.

GRUBS, TO REMOVE:

Grubs on orchard trees and gooseberry and currant bushes will sometimes be sufficiently numerous to spoil a crop; but if a bonfire be made with dry sticks and seeds on the windward side of the orchard, so that the smoke may blow among the trees, you will destroy thousands; for the grubs have such an objection to smoke that very little of it makes them roll themselves up and fall off; they must be swept up afterward.

GUESS GAME:

In this game some one goes out of hearing while the players fix on some object in the room. After this has been done he must ask them in turn the three following questions: "What is it like?" "Why is it like?" (the thing mentioned), and "Where would you put it?" To make myself clearer I will give an example. Supposing, for instance, A, B, C, and D to be playing, D to be the guesser, and a lump of sugar the thing chosen: D. "What is it like?" A. "Like snow." B. "Like a rock." C. "Like myself." D. "Why is it like a rock?" B. "Because of its shape." D. "Why is it like yourself?" C.

(1) Made from a plank 12 feet long, 11 inches wide and 2 1/2 inches thick.

"Because it and my temper possess the same qualities." D. "Where would you put it?" A. "On the table." B. "In the store-room." C. "In my mouth."

LAW MAXIMS, COMMON:

"Money paid on Sunday contracts may be recovered."

"Imbecility on the part of either the husband or the wife invalidates a marriage."

H

HAIR, CARE OF THE:

A young girl should learn the importance of forming habits of system. If she can regulate her duties in such a way as to have a particular day for sweeping, dusting, and arranging her room, another for mending and putting her wardrobe in order, a fixed time for study, reading, and letter-writing, etc., she will form a habit of regularity which will prove invaluable when the cares of womanhood come upon her. So also the personal habits should be regulated perfectly and attention given to them at a stated time.

A fine head of hair is a beautiful ornament, and it is well that every girl should be informed as to the best means of stimulating the growth and preserving the beauty of her hair. Left to care for itself, it will surely soon become coarse and unmanageable and lose all its beauty. I believe it is quite possible for nearly every young girl to possess a good head of hair if she is willing to bestow pains upon it.

Let me give a few simple rules which may be easily followed:

- The head should be washed occasionally with castile soap and warm water. Soap, if often used, may change the color or fade the hair.
- After washing the hair thoroughly, dry by rubbing it between 2 towels, and give it and the scalp a vigorous brushing with a moderately hard brush. Many ladies who have particularly fine hair spend 15 or 20 minutes in brushing it after disrobing for the night; others make a practice of cleansing the roots of the hair with a damp sponge every morning and brushing it thoroughly, as the hair is more pliable in the morning than at any other time. Frequent brushing with a perfectly clean brush is of the greatest use in giving a beautiful glossiness to the hair, and will subdue the coarsest and most refractory locks.
- Two brushes should be used, a moderately stiff one for cleansing and a softer for polishing. These brushes may be kept clean by washing them every few days in warm water and soda or in diluted ammonia. Do not use soap and hot water, as it will soon soften the bristles of the brush and render them useless. Soda will remove the grease and cleanse the brushes

with very little friction. Do not set them in the sun or near the fire to dry, but after shaking them well set them on the point of the handle in a shady place. Brushes may also be cleaned by rubbing them thoroughly with dry bran, which will leave the bristles stiff and firm.

- Occasionally dip a sponge in lukewarm sage tea, and thoroughly rub the head. It will preserve the color and give new life to the hair.
- Never use oils or pomades for the hair. Whatever obstructs the pores cannot but be injurious. All greasy preparations make the hair dry and harsh unless continually used, and nothing is more offensive than hair moist with oil.
- To prevent the ends of the hair from splitting and to hasten the growth clip them occasionally.

The preservation of the hair is important, not only out of consideration of beauty, but as a helpful bulwark against colds. Baldness is often hereditary. Moreover, certain parts of every man die before others. The scalp is often the first to atrophy, and the atrophic changes there produce baldness.

Cutting the Hair: It is very questionable whether frequent cutting of the hair is as favorable to its growth and beauty as it generally supposed. In fact, some of the most luxuriant heads of hair we have ever seen had never been touched by scissors. It is quite certain that the common practice of cropping, or shaving the head for the purpose of strengthening the growth of the hair, not only fails of this effect, but often produces the contrary result, and not seldom total baldness ensues where a small stock is sacrificed with the delusive hope of obtaining a great supply.

Growth of the Hair: At the root of each hair is a tiny bulb, in which the nutriment is supplied. As long as these bulbs (papilla) remain in a healthy condition the hair will continue to grow. It is of the first importance, therefore, that the scalp be kept clean, the pores open, and the processes of the nutritive supply free and active.

Why the Hair Falls Out: Hair falls out for want of nourishment. It dies just as a blade of grass dies in a soil where there is no moisture. This want of nourishment is only "functional," the papilla sacs and other apparatus remain, but are inactive. The mechanism which supplies it, the apparatus, is there to make it; but it is out of order, and makes it imperfectly; so the hair being imperfectly nourished, is dry, scant, or a mere furze, according the degree of the defective nourishment.

How to Prevent the Hair from Falling Out: As to men, when the hair begins to fall out, the best plan is to have it cut short, give it a good brushing with a moderately stiff brush while the hair is dry, then wash it well with warm soap-suds, then rub into the scalp, about the roots of the hair, a little bay rum or camphor water. Do these things at least once a week. The brushing of the scalp may be profitably done twice a week. Dampen the hair with water every time the toilet is made. Nothing ever made is better for the hair than pure soft water, if the scalp is kept clean in the way we have named.

How to Avoid Functional Baldness: If there is not that shining, glistening appearance, but a multitude of very small hairs, causing a "furziness" over the scalp, that is "functional" baldness; and two things are to be done. Keep the scalp clean with soap-suds, that is a "balm of a thousand flowers." More especially and principally seek to improve your general health by eating plain, substantial food 3 regular times a day, and by spending 3 or 4 hours between meals in moderate exercise in the open air or in some engrossing employment. A little turpentine or kerosene applied to the bald patches by means of sponges will hasten the first appearance of the hair, and the growth of the hair, when it re-commences, may be stimulated by constant shaving.

Avoid Hair-dyes: Hair-dyes, or so-called "hair-restorers," should be strenuously avoided, as they tend to fill the pores of the skin and almost invariably contain poisonous matters, which the system absorbs.

Caution in Using "Hair-oils:" The frequent use of "oils," "bear's grease," "arcturine," "pomades," "lustrals," "rosemary washes," and such-like greasy pomades are manufactured from lard-oil and simple lard. No "bear's grease" is ever used. If it could be procured readily it should not be applied to the hair, as it is the most rank and filthy of all the animal fats.

A Good Hair-dressing: There are many persons whose hair is naturally very dry and crisp; and in most families there is a want of some innocent and agreeable wash or dressing, which may be used moderately and judiciously. The mixture which may be regarded as the most agreeable, cleanly, and safe is composed of cologne spirit and pure castor-oil. The following is a good formula: Pure, fresh castor-oil, 2 ounces; cologne spirit, (95 per cent.), 16 ounces. The oil is freely dissolved in the spirit, and the solution is clear and beautiful. It may be perfumed in any way to suit the fancy of the purchaser.

Castor-oil for the Hair: A competent writer in the Boston Journal of Chemistry urges that the oil of the castor bean has for many years been employed to dress the hair, both among the savage and civilized nations, and it possesses properties which admirably adapt it to this use. It does not dry rapidly, and no gummy, offensive residuum remains, after taking on all the chemical changes which occur in all oils; upon exposure to light and air. It is best diffused by the agency of strong spirits, in which it dissolves, the alcohol or spirit rapidly evaporates, and does not in the slightest degree injure the texture of the hair. This preparation for dressing the hair of children or ladies will meet nearly or quite all requirements.

Utility of Beards: There are more solid inducements for wearing the beard than the mere improvement of a man's personal appearance, and the cultivation of such an aid to the every-day diplomacy of life. Nature combining, as she never fails to do, the useful with the ornamental, provides us with a far better respirator than science could ever make and one that is never so hideous to wear as that black seal upon the face that looks like a passport to the realms of suffering and death.

The hair of the mustache not only absorbs the moisture and miasma of the fogs, but it strains the air from the dust and soot of our great cities. It acts also in the most scientific manner, by taking heat from the warm breath as it leaves the chest, and supplying it to the cold air taken in. It is not only a respirator, but with the beard entire we are provided with a comforter as well; and these are never left at home, like umbrellas and all such appliances, whenever they are wanted.

Moffat and Livingstone, the African explorers, and many other travelers say that in the night no wrapper can equal the beard. A remarkable thing is, too, that the beard, like the hair of the head, protects against the heat of the sun; but, more than this, it becomes moist with the perspiration, and then by evaporation cools the skin.

To Strengthen the Hair: Dilute an ounce of borax and an ounce of camphor in 2 quarts of water, and wash the hair thoroughly twice a week, clipping the ends off occasionally. It will quickly grow long, thick, and even.

To Restore Hair when Removed by Ill-health or Age: Onions rubbed frequently on the part requiring it. The stimulating powers of this vegetable are of service in restoring the tone of the skin, and assisting the capillary vessels in sending forth new hair, but it is not infallible. Should it succeed, however, the growth of these new hairs may be assisted by the oil of myrtle-berries, the repute of which, perhaps, is greater than its real efficacy. These applications are cheap and harmless, even where they do no good; a character which cannot be said of the numerous quack remedies that meet the eye in every direction.

To Wash Hair-brushes: Hair-brushes, however dirty, may be washed and kept good for years, without loss of stiffness, by putting a small handful of soda into a pint jug of boiling water. When the soda is melted put in the brush and stir it about till clean. Rinse it in cold water, and dry in the sun or by the fire. The quicker it dries the harder the bristles will be.

To Curl the Hair: Take 2 ounces of borax, 1 dram of powdered gum senegal, 1 quart of hot water, (not boiling); mix, and as soon as the ingredients are dissolved add 2 ounces of spirits of wine strongly impregnated with camphor; on retiring to rest wet the hair with the above mixture and roll it in papers as usual; leave them till morning, when untwist and form into ringlets.

If an oil for the hair is desired the following are unobjectionable:

- *Rose Oil:* Olive oil, 1 pint; attar of roses, 5 to 16 drops. Essence of bergamot being much cheaper, is usually used instead of the more expensive attar of roses.
- *Red Rose Oil:* The same. The oil colored before scenting by steeping it in 1 dram of alkanet root with a gentle heat, until the desired tint is produced.

HAMMOCKS:

Hammocks are convenient during the warm months, and form comfortable beds or resting-places during the afternoons. They may be hung between two trees, or on the porch. The disposition of hammocks to sag can be obviated by placing sticks at each end with hooks along their length, which will catch in the meshes and spread them out flat.

(1) Take 4 yds. of strong, unbleached muslin; make a wide hem at each end; slip ropes through, fasten to a tree, and by changing your position a trifle you have an easy-chair, a bed, or cradle.

(2) Take a piece of manilla matting, from 2 to 3 yds. long and 1½ yds. wide; bind or hem the ends firmly; fasten each end to a piece of timber; these pieces should be 5 ft. long, 2 in. thick, and should have holes bored about 3 in. apart, the whole length; fasten by passing heavy twine from the matting to the hole, back and forth. For each end of the pieces of wood larger holes are bored, through which pass ropes to hang the hammock between two trees.

HANDS, CARE OF THE:

Take a wine-glassful of *eau-de-Cologne*, and another of lemon-juice, then scrape two cakes of brown Windsor soap to a powder and mix well in a mold. When hard it will be an excellent soap for whitening the hands.

To Keep White Hands: Our readers need not suffer from having their hands affected by water or soap-suds if the hands are dipped in vinegar-water or lemon-juice immediately after. The acid destroys the corrosive effect of the alkali, and makes the hands soft and white.

HANDS, GAME OF:

In this game the company generally divides into two parts, half being players, while the rest do the work of guessing. A thimble is then produced by one of the party, or something equally small, that may be easily held in the hand. Seated by the side of the table, the players begin passing on the article from hand to hand. When the working has been done sufficiently, the closed hands are all placed on the table for the opponents sitting opposite to guess in succession whose hand holds the treasure. As soon as the hiding-place is discovered the opposite side takes their turn.

HANGING BASKETS:

What looks more lovely than a plant suspended from a small rustic basket in the center of the upper part of the window? It interferes with nothing, and nothing interferes with it. There's an element of beauty in that simple fact. Plants which have slender branches, which naturally hang down, are at home in this situation. The mother-of-thousands; the wandering Jew, with its pretty marked leaves; the lobelias, and some of the trailing campanulas or bell flowers; the well-named rat-tailed cactus, and the so-called ice-plants are more at home when suspended than when grown in any other position.

Some families who have hard work to buy their daily bread may think they cannot afford to purchase a hanging-pot and its accompaniments; well, then, fill an old fruit-can with earth, bore 2 holes opposite near the top, then fasten a cord to it, set your slips, and suspend from a nail driven in the center of the upper casing of the window. After the lapse of a few months it would puzzle any one to tell whether your hanging-pot cost $5 or five cents, so thickly will it be covered with vines. By all means place hanging plants in your windows. They beautify home.

To Water: Plants in hanging-baskets are with difficulty kept moist enough when watered in the ordinary way. It has been recommended to immerse the basket in a tub of water for a few minutes, then take it out and allow it to drip before returning it to its usual place.

HANGING ORNAMENTS:

- Take a common pine cone and plant in its crevices a few canary seeds; place this half way in a hyacinth water-glass, and the seeds will sprout and throw out delicate little green feathery blades, shortly filling the whole upper portion with a little festoon of verdure(1).
- Take a large turnip and scrape out the inside, leaving a thick wall around. Fill the cavity with earth, and plant in it some clinging vine or morning-glory. Suspend the turnip with cords, and in a little time the vines twine around the strings, and the turnip, sprouting from below, will put forth leaves and stems that will turn upward and gracefully curl around the base.

(1) The green color of growing things.

- Take a common tumbler or fruit-can and fill it nearly full of soft water. Then tie a bit of coarse lace or cheese-sacking over it, and press down into the water covered with a layer of peas. In a few days they will sprout, the little thread-like roots going down through the lace into the water, and the vines can be trained up to twine around the window; or, what is prettier, a frame may be made for the purpose.
- The sweet-potato vine is also a curiosity; few would believe until they have tried it how pretty a sight may be made of it. Put a sweet potato in a tumbler of water, or any similar glass vessel; keep the lower end of the tuber about 1 or 2 in. from the bottom of the vessel; keep on the mantel shelf; sun it for 1 or 2 hours each day and soon little roots will appear—they will throw up a pretty vine, and grow rapidly over any trellis-work above.

HARNESS, TO CARE FOR:

A harness that has been on a horse's back several hours in hot or rainy weather becomes wet; if not properly cleaned the damage to the leather is irreparable. If, after being taken from the horse, it is hung up in a careless manner, traces and reins twisted into knots, and the saddle and bridle hung askew, the leather when dried retains the same shape given it when wet, and when forced into its original form damage is done to the stitching and leather.

The first point to be observed is to keep the leather soft and pliable. This can be done by keeping it well charged with oil and grease; water is a destroyer, but mud and saline moisture from the animals are even more destructive. Mud in drying absorbs the grease and opens the pores of the leather, making it a prey to water, while the salty character of the perspiration from the animal injures the leather, stitching, and mountings.

It therefore follows that to preserve the harness the straps should be washed and oiled whenever they have been moistened by sweat or soiled by mud. If the harness is thoroughly cleaned twice a year, and, when unduly exposed, treated as we have recommended, the leather will retain its softness and strength for many years.

HARNESS WOUNDS ON HORSES:

The best cure for harness wounds on horses is burned leather. Rub the ashes on the sore and a cure is soon effected.

HARVEST DRINK:

Mingle together 5 gallons of pure water, 1/2 gallon molasses, 1 quart vinegar, and 2 ounces of powdered ginger. This drink is very invigorating.

HAY-FEVER, PERSONS AFFECTED:

In a book entitled *Experimental Reseaches on the Causes and Nature of Catarrhus Æstivus*, (Hay-fever or Hay-asthma), Mr. Blackley published some very interesting conclusions respecting this singular disease. He finds that it is peculiar to the educated classes, but is not aristocratic, like the gout, being more common in proportion to the spread of mental culture and the intensity of intellectual occupation.

Causes: As to the actual inciting cause of the disease, it has been referred to summer heat, dust, ozone, the odors of flowers, the pollen of blossoms, and especially of grasses. The author's experiments led him to the conclusion that it is to the pollen of flowering plants (including grasses) that the disease is due. As to the places least likely to be affected by the disease, the author found hay-fever least common in the centers of large cities, and the sea-shore, and high-lying districts given up to pasturage.

Remedies: Dr. George M. Beard expresses the opinion that the disease is not amenable to any specific remedy; that the leading indications are prevention: avoidance of heat, light, worry, dust, vegetable and animal irritants, and other exciting causes, fortifying the system by tonics, before and during the attack, and relieving the symptoms by sedatives and anodynes(1); indications which are best met by resort to the sea-shore or to a sea-voyage, high latitudes, and—for those who cannot avail themselves of such changes—cool, closed, dark rooms.

HAY FOR HOGS:

Very few are aware of the fact that hay is very beneficial to hogs; but it is true nevertheless. Hogs need rough food as well as horses, cattle, or the human race. To prepare it you should have a cutting-box, (or hay-cutter), and the greener the hay the better. Cut the hay short and mix with bran, shorts, or middlings, swill or other slop food; it is highly relished by them. In winter use for hogs the same hay you fed to your horses, and you will find that, while it saves bran, shorts, or other food, it puts on flesh as rapidly as any thing that can be given them.

HEAD, CLOTHING THE:

The most desirable thing to consider in covering the head is not so much cold as baldness. Colds come from baldness, not wholly, but often. Of course the first principle would be to go with the head bare. The noble red man fades into the natural emaciation of age with a full head of hair merely because he wears no hat. If you must wear a hat, wear a soft hat. It binds the head and arrests the circulation less than a stiff hat. If a stiff hat is regarded as necessary, the stovepipe is of the most rational sort. It gives

(1) Pain relievers.

more air for the top of the head to breathe in. Hence caps which fit closely all over are not good.

HEADACHE, CAUSES OF:

Probably one of the most common headaches, if not the most common, is that called nervous. The class of people who are most subject to it are certainly not outdoor workers. The worst form of headache is the periodic.

We note some of the most ordinary causes of nervous headache: Overwork indoors; overstudy; work or study indoors, carried on in an unnatural or cramped position of body. Literary men and women ought to do most of their work at a standing desk, lying down now and then to ease brain and heart and permit ideas to flow. They should work out of doors in fine weather—with their feet resting on a board, not on the earth—and under canvas in wet weather.

Neglect of the ordinary rules that conduce to health; want of fresh air in bedrooms; want of abundant skin-exciting exercise; neglect of the bath; over-indulgence in food, especially of a stimulating character; weakness or debility of body; however produced, (this can only be remedied by proper nutriment); nervousness, however induced; the excitement inseparable from a fashionable life.

Three Remedies:

(1) Much sick-headache is caused by overloading the stomach—by indigestion. It may be relieved by drinking very freely of warm water, whether it produces vomiting or not. If the feet are cold, warm them or bathe them in water as hot as you can bear it. Soda or ashes in the water will do no good. If the pain is very severe apply a warm cloth wrung out of hot water to the head—pack the head as it were. In some cases medicine is necessary; but if the above is properly carried out almost immediate relief is experienced.

(2) One forth of a grain of ipecac(1), repeated every half hour or hour, has relieved many cases of nervous sick-headache, and if the ipecac is continued in 1 to 3 grain doses 3 or 4 times daily a cure will frequently result—at least intervals will be prolonged.

(3) Another class of sufferers may be relieved by turpentine. Frontal headaches, most apt to occur after prolonged mental effort, may likewise be induced by unduly sustained physical exertion. A cup of very strong tea often relieves this form of headache, but this remedy with not a few is perilous, for bringing relief from pain it may produce a general restlessness, and, worst of all, banish sleep.

(1) Ipecacuanha. A medicine from the dried roots from a Brazilian plant used as a counter-irritant and to induce vomiting.

Turpentine in doses of 20 to 30 minims(1), given at intervals of 1 or 2 hours, will entirely remove the headache.

HEAD AND FACE, PAINS IN THE:

A friend assures us that he was cured of a severe attack of tic-douloureux by the following simple remedy:

Take 1/2 pint of rose-water, add 2 tea-spoonfuls of white vinegar to form a lotion. Apply it to the part affected 3 or 4 times a day. It requires fresh linen and lotion each application; this will, in 2 or 3 days, gradually take the pain away.

HEADS, JADED:

These are caused by overwork and want of exercise. Man has it in every rank of life; but it is chiefly found among the persons of sedentary pursuits and among both sexes and almost all ages above 14. Generally the first symptom of the malady is discomfort during headwork in the back of the head and in the upper part of the spinal region. Meet this symptom with rest, and seek in sun-light and fresh air some fresh investment for the nervous system. Alcohol and all sleep-producing drugs are dangerous in the highest degree, for they mask the malady without curing.

HEALTH NOTES:

Pine Woods and Health: The pleasant odor emitted by fir-trees in a sunny atmosphere has long been thought serviceable to invalids, and the vicinity of pine woods has been declared salubrious.

Danger of Cold Water in the Face: It is dangerous to wash the face in cold water when much heated. It is not dangerous, but pleasantly efficacious, if warm water is used.

A Refreshing Bath: Sun-baths cost nothing and are the most refreshing, life-giving baths that one can take, whether sick or well.

To Prevent Harm from Drinking Cold Water: It is a very safe rule to wet your wrists before drinking cold water if at all heated. The effect is immediate and grateful, and the danger of fatal results may be warded off by this simple precaution.

Position after being Tired: If very tired physically, lie on the back, knees drawn up, the hands clasped above the head or resting on the elbows, the fore-arms at right angles, and the hands hanging over by the bend of the wrists.

(1) The smallest liquid measure; generally a single drop.

Pie-crust and Dyspepsia: Whoever eats heavy pie-crust commits a crime against his physical well-being, and must pay the penalty. The good housewife should see to it that all pastry and cakes are light; no other should be eaten.

Eating at Certain Intervals: After 50 yrs. of age, if not a day-laborer, and sedentary persons after 40, should eat but twice a day—in the morning and about 4 in the afternoon; persons can soon accustom themselves to a 7-hours' interval between eating, thus giving the stomach rest, for every organ without adequate rest will "give out" prematurely.

Cold or Warm Drinks: Of cold or warm drinks the former are the most pernicious. Drinking at meals induces people to eat more than they otherwise would, as any one can verify by experiment, and it is excess in eating that devastates the land with sickness, suffering, and death.

Most Healthful Seat in a Car: Other things being equal, the forward seats in a street or railway car are the most healthful. The forward motion of the car causes a current of air backward, carrying with it the exhalations from the lungs of the forward passengers. In all cases avoid as much as possible inhaling another's "breath."

Spread of Pestilence: Spread of pestilence is possible through the rag-picker who takes contagion to the very door of the rich man. The breath of the wretched beggar craving alms of the lady at her carriage-step may waft to her in the seeds of death. The little street-wanderer, in brushing past your child, may render vain the anxious care of years. The highly recommended nurse-maid may carry the infant into scenes and atmospheres the most dangerous.

Improper Sitting and its Evils: Consumptive people and all afflicted with spinal deformities sit habitually crooked in one or more curves of the body. There was a time in all these when the body had its natural erectness, when there was not the first departure on the road to death. The make of our chairs, especially that great barbarism, the unwieldy and disease-engendering rocking-chair, favors these diseases, and undoubtedly, in some instances, leads to bodily habits from which originate the ailments just named, to say nothing of the piles, fistula, and the like. The painful or sore feeling which many are troubled with incessantly for years at the extremity of the backbone, is the result of sitting in such a position that it rests upon the seat of the chair at a point several inches forward of the chair-back.

Chewing between Meals: The habit of chewing substances of any kind between meals is always harmful to health. The chewing overtaxes the organs which secrete the saliva, and exhaust them so that the chief agent in promoting the digestion of food is diminished in quality and efficiency. The act of chewing always excites the flow of saliva. Persons who chew gum soon become sensible of the exhaustion and fatigue of the salivary glands. The same is true of those who chew tobacco. In order to promote the best condition of these glands they should rest "between meals."

Cause and Cure of Leanness: Leanness may be caused by insufficient food or over-exertion, or both. But the usual cause is disease; the vital powers being more occupied in removing impurities and poisons and overcoming abnormal conditions, than in digesting and assimilating nutrient material. The patient should eat all the plain nutritious food that he can assimilate. Those lean persons who are not accustomed to fruit will find baked sweet apples a good addition to each meal to begin with. Oatmeal mush, with a slice of wheat-meal bread, and 2 or 3 baked apples make a breakfast with which any lean individual may be justly content.

To Cool a Room: Wet a cloth of any size, the larger the better, and suspend it in the room. Let the ventilation be good, and the temperature will sink from 10 to 20 degrees in less than a hour.

Inflation of the Lungs: Five minutes spent in the open air after dressing, inflating the lungs by inhaling as full a breath as possible, and gently pounding the breast during the inflation, will greatly enlarge the chest, strengthen the lung power, and very effectually ward off consumption.

Eating, Sleeping and Speaking—Simple Precautions:

- Never eat hurriedly, because it tends to cause indigestion. Never dine in excitement, because the blood is called to the brain which ought to aid in the process of digestion.
- Never swallow food without thorough chewing, because it brings on dyspepsia. Never eat when you do not want it, because when you shall want you cannot eat.
- Never sleep with your mouth open, because the air breathed with carbonic acid disturbs the mucous membranes.
- Never go to rest without washing the hands and face, because more dirt accumulates on the skin in the day than in the night, and is re--absorbed during the night.
- Never begin a journey until breakfast is eaten.
- After speaking, singing or preaching in a warm room in winter do not leave it immediately. In leaving close the mouth, put on the gloves, wrap up the neck and put on a cloak or overcoat before passing out of the door. The neglect of these simple

precautions has laid many a good and useful man into a premature grave.

- Never speak under a hoarseness, especially if it requires an effort or painful feeling.

Danger from Wet Clothes: Few persons understand fully the reason why wet clothes exert such a chilling influence. It is simply this: Water, when it evaporates, carries off an immense amount of heat, in what is called the latent form. One pound of water in vapor contains as much heat as 9 or 10 lbs. of liquid water, and all this heat must, of course, be taken from the body. If our clothes are moistened with 32 lbs. of water—ie., if by wetting they are 3 lbs. heavier—these 3 lbs. will, in drying, carry off as much heat as would raise 3 gallons of ice-cold water to the boiling point.

Concerning the "Tea-pot:" When any tin-lined vessel, especially the tea-pot, becomes rusted or blackened inside there is danger in its use. The acid contained in the tea combines with the iron of the exposed portions of the vessel, and forms a chemical compound, not unlike ink. It corrodes and darkens the teeth, and cannot be inoffensive to the stomach. I have seen the discoloration both of natural and artificial teeth prove so obstinate from this cause as to require several scourings with soap and ashes with a stiff brush to remove it. When housekeepers hear any of the family remarking, "This tea tastes like ink," it is time to examine, possibly to throw away, the tea-pot. "The most palatable and wholesome tea is made by steeping in a bright tin or porcelain cup, then pouring into a freshly scalded earthen tea-pot. Thus treated it will never acquire the astringent quality so deleterious to the teeth and to health."

Concerning Ice-cream: An eminent physician in France has investigated the article known in cities as street-corner ice-cream, and finds it to contain poisonous colored matter, which produces serious symptoms when taken in a continued course, and is a prolific cause of scrofulous eruptions and dropping out of the hair among the lower classes.

Carrying Lead-pencils: There is often danger in carrying lead pencils in the pocket. Several cases of deaths are recorded of persons who were pierced by pencils carried in the pocket. We should be careful to place the pencil, or other sharp instrument, in such a way in the pocket as to provide against such danger.

Visiting Infected Rooms: Avoid entering a sick-room while in a state of perspiration, because in cooling off the pores absorb freely; nor should a person sit between the sick and the fire. Do not approach contagious diseases with an empty stomach.

Dangerous Medicines: *Thousands of deaths take place every year from the unauthorized use of dangerous medicines. They often occur on this wise:*

A person is suffering, the family physician is called; he writes a prescription, it is taken; grateful relief is experienced; patient desires to know the name of the marvelous remedy, bears it in mind, and if there is something similar he ventures to send for it (the remedy) direct to the druggist. On being relieved again he becomes enthusiastic, and volunteers advice to his friends. They are relieved—sometimes—and forthwith he begins to think he knows "about as much as any of the doctors." A little later it is not unusual to see a record in the newspapers that Mr.— — was "found dead in his bed this morning." Remember, that a prescription providing a remedy for one disease may prove perilous in another.

How to Escape Fever Infections: In a properly chosen, well-lighted, well-aired, well-scrubbed dwelling with thoroughly washed inmates, there is comparatively little fear of infectious poisons. But it is well for every one to be acquainted with some of the easiest means of resistance and of escape when the gigantic evil approaches, or when duty compels us to go within its range. Knowledge of the reality will prevent foolish exaggerations, and diminish useless fear.

Fever Infections: All infectious fever (typhus, scarlatina, small-pox, etc.) arise from the reception of a subtle poison into the blood, which, spreading through the system, is exhaled from it principally by the skin and lungs. This poison has been actually condensed out of impure air poisoned by filth and decay, and appears in the form of a dirty-looking, half-solid, half-fluid, half-gelatinous stuff, a few drops of which inserted into the veins of a dog will inoculate that dog with typhus fever.

Ventilation: The poisonous infection is lighter than air and ascends. If we allow it to escape at the top of the room the air below is safe. This is the reason why in fever-wards few cases of infection occur; without the ventilators in the ceiling they would be the dens of death. The circulation of fresh air in a fever-chamber by open doors and windows must be produced several times a day, (care being taken that the patient be not directly exposed to the draught,) or, still better, let the upper part of a window be kept permanently open, and if the patient be in a box-bed let there be several holes bored through the roof of the bed, to allow the exit of infectious vapor in the direction of the open window.

Fever Infection and Fear: As far as possible avoid fear. Fear is also a fruitful source of infection, for it weakens the pulse and the whole frame. Travelers in the East have told that when a dog is suddenly bitten by a rattlesnake the wound is not considered half so deadly as when the dog has seen the reptile and stood trembling before it; fear in this case aids and quickens the poison. Charms and amulets, met with occasionally among the poor of our country, and frequently in foreign ones, may thus actually be useful by inspiring confidence, although it is the confidence of superstition.

Poisonous Soap: A common and annoying form of skin-disease, "eczema," is sometimes produced by bad soap. The soap that seems to suffer most in analytical experiments is the cheaper kind of "old Brown Windson," which is made from putrid animal matter extracted from heaps of decaying bones, which are described as emitting a stench that is intolerable. The brown color which is given to the higher-priced Brown Windsor by artificial means, this cheaper soap gets quite sufficiently from the filthy fat from which it is made; and the stench, which even the saponifying(1) process does not quite remove, is disguised by the perfume which is afterward added.

Orange-peel Poisonous: Fatal consequences may follow the swallowing of the rind of oranges. The oil of the rind is highly acrid, and adds greatly to the noxious quality of the indigestible mass.

Danger in Carrying Matches: Many persons have the habit of carrying friction matches loosely in their pockets, and using these at the same time quite indiscriminately for carrying tobacco, candles, cakes, and other eatables. Aside from the danger of ignition of the matches, which might cause serious burns, a greater danger arises from the fact that the tips of the matches, highly charged with phosphorus, are liable to break off and mix with those eatables in the pocket, and in that way find their way into the stomach, and occasion fatal accidents of poisoning.

Poisonous Candies: In no class of articles intended for consumption is the use of poisons so free as in candies and confections. Arseniate of copper, copperas, white-lead and litharge, (or red-lead) and the aniline colors, red, green, or blue, and other poisons, mineral and vegetable, are frequently employed in the manufacture of candies. There are confectioners who do not use such dangerous drugs, or who use them so sparingly that they work no immediate appreciable harm to the consumer; but others are neither so scrupulous nor so well-informed about the real nature of the poisons which impart the desired vividness of color or fineness of flavor to their products. Bright, highly colored, handsome candies always sell better than dull, plain varieties. The beautiful tints can be had most cheaply and satisfactorily by the use of the virulent mineral poisons—chiefly arseniates and preparations of copper and lead.

Be cautious, therefore, in purchasing candies to buy only of manufacturers or dealers who are scrupulously careful in their preparation.

(1) The conversion process of a fat into a soap.

Care Concerning Ice-cream: Ice-cream may be colored as freely as any other confections. The brilliant red tint of strawberry cream may be attained by litharge or rosaline; the splendid green tint of pistachio cream (so-called) may be derived from arseniate of copper more economically than from the pistachio nut or spinach-water.

Poisonous Vegetables: There are many beautiful and innocent-looking forms of vegetable life to be met with in our gardens and hedges which are yet full of deadly poison, while others, from their close resemblance to nutritious articles of food, are often partaken of by mistake, and fatal accidents are consequently of too frequent occurrence. Here is a partial list of them: "Monkshood," or aconite; "fool's parsley," a species of hemlock; buttercups, (often poisonous to children's hands); laburnum seeds; deadly-nightshade, (half a berry of the dark purple has caused death); belladonna, (poison lies in the fruit answering to the potato apple); leaves of the common laurel; the wild arum; and mushrooms.

HEART, FATTY DEGENERATION OF THE:

A term used to denote a change of the substance of the heart from muscle to fat. Another disease, sometimes called ossification of the valves of the heart or of the arteries, consists in a simple change into a limy substance, and is properly denominated calcareous degeneration of the heart. In these cases there is much weakness in the heart itself, as well as in the circulation and in the whole general physical system. A reputable physician should be consulted.

HEATED BODY, TO COOL:

During very hot weather keep cool. Just before retiring take a cool bath, after which don the night-dress without drying the body, and lie down. The result is much like that produced by sprinkling water on the floor in the evening. The water absorbs the heat, and as it evaporates throws the heat off with it, leaving the body dry and cool. Avoid heating food. Do not increase the temperature by alcoholic beverages. Sleep regularly; resist the temptation to sit up late because the evening is cool.

HEAVES IN HORSES:

(1) A correspondent recommends sunflower seed as a cure for the heaves in horses. He had 1 bushel of the seed ground with 2 bushels of oats, and gave a horse 2 quarts of the mixed meal, wet in warm water, 3 times a day. He took the time when the horse was not used at hard work. In 2 weeks not a sign of the heaves could be observed, and the horse looked as sleek and bright as if his hair had been oiled. He had cured 2 horses of his own of this distressing complaint, and recommended it to others, who had experienced a

like result. In cases of horse distemper and coughs it is an excellent remedy.

(2) Very bad cases of heaves have been cured by simply feeding the animal upon cut and moistened feed, of very good quality and in small quantities, 3 times a day; for instance, 4 lbs. of timothy hay and 3 quarts of feed made of equal quantities of oats, corn, and wheat bran ground together. With this was mixed a small quantity of salt, and twice a week 1 dram of sulphate of iron and $^1/_2$ ounce of ground gentian root were given in the feed. A liberal bran mash every evening will also be very useful. A horse that cannot be cured by this treatment is of no value, and may be considered past cure.

HEMORRHAGE, TO RELIEVE:

To stop hemorrhage of the lungs, cord the thighs, and arms above the elbow, with small, strong cords tightly drawn and tied. It will stop the flow of blood almost instantly, as it has done for the writer many times. It was recommended by a physician of experience.

HENS, HOW TO MAKE LAY:

While on a visit in the fall to a friend we were surprised to see the number of eggs he daily obtained. He had but 16 hens, and the product per diem averaged 13 eggs. He was in the habit of giving on every alternate day $1^1/_4$ tea-spoonful of cayenne pepper mixed with the soft food, and took care that each hen obtained her share. The experiment of omitting the pepper was tried, when it was found that the number of eggs was reduced each trial from 5 to 6 daily. We believe that the moderate use of this stimulant not only increases the number of eggs, but effectually wards off diseases to which chickens are subject.

HEREDITY:

The great Froebel's motto was, "Let us live for our children." In health of body, as well as of morals and mind, every parent should recognize this as a solemn duty. Parents owe it to their children to bequeath to them healthy bodies and minds, and this can only be done by themselves from the first observing the laws of health.

HICCOUGH, RELIEF FROM:

The following simple directions have proved successful in the numerous cases, and bear the indorsements severally of responsible names:

(1) Holding the breath as long as possible.

(2) Drinking as many successive swallows as possible without breathing.

(3) Startling the patient by a sudden motion or communication.

(4) Sugared water is often given to infants by their nurses as a sure cure.

(5) Concentrating the mind intensely upon some subject.

(6) Hold up the right arm, extending the hand as far as possible, and look at it.

(7) Take a small piece of lump sugar into the mouth and let dissolve very slowly, or drink any liquid very slowly, and the hiccoughs will cease.

HIGH TEAS:

These are the revival of an old fashion. The chief modern improvement is that the ladies and gentlemen present are seated in pairs at the table. Fried chicken, hot cakes, sweet-meats, etc., are in order, and even roast turkey. No wines are permitted at the high tea, which must not be later than 7 P.M. Only good conversationalists are admitted, as, after adjourning from the *salle a manger*, the guests are expected to amuse them-selves. Some amateur music is occasionally rendered; but the portfolio of engravings, the ceramics on the *etagère*, pictures, books, etc., are depended upon to afford interest. At the high tea the guests sit at one table. Costumes of velvet and satin, or such handsome dresses as may be worn on the street, are all that is required. A few natural flowers are added, and in many cases a small bouquet or basket of fresh blossoms at each plate. High teas are in general favor during early spring

HILLS, DRAINS FOR:

When the site is on the side or foot of a hill it is generally necessary to cut off the water that drains from the higher level by constructing drains across the hill and connecting these with the drains at right angles running down through the hillside. Where the spring has naturally formed itself an outlet, it may frequently only be necessary to bore into it, or render it larger and of more depth, which, by affording the water a more free and open passage, may evacuate and bring it off more quickly or sink it to a level so greatly below that of the surface of the soil as to prevent it from flowing into or over it.

HISS AND CLAP, GAME OF:

In this game the gentlemen are all requested to leave the room, when the ladies take their seats, leaving a vacant place on the right side of every one for the gentlemen of their choice. Each gentleman in turn is then summoned and asked to guess which lady he imagines has chosen him for her partner. Should he guess rightly he is allowed to take his seat by the lady who has chosen him, while the company loudly clap hands, in proof of their congratulations on his success; but should he guess wrongly, he will be only too glad to disappear from the scene, so loud will be the hisses of his friends.

HOARSENESS, REMEDIES FOR:

(1) Horse-radish will afford instantaneous relief in most obstinate cases of hoarseness. The root, of course, possesses the most virtue, though the leaves are good till they are dry, when they lose their strength. The root is best when it is green. The person who will use it freely just before beginning to speak will not be troubled with hoarseness. I would like to add that the root boiled down and sweetened into a thick syrup will give relief in the severest cases. It was formerly used in this way in our family, and though very bad to take never failed to give relief.

(2) When the voice is lost, as is sometimes the case, from the effects of a cold, a simple, pleasant remedy is furnished by beating up the white of 1 egg, adding to it the juice of 1 lemon, and sweetening with white sugar to taste. Take a tea-spoonful from time to time. It has been known to effectually cure the ailment.

(3) Boil 2 ounces of flaxseed in 1 quart of water, strain, and then add 2 ounces of rock-candy, 1/2 pint of syrup or honey, and the juice of 3 lemons; mix and then boil together. Let it then cool, and bottle for use. Take 1 cupful before going to bed—the hotter you drink it the better.

(4) *Miss Parloa gives this cure for hoarseness:* Bake a lemon or sour orange for 20 minutes in a moderate oven, then open it at one end and dig out the inside, which sweeten with sugar or molasses, and eat. This will cure hoarseness and remove the pressure from the lungs.

HOEING:

Plants grow and mature better when the ground is hoed frequently. The loosening of the soil in the operation of hoeing is as beneficial to the plants as the destruction of weeds. The cultivated soil being made porous, immediately conveys to the roots of the plants the moisture and attracts a heavier fall of dew. When the surface is kept loose it acts as a mulch, affords actual resistance to the rays of the sun, and keeps the roots of the plants cool; but when it is hard it becomes a good conductor of heat, which deeply penetrates it.

In the cultivation of corn, potatoes, and similar crops, stirring the soil among the plants can scarcely be repeated too frequently during the early part of the season; in fact, these operations may be continued until the crop is well on toward maturity. The sprouting weeds are thus destroyed in the germ, and the work is comparatively easy all the season afterward.

HOME REMEDIES, SOME SIMPLE:

Half a tea-spoonful of common table salt dissolved in a little cold water and drank will instantly relieve "heartburn" or dyspepsia. If taken every morning before breakfast, increasing the quantity gradually to a teaspoonful of salt in a tumbler, it will in a few days cure any ordinary cases of dyspepsia, if at the same time due attention is paid to the diet. There is no better remedy than the above for constipation. As a gargle for sore throat it is equal to chlorate of potash, and is entirely safe. It may be used as often as desired, and if a little is swallowed each time it will have a beneficial effect on the throat by cleansing it and allaying the irritation. In doses of 1 to 4 tea-spoonfuls in 1/2 pint to 1 pint of tepid water it acts promptly as an emetic, and, in cases of poisoning, is always on hand. It is an excellent remedy for bites and stings of insects. It is a valuable astringent in hemorrhages, particularly for bleeding after the extraction of teeth. It has both cleansing and healing properties, and is therefore a more excellent application for superficial ulcerations.

Mustard is another valuable remedy. No family should be without it. Two or 3 tea-spoonfuls of ground mustard stirred into 1/2 pint of water acts as an emetic very promptly and is milder and easier to take than salt and water. Equal parts of ground mustard and flour of meal made into a paste with warm water and spread on a thin piece of muslin with another piece of muslin laid over it, forms the indispensable "mustard plaster." It is almost a specific for colic when applied for a few minutes over the pit of the stomach. For all internal pains and congestions there is no remedy of such general utility. It acts as counter-irritant by drawing the blood to the surface; hence in severe cases of croup a small mustard plaster should be applied to the back of the child's neck. The same treatment will relieve almost any case of headache. A mustard plaster should be moved about over the spot to be acted upon, for if left in one place it is liable to blister. A mustard plaster acts just as well when at a considerable distance from the effected part.

An excellent substitute for mustard plasters is what is known as "mustard leaves." They come a dozen in a box, and are about 4 by 5 in. They are perfectly dry, and will keep for a long time. For use it is only necessary to dip one in a dish of water for a minute and then apply it.

Common baking-soda is the best of all remedies in cases of scalds and burns. It may be used on the surface of the burned place either dry or wet. When applied promptly the sense of relief is magical. It seems to withdraw the heat and with it the pain, and the healing process commences. It is the best application for eruptions caused by poisonous ivy and other poisonous plants, as also for bites and stings of insects.

HOMESTEAD, TO KEEP HEALTHY:

A healthy house makes healthy people. It should be dry, warm, airy, and free from smoky chimneys. To be dry it must be well drained, and should be free from dense, overshading foliage. Do not scour the floors too often, for fear of dampness. It is not necessary to sleep in a cold room to get fresh air. The cold air of the external atmosphere should be made to enter the room to get fresh air. The cold air of the external atmosphere should be made to enter the room in such a manner that it is thoroughly warmed. Let plenty of light into the room. Throw open the blinds and draw aside the curtains. Pale cheeks touched by sunlight will acquire a deeper hue.

Look well to the cellars. In too many cellars will be found rotten apples, cabbages, turnips, onions, etc. In some will be found old brine, with pieces of decayed meat, sending forth an odor, when the cover of the barrel is taken off, which is vile enough to wrench the stomach of a pig. In others there will be musty cider-barrels, possibly vinegar-casks, in which the vinegar has passed on to the putrefactive stage, disseminating the spores of decay and death.

Decaying wood generates one of the most subtle poisons, because the odor is not particularly offensive. Rotten timbers in the cellars and moldy wood or chips in the wood-house fill the air with spores, which, inhaled by one whose blood is low, may generate disease. Under the cider and vinegar-barrels, and around potato-bins, may often be found old timbers and boards that are full of dry-rot, ready to propagate itself whenever the rotten particles may find a lodgement.

In the well, also, rotten wood is a subtle poison, more dangerous than a decomposing toad, as the later makes his presence known, while few tastes are so keen as to detect the presence of decaying wood.

Probably the most prolific source of disease around the house is the cess-pool into which pass the kitchen and chamber slops. In the cities and large villages these are carried off in the sewers, but seldom does a farmhouse have any system of sewerage. The slops are too often thrown out of the kitchen door and left to generate vile odors on the surface of the ground. To keep the air of the cellar around the house pure and sweet, resort to free sprinkling, as occasion may demand, or dry, slaked lime.

HORSES, HOW TO JUDGE:

If the color be light sorrel, or chestnut, his feet, legs, and face white, these are marks of kindness. If he is broad and full between the eyes, he may be depended upon as a horse of good sense, and capable of being trained to do any thing. As respects such horses, the more kindly you treat them the better you will be treated in return. Nor will a horse of this description stand a whip, if well fed.

If you want a safe horse avoid one that is dish-faced. He may be so far gentle as not to scare, but he will have too much go-ahead in him to be safe with every body. If you want a fool, but a horse of great bottom, get a deep bay, with not a white hair about him. If his face is a little dished, so much the worse. Let no man ride such a horse that is not an adept in riding—they are always tricky and unsafe. If you want one that will never give out, never buy a large, overgrown one.

A black horse cannot stand heat, nor a white one cold. If you are particular to procure a gentle horse get one with more or less white about the head; the more the better. Many people suppose the parti-colored horses belonging to the circuses, shows, etc., are selected for their oddity. But the selections thus made are on account of their great docility and gentleness.

HORSES, TO TELL THE AGE OF:

Every horse has 6 teeth above and below. Before 3 yrs. old he sheds his middle teeth; at 3 he sheds one more on each side of the central teeth; at 4 he sheds the 2 corner and last of the 4 teeth. Between 4 and 5 the horse cuts the under tusks; at 5 he will cut his upper tusks, at which time his mouth will be complete. At 6 yrs. the grooves and hollows begin to fill up a little; at 7 the grooves will be well-nigh filled up, except the corner teeth, leaving little brown spots where the dark-brown hollows formerly were. At 8 the whole of the hollows and grooves are filled up. At 9 there is very often seen a small bill to the outside corner teeth; the point of the tusk is worn off, and the part that was concave begins to fill up and become rounding; the squares of the central teeth begin to disappear, and the gums leave them small and narrow at the top.

HOT-BEDS, TO MAKE:(1)

There is no mystery about a hot-bed, yet farmers and many others do without this convenience from some supposed difficulty in making and caring for it. Sashes, a few boards, and some horse manure are the materials required. Regular hot-bed sashes are 3 by 6 ft., and may be bought ready glazed at the sash and blind factories; old window-sashes will answer as a makeshift, but are far less convenient. Select a place sheltered by a building or fence from cold winds; dig a pit 2$^1/_2$ ft. deep, wide as the sashes are long, and as long as the number of sashes to be used require. Line this pit with rough boards nailed to the posts driven down at the corners. The rear board should extend a foot above the surface, and the front one 4 in. above. The front or lower side should face the south. Nail strips from front to rear for the sashes to slide upon.

HOT DRINKS:

The temperature of milk is of great importance to all persons. Hot liquid stimulates every digestive agency, and cold liquid has the reverse effect. This is the whole secret of the hot-water cure, and it applies with particular force to milk. There is much in that for the stomach to digest, and therefore it needs to be assisted rather than hampered.

HOTEL, ETIQUETTE AT:

- When a lady arrives at a hotel alone it is best to be provided

(1) Compost pile.

with a letter of introduction. She should, upon arrival, present her letter and mention the time for which she desires a room.

- She should wear the most modest dress appropriate to the hour of the day. Full dress must not be worn unless she has an escort.
- She should never go alone to the supper-table at a late hour, but should have that meal sent to her room in such case.
- A lady should lock her trunks before leaving her room and give most of her money and jewelry into the care of the proprietor on her arrival, ringing for them if she requires them during her stay.
- Guests should not use the piano of a hotel uninvited if there are others in the room. It is still worse to sing.
- A lady should never go to the door of a hotel to call a hack. Ring for a servant, and he will bring the hack to the ladies' entrance.
- No lady should stand or linger in the halls of a hotel, but pass through them quietly; nor stand alone at the front windows of a parlor, or walk out alone on the porch or any conspicuous place.
- She is not expected to recognize friends across the dining-room of a hotel.
- No scolding of servants is permissible. If they are negligent or disrespectful, complain to the housekeeper, head waiter, or landlord.
- Do not take any paper, book, or music in a hotel parlor to your own room.
- Lounging in a public parlor can never be permitted.
- A lady should not touch any of her baggage in a hotel after it is packed. Servants should carry to the hack even the traveling-shawl, satchel, or book.
- No lady should pass in or out at the public entrance of a hotel.

HOUSE-CLEANING:

Before beginning on a general house-cleaning see that you have an ample supply of water and fuel provided, so that you may not be stopped or delayed by a lack of these. As fast as the kettles and boilers are emptied fill them up again.

Always begin up-stairs first, so the dust can fall where it has to be cleaned up any way. Undertake one room at a time, as it makes too much confusion and discomfort to attempt to clean several at a time, and entails too much fatigue on the housekeeper.

Take down the curtains and lambrequins(1), remove the ornaments, and have every mattress and spring carried into the open air; then have the carpet taken up, thoroughly shaken outdoors, folded up smoothly and put away with tobacco between the folds. The floor may then be swept, and afterward the walls and furniture should be vigorously dusted. A soft old towel is better for this purpose than feathers. Go over every piece of furniture in the room. Reach up to those strongholds of dust, the tops of the bed, wardrobe, and bureau.

Next go to the bed; have the slats removed, and with a feather dive into every hole and crevice with nitrate of silver mixed with the beaten white of an egg. Keep the children out of the way, as nitrate of silver is very poisonous. If you have not this article, wash over the bed with cold water and salt, and then apply a mixture of kerosene oil and spirits of turpentine in equal parts. Look into the corners of the mattress and the rosettes with which it is tacked.

Then wash the windows, polishing them off with old flannel when dry. If you have oil-cloth or matting on the floor, it may be readily cleaned by wiping it over with it thoroughly scoured with hot buttermilk or with cold water and salt.

If the floor is bare, have water and concentrated lye. Use a brush, as the lye is apt to hurt one's hands. If you wish to stain the floor you can do by washing it with a decoction made of red-oak or black walnut.

HOUSEHOLD HINTS:

- Do not deposit wood ashes in a wooden vessel or upon a wooden floor.
- Never use a light in examining a gas-meter.
- Never take a light into a closet.
- Never read in bed by candle or lamp light.
- Never leave clothes near a grate or fire-place to dry.
- Be careful in making fire with shavings, and never use any kind of oil to kindle a fire.
- Keep all lights as far from curtains as possible. Always fill and trim your lamps by daylight, and never near a fire.
- Good nice pie-crust can always be made by observing the following rule: One quarter of a cup of shortening to every cup of flour used; to be mixed as dry as possible with cold water, and mixed only with a knife.
- Take sweet butter only for baking purposes, and never fail to

(1) A drapery covering the upper part of a window or door or hanging from a shelf.

thoroughly beat together your butter and sugar, if you would be sure of good results in cake baking.

- Have metal or earthen vessels for matches, and keep them out of reach of children. Wax matches are not safe.
- Ground mustard mixed with a little water is an excellent agent for cleansing the hands after handling odorous substances.
- Cut hot bread or cake with a hot knife, and it will not be clammy.
- Salt extracts the juices of meat in cooking. Steaks ought therefore not to be salted until they have been broiled.
- In broiling dumplings of any kind, put them in the water one at a time. If they are put in together they will mix with each other.
- Do not cut lamp-wicks, but trim them by wiping off with a scrap of paper.
- Never boil vegetables with soup stock, for if you do it will certainly become sour in a short time.
- Boil cream for coffee, and see if the coffee will not taste better, as well as keep hot longer.
- Pin-cushion covers made of cheese-cloth embroidered and trimmed with lace wear well, and keep their looks.
- Some one says that leaves of parsley eaten with a little vinegar will destroy the odor of breath tainted by onions.
- Hot liquid lye is recommended for removing obstructions in waste-pipes. Or let the potash dissolve over the night in the pipes.
- To wipe dust from papered walls take a clean, soft piece of flannel. Of course it must not be damp, but the dry flannel will remove the dust.
- Varnish the soles of your shoes and it will render them impervious to dampness, and will also make them last longer.
- *This is a good plan:* Clean the mica in stove doors with vinegar. Take clinkers out of stoves by putting a few oyster-shells into the grate, when they will become loosened and may be removed without injuring the lining.
- Save the droppings from spermaceti candles, tie them in a cloth, and keep to smooth rough flat-irons.
- Never starch napkins. An old black bunting or cashmere dress may be made to serve a further period of usefulness by being made into a petticoat.

- Between two evils choose neither.
- Writing a will does not shorten life, and yet many men fear it will.
- Save old suspender rings and sew them on the corners of kitchen holders to hang them up by. It will be easy then to flip them on to a nail, and they will not be so likely to get lost.
- Powdered borax, with a little sugar, blown into the cracks and crevices with a small bellows, will drive away house-ants.
- Have a high stool in the kitchen to sit on when tired, to continue your work if necessary. Perched on its top you can wash dishes or iron with ease. A low soft sheep-skin mat is restful to stand upon.
- There is nothing better for cleaning brass or copper than coal ashes. They are also good to scour knives and forks with. For tin whiting or fine sand is best. To cleanse jars or jugs or any earthen vessel slaked lime is good, or warmed lye.
- To keep a stove smooth take a coarse and pretty large piece of flannel, roll it hard, and dip it in fine sand. Proceed to rub your stove when ever you are through cooking. Almost any stove will look better for being done the same way occasionally. Boiled starch is also very good to keep a stove looking well; put it on where it will not burn off—around the back and sides where it does not get very hot.

HOUSE-PAINTING DIRECTIONS:

Priming: Apply as thick as the paint will spread easily, rubbing out well with the brush. Use litharge(1) as a dryer. After sand-papering and dusting, putty up all the nail-heads and cracks with a putty-knife.

Outside Second Coat: Mix your paint with raw oil, using it as thick as possible consistent with easy spreading. After it is applied cross-smooth the work until it is level and even, then finish lengthwise with long light sweeps of the brush.

Outside Third Coat: Make a little thinner than the last, rub out well, cross-smooth, and finish very lightly with the tip of the brush.

Inside Second Coat: Mix your paint as thick as you can work it, using equal parts of raw oil and turpentine; rub this out well and carefully with the brush, cross-smooth, and finish even and nice.

(1) Lead protoxide.

Inside Third Coat: Mix with 3 parts turpentine and 1 part of raw oil; rub out well and smooth off with great care.

Fourth Coat, Flatting: Mix with turpentine alone thin enough to admit of spreading before it sets. Apply quickly without cross-smoothing, and finish lengthwise with a light touches of the tip of the brush, losing no time, as it sets rapidly.

Drawn Flatting: Ground white-lead is mixed with turpentine almost as thin as the last-named mixture. The lead will soon settle and the oil and turpentine rise to the top; pour it off, and repeat the mixture until what rises to the top is clear turpentine. The oil being all withdrawn by this process, with great care. This is used as a fourth coat, and the room must be kept shut and free from draught, as the color sets as fast as it is put on.

Plastered Walls: Give them a coat of glue size before painting oil.

Killing Smoky Walls or Ceilings: Wash over the smoky or greasy walls with niter, soda, or thin lime whitewash—the last is the best.

HOUSE-PLANNING:

"The wise woman buildeth her house," and the first thing to be settled is its site. This should be, if possible, on a sufficient elevation to secure a dry cellar and perfect drainage. In choosing the site regard should be had to the lighting and ventilation of the house, to its protection from wintry storms and winds, and its exposure to the sun.

In cities and towns, where land is costly, houses of many stories are a necessity, but in the country why not spread out on the ground instead of climbing so high into the air? One flight of stairs is endurable, 2 are wearisome, and 3 are intolerable, save to young people. Basement kitchens are necessary in the city, but entirely out of place in the country. The best place for a kitchen is in an ell, with laundry, store-room and drying-room for clothes joining, and with children's play-room and drying-room for clothes in winter in the story above.

The first rooms planned should be the kitchen, dining-room, and sitting-room. Beginning with the kitchen, let the designer decide upon its size, and then settle upon the places for the chimney, sink, pantry, work-table, cellar door, wood-house door, and the door into the dining-room. Let the windows of the kitchen face south, if possible, and have a door opening toward the south and on to a piazza running the length of the kitchen. If there are young children in the family this piazza will give them an open air play-room on sunny days in the winter, where they can be under the eye of the house-mother while she is about her work.

The kitchen planned, the dining-room, sitting-room, parlor, and the bed-rooms follow. Regard should continually be had to the furnishing of these rooms, for it is no unusual thing to find a dining-room with no suitable place for an extension-table, to find a parlor with no convenient place for the piano or sofa, to find bed-rooms with no place for the bed where it will be out of the draught when the doors and windows are open, and so situated that the occupants will not be compelled to open their eyes in the morning directly upon the windows. This last point can be made by the use of screens near the bed.

A house for a family of young children, where the mother expects to care at the same time for her children and her house, should have the nursery on the same floor as the kitchen and the dining-rooms, not only to save running up and down stairs, but to prevent the children from falling down stairs, and to enable the mother to be near them while at her work. The nursery should command all the sunshine possible. If an invalid or aged person is a member of the family, his room should be, if possible, on the first floor.

HOUSE-WIFE, RULES FOR THE YOUNG:

General Order of Working for Every Day:

- Before leaving your room throw open windows, top and bottom; lay pillows in the sun, bed-clothes to air, and turn back mattress.
- As soon as you come down stairs open blinds and windows.
- Light kitchen fire, take up ashes, sift them.
- Brush off the stove, rinse and fill the kettle.
- Sweep the kitchen, the stoop, or piazza, beating all mats thoroughly.
- Remove stale flowers from parlor and dining-room, and dust.
- Prepare for breakfast, putting biscuits or muffins to bake while you lay the table.
- Close blinds on sunny side.
- After breakfast clear the table as soon as possible, putting milk and butter away at once, instead of allowing them to remain in the hot kitchen.
- Do not leave the white table-cloth on a moment longer than necessary, as it attracts flies.
- For the same reason remove the crumbs from the floor.
- Wash and put away breakfast dishes.
- Darken the dining-room, pantry, and all unused rooms.
- Make beds, empty slops, wash soap-dishes, fill water-pitchers,

fold dry towels, take away soiled ones—but, if damp, dry them before putting into the soiled clothes-hamper, as every thing quickly mildews in hot weather.

- Darken rooms after having put them in perfect order.

HUNT THE RING, GAME OF:

The game of *Hunt the Ring* is, perhaps, better liked than *Hunt the Slipper,* on account of its being in the estimation of most people more convenient and manageable. Either a ring or a small key may be used for the purpose. Whichever it is, a string must be passed through it, and the ends fastened in a knot, forming thus a circular band. The company then stand in a circle, allowing the string to pass through the hands of each person, and enabling every one to slide the ring easily along from one to the other. The object of the player standing inside the circle is to stop it in its progress, which, in most cases, he finds a rather difficult task. The game is also frequently played without any string, when every one tries, of course, to pass the ring around very rapidly, without being detected by the hunter.

HUNT THE WHISTLE, GAME OF:

This game is always successful, and a source of very great amusement if only some one ignorant of the secret can be found who will volunteer to act as hunter. Such person is first requested to kneel down while some lady goes through the ceremony of conferring upon him the order of knighthood. During the process the whistle, attached to a piece of ribbon, is pinned to the coat of the newly made knight. He is then told to rise and go in quest of the whistle, which is in the possession of one of the party.

The hunt now begins, the players all trying to deceive their victim in every way imaginable, and to make him think that they are passing the whistle from one to another. On every possible occasion, of course, the whistle should be sounded, until the deluded knight has made the discovery that the object of his search is fastened to himself.

HYPO, OR HYPOCHONDRIAS:

This is the depression of spirits or "blue devils." It chiefly affects persons of the melancholic temperament, and is commonly induced by hard study, irregular habits, want of proper social intercourse, living in close apartments, and insufficient out-of-door exercise.

Treatment: Similar to that recommended for dyspepsia, observing, however, that success depends more on engaging and amusing the mind, than in administration of medicine.

HYSTERICS:

The fit may be prevented by the administration of 30 drops of laudanum, and as many of ether. When it has taken place open the windows, loosen the tight parts of the dress, sprinkle cold water on the face, etc. A glass of wine or cold water when the patient can swallow. Avoid excitement and tight lacing.

An attack is generally preceded by depression of spirits, restlessness, etc. It is sometimes marked by convulsions or fits. At times the attacks are local, manifested by spasms in the throat, the patient feels a ball rise there, her heart beats violently and she laughs and cries by turns.

In the worst cases the limbs are thrown into spasms; the patient struggles violently, rising up in a sitting posture, and throwing herself back, twisting the body from side to side, clenching the hands, and throwing the arms about, so that she is with difficulty held.

Quinine will be found a good tonic, 1 grain 3 times a day, in the form of pill, or in a little sweetened milk.

I

"I APPRENTICED MY SON," GAME OF:

The shortest way of describing this game will be to give an illustration of the manner in which it is played. John: "I apprenticed my son to a grocer, and the first thing he sold was a half a pound of C."

Nellie: Coffee? - No. Sam: Cocoa? - No. Tom: Cayenne pepper? - No. Edith: Chicory? - Yes.

Edith, being the guesser of the right article, is entitled to be the next to apprentice her son. One guess only in turn is allowed to each player.

ICE, TO KEEP:

(1) Small quantities of ice may be preserved in summer by making a small bag large enough to hold the ice; then make another much larger bag, and fill the space between with sawdust or feathers.

(2) Cut a piece of flannel about 9 in. square, and secure it by ligature round the mouth of an ordinary tumbler, so as to leave a cup-shaped depression of flannel within the tumbler to about half its depth. In the flannel cup so constructed pieces of ice may be preserved many hours; all the longer if a piece of flannel 4 or 5 in. square be used as a loose cover to the ice cup; cheap flannel with comparatively open meshes is preferable, as water easily drains through it, and ice is thus kept quite dry; when good flannel with close texture is employed, a small hole must be made in the bottom of the flannel cup, otherwise it holds water and facilitates the melting of the ice.

ICE-WATER AND HEALTH:

Ice-Water Hinders Digestion: Cold water is a less rapid solvent than warm water, as cold air is a better preservative than warm air. So ice-water taken into the stomach chills the coats and contents of that organ, and thus suddenly checks and hinders the digestion of the food.

Iced Drinks Affecting the Head: An intelligent and influential medical journal says very sensibly, "Drinks should be sipped, not gulped" and adds: "The intimate connection between stomach and brain is known to every body, and it must be obvious that to pour an iced draught into the stomach must at once send the blood to the head. Very few who have indulged in the rapid drinking of these beverages have failed to notice that a sudden pain in the head was the result. It may have been a sharp shoot, or a mere feeling of dullness, and it may have been passed off in a moment, but it was at least incipient congestion of the brain."

Evils of Iced Drinks: Another eminent hygienic authority urges that "no well man has any business to eat ices or drink iced liquids in any shape or form, if he wants to preserve his teeth, protect the tone of his stomach, and guard against sudden inflammations and prolonged dyspepsia. It is enough to make one shudder to see a beautiful young girl sipping scalding coffee or tea at the beginning of a meal, and then close it with a glass of ice-water, for at 30 she must either be snaggle-toothed or wear those of the dead or artificial."

Caution about Ice: Dr. W. W. Hall, in one of his health tracts, has these suggestive words: "If the reader is down town or away from home on a hot day and feels as if it would be perfectly delicious to have a glass of lemonade, soda-water, or brandy toddy, by all means let him resist the temptation until he gets home, and then take a glass of cold water, a swallow at a time, with a second or two interval between each swallow.

Several noteworthy results will most assuredly follow. After it is all over you will feel quite as well from a drink of water as if you had enjoyed a free swig of either of the others. In 10 minutes after you will feel a great deal better. You will not have been poisoned by the lead or copper which is most often found in soda-water. You will be richer by 6 cents, which will be the interest on a dollar for a whole year. You will not have fallen down dead from the sudden chills which sometimes result from drinking soda, iced-water, or toddy in a hurry."

How to Cool Drinking-water without Ice: Fresh spring- or well-water is abundantly cool for any drinking purpose whatever. In cities where water is artificially supplied the case is somewhat different; but even then there is no good excuse for drinking ice-water, because, even if the excuse were good in itself, the effects on the stomach and teeth are the same.

Make a bag of thick woolen doubled, lined with muslin; fill it with ice; have in a pitcher an inch or two of water above the faucet, and let this bag of ice be suspended from the cover within 2 in. of the surface of the water. The ice will melt slowly and keep the water delightfully cool, but not ice-cold. A still better effect will be produced if the pitcher is also well enveloped in woolen.

Again, water almost as cool as it can be, unless it has ice actually in it, may be had without any ice at all by enveloping a closed pitcher partially filled with water with several folds of cotton, linen, or bagging, and so arranging it that these folds are kept wet all the time by water dropping from another vessel, on the principle of evaporation. Water which is not iced may be drank freely throughout the meal, as the natural thirst demands.

INDIA-INK MARKS, TO REMOVE:

There is no method known of removing India-ink markings that have been pricked into the skin save by the process by which they were introduced. The superficial application of any remedy to remove it will be utterly useless. The only method that will prove efficacious is the painful and tedious one of pricking the skin as was done when the markings were made, and squeezing out the solid particles of coloring matter with the blood. If this be done carefully and thoroughly the marks may be removed; but in no other way can it be done, except by actually cutting out the marked piece of skin.

INDIGESTION REMEDIES:

(1) Many of the Welsh peasants live almost wholly upon oatmeal-cakes and buttermilk, and seldom suffer from indigestion. The acid (lactic acid) in the buttermilk is regarded as a promoter of digestion.

(2) Dyspepsia(1) is cured by muscular exercise, voluntary or involuntary, and in no other way can it be cured, because nothing can create or collect the gastric juice except exercise; it is a product of the human machine. Nature only can make it.

(3) *A Southern gentleman says:* "For something near two yrs. I had suffered with dyspepsia and soreness of the gastric organs. During that time I used several different preparations, and advised with every physician I met, but still could get no permanent relief. Four or five months ago I commenced to the use of a remedy that has proved very beneficial to me. *Here it is:*

"Every night before I retire, and every morning just as soon as I rise, I give myself a good pounding all over the breast and stomach, breathing long, full breaths frequently during the operation, and throwing my arms in every direction. I followed this course energetically for some time. Now I have no symptoms of dyspepsia, and the soreness in my stomach, which gave me an untold amount of annoyance, has almost entirely disappeared. Of course, the pounding must be light and moderate at first. This remedy is simple, and can be used by all."

INFANTS, FOOD OF:

Happy indeed is the child who, during the first period of its existence, is fed upon no other aliment than the milk of its mother or that of a healthy nurse. If other food becomes necessary before the child has acquired teeth, it ought to be of a liquid form; for instance, biscuits or stale bread boiled in an equal mixture of milk and water, to the consistency of a thick soup; but by no means even this in the first week of its life. Flour or

(1) Indigestion.

meal ought never to be used for soup, as it produces viscid humors, instead of wholesome nutritious chyle(1). Potatoes should be allowed only in moderation and not to be eaten with butter, but rather with other vegetables, either mashed up or in broth.

The following order of giving food to children has been found proper and conducive to their health: After rising in the morning, suppose about 6 o'clock, a moderate portion of lukewarm milk with well-baked bread, which should by no means be new; at 9 o'clock, bread with some fruit, or, if fruit be scarce, a small quantity of fresh butter; about 12 o'clock, the dinner, or a sufficient quantity; between 4 and 5 o'clock some bread with fruit, or, in winter, the jam of plums as a substitute for fruit.

Children should be allowed to eat till they are satisfied, without surfeiting themselves, that they may not crave for a heavy supper, which disturbs their rest and is productive of bad humors; lastly, about 7 o'clock, they may be permitted a light supper, consisting either of milk, soup, fruit, or boiled vegetables and the like, but neither meat or mealy dishes, nor any article of food which produces flatulency; in short, they ought then to eat but little and remain awake at least an hour after it.

It has often been contended that bread is hurtful to children; but this applies only to new bread, or such as is not sufficiently baked; for instance, our rolls, muffins, and crumpets, than which nothing can be more hurtful and oppressive. Good wheaten bread is extremely proper during the first years of infancy; but that made of rye, or a mixture of wheat and rye, would be more conducive to health after the age of childhood.

Physicians are decidedly against giving drink to children in large quantities, and at irregular periods, whether it consists of the mother's milk or any other equally mild liquor. Many children acquire a habit of drinking during their meals; it would be more conducive to digestion if they were accustomed to drink only after having made a meal. This useful rule is too often neglected, but it is certain that inundations of the stomach during the mastication and maceration of the food not only vitiate digestion, but may be attended with other bad consequences, as cold drink when brought in contact with the teeth previously heated may easily occasion cracks or chinks in these useful bones, and pave the way for their decay.

INFANTS' BANDS:(2)

To make unnecessary the use of pins in a baby's wardrobe the bands and waists may be thus made:

Make the band the usual length—5 fingers—then sew strips of tape long enough to tie around the infant on one end of the band two-thirds in. from the top and bottom. The tape should be sewed in the middle of its

(1) The fluid of the lacteal vessels.
(2) A swaddle or swaddling–band, a secure wrap for an infant.

length, so that the two ends will be of equal length. At 3 in. from the other end of the band work 2 holes for the tapes to pass through. This to be tied in front. Or, make an oval 25 in. in length and 7 in. in width. Attach to each end tapes 12 in. long and three-fourths in. wide; 7 1/2 in. from one end make an opening up and down 4 in. in length through which the tape at the other extreme of the oval is to be drawn. For waists this shape is made wider; arm-holes are cut out, and strips of wide tape are sewed on for straps. A child is not likely to outgrow a waist made in this way before it is worn out. It may be tied behind or before.

INGROWING TOE-NAIL:

This affection is of more consequence than is usually supposed. It is sometimes a serious matter to the patient and causes much pain. One principal cause comes from the fashion of wearing very small-toed boots, and another from wearing much-darned stockings. It is not usually the nail that is in fault, but the skin surrounding it. This becomes thickened and ulcerated, and gradually the nail becomes overlapped. The nail then becomes bent and grows irregularly, but it is the highly sensitive skin that gives the pain.

Remedies:

(1) Mr. Wood, surgeon of King's College Hospital, recommends broad-toed boots, also scraping the center of the nail thin with a piece of glass. A plug of cotton under the edge of the nail will aid in restoring it to proper shape and position.

(2) A Liverpool physician has for the past 20 yrs. employed compressed sponge very successfully in the treatment of ingrowing nails. His method is to render the sponge compact by wetting, and then tying it tightly until it is thoroughly dry. A bit of the sponge, in size less than a grain of rice, is placed under the nail and secured by strips of adhesive plaster. In this way the point of the nail is kept up from the toe until the surrounding soft parts are restored to their normal condition by appropriate means. Of course, there is no pain in this remedy, and its application requires only ordinary skill.

(3) It is stated that cauterization by hot tallow is an immediate cure for ingrowing nails. Put a small piece of tallow in a spoon, and heat it over a lamp until it becomes very hot, and drop 2 or 3 drops between nail and toe.

INK, HOW TO MAKE:

Take 1/4 lb. of extract of logwood, 1 gallon clear, soft water; heat it to the boiling point in a perfectly clean iron kettle; skim well, stir, then add

90 grains of bichromate of potash, 15 grains prussiate of potash(1), dissolved in 1/2 pint of hot water; stir well for 3 minutes; take off and strain. The above will make 1 gallon of the best ink which I have ever used.

INK, INDELIBLE MARKING:

One and a half drams of nitrate of silver, 1 ounce of distilled water, 1/2 ounce of strong mucilage of gum arabic, three-fourths dram of liquid ammonia. Mix the above in a clean glass bottle, cork tightly, and keep in a dark place till dissolved, and ever afterward. Directions for use: Shake the bottle, then dip a clean quill pen in the ink and write and draw what you require on the article; immediately hold it close to the fire, (without scorching), or pass a hot iron over it, and it will become a deep and indelible black, indestructible by either time or acids of any description.

INK, WAYS TO REMOVE FROM LINEN:

(1) To take ink out of linen, dip the ink-spot in pure melted tallow; then wash out the tallow, and the ink will come out with it. This is said to be unfailing.

(2) Milk will remove ink from linen or colored muslins, rub and rinse in cold water.

(3) An inkstand was turned over upon a white table-cloth; a servant threw over it a mixture of salt and pepper plentifully, and all traces of it disappeared.

(4) Rub the spot well with the end of a clean mold candle, leaving some of the tallow in lumps upon it for 24 hours; then wash the article in boiling water, and the ink will disappear.

(5) Take 1 ounce sal-ammoniac(2), 1 ounce salts of tartar, wine-bottle of cold soft water. Well mix the above; wet the linen thoroughly with the mixture, and repeat the process till the spots disappear.

INK SPOTS, TO REMOVE:

To remove iron-rust or ink-spots, moisten the spots and apply salts of lemon until they disappear, and then rinse well. Salts of lemon are made of equal parts of oxalic acid and tartaric acid. Another way is to moisten with lemon-juice, sprinkle well with salt, and lay in the sun. If ink is spilled on colored goods that will not bear acids soak them immediately in sweet milk boiling hot. Hot melted tallow poured through ink-spots will also remove them.

INK-STAINS, TO REMOVE FROM SILVER:

The tops and other portions of silver inkstands frequently become

(1) Potassium cyanide.
(2) Ammonium chloride.

deeply discolored with ink, which is difficult to remove by ordinary means. It may, however, be completely eradicated by making a little chloride of lime into a paste with water, and rubbing it upon the stains. Chloride of lime has been misnamed "the general bleacher," but it is a foul enemy to all metallic surfaces.

INK-STAINS, TO REMOVE FROM THE HANDS:

Indexical pumice-stone soap will instantly remove ink-stains from the hands.

INSANITY:

The studious, very nervous, and those who are engaged in sedentary or indoor occupations or who indulge in irregular or vicious habits, as well as fast livers, are the most liable to this affection. It also frequently arises from disordered physical health. It is sometimes inherited.

Treatment: Change of scene, outdoor exercise, agreeable company, pleasing mental occupation, and due attention to diet, clothing, ventilation, etc., with the judicious use of some mild aperient medicine and tepid bathing, will generally alleviate and frequently effect a cure.

INSECT-POWDER, PERSIAN:

The powder is the pulverized flowers of pyrethrum, carneum, and roseum, growing on the Caucasian Mountains. It is not poisonous to man unless inhaled or swallowed in large quantities, but it is known to be death to insect life in all its forms, first stupefying and then killing. Scattered over the bedstead and clothing, or the person, it destroys bed-bugs, lice, etc.

For flies and mosquitoes the best way to apply it is to burn it. Take a tea-spoonful of the powder in a dish of any kind, and set fire to it. A dense smoke arises which is certain destruction to all insects with which it comes in contact. A tincture prepared by placing 1 part of the powder in 4 of alcohol, distilled with 10 times its bulk of water, and applied to the body, is said to be a perfect protection against vermin of all kinds. White hellebore answers to the same purpose and is cheaper.

INSECTS ON PLANTS, TO DESTROY:

Insects are a very serious drawback to healthy and vigorous plants, and most vigilant watch should at all times be set for them; but, in spite of all our care, they will appear and increase with such rapidity that no time should be lost in destroying them. No plants, however, should be taken into the house until thoroughly cleansed. Cultivated plants seem to furnish food for several different species of insects, and the treatment necessary to destroy one form will not answer for another.

The black or green fly, or aphis, are always the most numerous, and are first seen on the new growth of houseplants; but in an amazingly short time spread to the older leaves, especially to the soft wooded ones, as well as flowers, absorbing the juice and vitality of the plant. It is easy enough to fumigate the greenhouse to destroy insects, which, of course, could not be done in our dwellings, and many plans have been recommended.

One says, sprinkle Scotch snuff on the foliage and let it remain 2 or 3 days; another says, a weak solution of carbolic acid, applied with a swab or feather; and still another says, take a little coal-oil, just enough to make a colored scum on the surface of a tub of water, and dip the inverted plant into it, not allowing the pot to touch it.

Others recommend hot water, and we have found that to be the least objectionable. Our plan is to dip the plant in a tub of water that will register 120 degrees with a thermometer, repeating it the following day. Of course, the plant must not remain in the hot water, as it would be soon cooked.

To destroy the green fly in greenhouses or conservatories the most approved method is fumigating, which is done by placing on a pan of live coals a quantity of damp tobacco stems, filling the house with a dense smoke, and keeping it closed until morning; but, as heliotropes, etc., are liable to be injured by smoke, spread paper over the plants while fumigating. It is better, however, to fumigate 2 or 3 nights in succession than to risk too dense smoke.

But the most destructive and least known insect is the red spider. It is too small to be readily seen, but its presence is easily detected by gray or yellowish spots on the apparently dying leaves. The little insect lives upon the under side of the leaf, and not only absorbs its vitality, but weaves a fine web, which closes the pores through which the plant breathes. They delight in hot, dry atmosphere, just such a one as our sitting-room affords; but are readily destroyed by syringing the plant often with clear, warm water, or a good bath in the tub, and then sprinkle with sulphur. But if small plates of bright tin or glass, with a little sulphur on them, are placed under the plants, in the full rays of the sun, no red spiders will trouble them, as the sulphur flumes kill them. A weak solution of whale-oil soap is excellent; but it must be very weak, or it would not only kill the foliage, but the plant also.

The mealy bug is also very destructive to hot-house plants, but is really the easiest to exterminate of any in this list. They are a large, white, woolly looking lump in the axil of the leaf, and are easily kept down by frequent syringing with warm, greasy water, to which a little sulphur should be added. But if full grown they should be picked off by hand or a small, sharp-pointed stick.

INSOMNIA:

The sufferings, experience, and subsequent relief of a chronic sufferer from insomnia are detailed in the following paragraph: It was originally published in the Pall Mall Gazette, *and attracted a great deal of attention because the writer had experimented with every known remedy, every fad, and logical idea that suggested itself to him. Because his memoirs of the terrible ordeal he went through are so complete, it is well to summarize them.*

In the first place, he found no reason to forego food just before retiring. He dined at 7, and took a biscuit and butter at 11 or 12 o'clock. He always kept a biscuit in his room to eat if he failed to sleep, and he says that when his malady was acute he found a sandwich better. One remedy that he tried was rubbing the nape of his neck with acetic acid just before going to bed. It produced not the slightest effect in the several times that he tried it. He got a hop pillow, but the smell was so nauseating after a while that he gave it up. Then he ate spring onions at night, but they did no good. He next slung an onion cut in two around his neck at night, but that did not help him. He was told that if he spent every day on the water he would woo sleep back to his bed, but it was a false endeavor. He tried whisky and water, but that kept him awake the entire night and gave him a splitting headache as well. He tried reading and smoking in bed, sponging with cold water, and rubbing with a flesh-brush, but with out good effect. He tried a compress around his stomach, then on the back of his head, and then around his legs—the latter with a simultaneous dose of wine of coca. He found that the coca without the compress was of some little avail. At last some one gave him more relief than he had felt before by suggesting that his ailment lay in his liver. He got some sleep when he began treating his liver. He found, too, that the tobacco used in Manilla cigars had a more soporific effect than any other tobacco, and smoking those cigars added to his sleeping powers. Next he heard of the theory of Prof. Wilhelm Schmoele, that lemon-juice is such an elixir of life that a person may indefinitely prolong his existence if he takes the juice of a lemon every day. Experimenting with lemon-juice—the real juice of fresh lemon—improved his indigestion, corrected his liver, and greatly induced sleep.

So that this sufferer says his first precept to the sleepless, "See that your liver is in order." He is equally emphatic against recourse to alcohol, which heats the blood and accelerates its circulation. Next he declares that it is a good thing when one awakes at night to light a candle, eat a biscuit, and take a book—not an exciting book, but one calculated to put the thoughts into a quiet train. He also cautions every one against having too many bed-clothes. A light sleeper should accustom himself to as few bed-clothes as possible, and to be sure to leave the window open.

INVITATIONS:

All invitations, excepting dinner invitations, are issued in the name of the gentleman and lady of the house, or, when extended to gentlemen only, in the name of the host. Answers to invitations, excepting such diner invitations as are issued in the name of the gentlemen only, must be addressed to the lady of the house.

In the height of a fashionable season send invitations at least a fortnight beforehand. For a small company a week's notice is sufficient. For a costume ball or any occasion when elaborate dresses are needed a month should be given.

Printed cards of invitation are *en règle* for large gatherings, private and public, but not for small parties. For the last whole sheet of small written note is appropriate, and may have the initial letter or monogram upon it and the envelope. Any more decoration is in bad taste. It is the best to send invitations to private parties by special messenger.

The proper form for a dinner invitation is:

Mr. and Mrs. Clover request the favor of Mr. and Mrs. Leighton's company at dinner on Tuesday the 8th of January, at 5 o'clock. R.S.V.P.

The letters at the bottom are placed there whenever an answer is desired. They stand for the French words, "Respondez s'il vous plait"— "An answer, if you please." The answer accepting the invitation should run as follows:

Mr. and Mrs. Leighton have much pleasure in accepting Mr. and Mrs. Glover's kind invitation to dinner on the 8th of January.

If declined, the following form must be used:

Mr. and Mrs. Leighton regret that a prior engagement (or other reason stated) will prevent their accepting Mr. and Mrs. Glovers's kind invitation to dinner on the 8th of January.

Persons moving in one circle of society should not, as a general rule, be invited to meet those who move in another circle. A man of strong political or religious bias in one direction should not be invited to meet another opposed to his views.

IRONING:

The irons should be scrupulously clean. They should always be perfectly wiped before putting away, and kept in a dry place. If the starch sticks to the flat-iron take a bit of beeswax, put it between two sheets of paper, and then rub the warm flat-iron over it; or keep it tied up in a rag to rub on the irons; then, if covered with brown starch, scrape it off with a knife and rub the flat-iron on the oiled paper; this gives linen a fine gloss. The warmth and heaviness of the iron should be regulated by the articles to be ironed.

A shirt-board for ironing is a necessity in every well regulated family. This should be covered with at least two thicknesses of blanket, and have the ironing sheet, also double, smoothly pinned over it so that it cannot slip. Iron-holders should have a cover of white cotton cloth, made to fit nicely, and fastened on with buttons, and when it becomes soiled it can be removed, washed, and replaced. To keep your ironing-board clean and free from dust, take two breadths of calico, (an old dress skirt may be used), and make a bag to slip the board in when you put it away.

Muslins and laces require to be ironed twice, gently pulling them out after the first ironing. Embroideries should be ironed over several thicknesses of flannel. As a general rule all fine muslin work should be ironed first under a piece of old cambric, as it clears the muslin from the starch and prevents it from being scorched. The bosoms and cuffs of gentlemen's shirts should also be ironed in similar manner.

In ironing pocket-handkerchiefs the flat-iron should be passed over each side before the middle is touched, slightly pulling each corner with the left hand while you iron with the right.

To iron plaits(1) neatly the frills should be laid straight in front of the ironer, while she makes the creases of the desired width with the right hand, holding the point of the hem with the left hand till the iron has pressed it down. All plaits must be laid even to the thread to look well.

Laces are to be carefully brought into shape, and all the edge or purling pulled out like new.

In ironing silks, cover them over with paper on fine cotton, and use openly a moderately heated iron, taking great care that the iron does not touch the silk at all, or it will make it look glossy and show that it has been ironed. Any white article if scorched slightly can be in part restored, so far as looks go; but any scorching injures the fabric.

IRON POTS, TO MEND:

Iron pots and utensils can easily be mended by using the following preparations:

Take 2 parts of sulphur and one part (by weight) of fine black-lead; put the sulphur in an old iron pan, holding it over the fire until it shall begin to melt, then add the lead; stir well until all shall be mixed and melted; then pour out on an iron plate or smooth stone. When cool break in small pieces. A sufficient quantity of this compound being placed upon the crack of the iron pot to be mended, it can be soldered by a hot iron in the same way a tinsmith solders his sheets. If there be a small hole in the pot drive a copper rivet in it, and then solder over it with this cement.

IRON-RUST STAINS:

These may be removed by the use of lemon-juice and salt, or with oxalic acid. Moisten the stain with a solution of oxalic acid, lay in the sun, and when the stain is out rinse thoroughly. The acid should not come in contact with any abraided surface of the hands, and should be labeled "Poison."

(1) Pleats.

ITCHING OR PRURITUS:

Caused by a morbid sensibility of the nervous system, similar to what exists in hysteria. No local disorder is perceptible; the skin retains its wonted appearance, yet its nervous excitability occasions unspeakable torment.

Treatment: Tonics and anodynes are required; give 10 drops of Fowler's solution of arsenic in 1/2 ounce of water 3 times a day, after meals, and 1/2 dram of McMunn's elixir of opium in a little sweetened water once in 3 days. Apply locally lemon-juice or vinegar mixed with an equal quantity of water; or chloral hydrate, 1/2 dram; water, 4 ounces; mix.

IVORY, TO BLEACH:

Take 2 handfuls of lime, slake it by sprinkling it with water; then add 3 pints of water, and stir the whole together; let it settle 10 minutes, and pour the water into a pan for your purpose. Then take your ivory and steep it in the lime-water for 24 hours, after which boil it in a strong alum-water 1 hour and dry it in the air.

IVORY, TO GILD:

Immerse it in a solution of nitro-muriate of gold, and then expose it to hydrogen gas while damp. Wash it afterward in clean water.

IVORY, TO POLISH:

Remove any scratches or file-marks that may be present with finely pulverized pumice-stone, moistened with water. Then wash the ivory and polish with prepared chalk, applied moist upon a piece of chamois leather, rubbing quickly.

IVORY, TO SILVER:

Pound a small piece of nitrate of silver in a mortar, add soft water to it, then mix well together, and keep in vial for use. When you wish to silver any article, immerse it in this solution, let it remain till it turns of a deep yellow; then place it in clear water, expose it to the rays of the sun. If you wish to depicture a figure, name, or cipher on your ivory, dip a camel's-hair pencil in the solution, and draw the subject on the ivory. After it has turned a deep yellow, wash it well with water and place it in the sunshine, occasionally wetting it with pure water. In a short time it will turn of a deep black color, which if well rubbed, will change to a brilliant silver.

IVORY, TO WHITEN:

Slake some lime in water, put your ivory in the water, after being decanted from the grounds; boil it till it looks quite white. To polish it afterward set it in the turner's wheel, and, after having worked, take brushes and pumice-stones, subtle powder with water, and rub it till it looks perfectly smooth. Next to that heat by turning it against a piece of linen or sheepskin leather, and when hot rub it over with a little dry whiting diluted in oil of olive, then with a little dry whiting alone, finally with a piece of soft white rag. When all this is performed as directed the ivory will look very white.

IVORY ORNAMENTS, TO CLEAN:

To clean ivory ornaments, rub them well with fresh butter, i.e., without salt, and put them in the sunshine. Discolored ivory may be whitened by rubbing with a paste composed of burned pumice-stone and water, and then placing it under glass in the sun.

IVY, ENGLISH, TREATMENT OF:

The use of the English ivy cannot be too strongly recommended as a decoration in our rooms during the winter season. A lady noted for the beauty and freshness of her ivies was asked the secret of her success, which was simply putting a small piece of beefsteak at the roots of the plants every spring and fall. It is also said that to tightly rub each leaf on both sides with sweet-oil will preserve a fresh, vigorous appearance of ivies, in spite of furnace heat and gas, usually so injurious to all house plants. These simple measures are well worth trying.

IVY, POISONING, CURE FOR:

Bathe the parts affected with sweet spirits of niter(1). If the blisters are broken so that the niter be allowed to penetrate the cuticle, more than a single application is rarely necessary; and even where it is only applied to the surface of the skin 3 or 4 times a day there is rarely a trace of the poison left next morning.

(1) Potassium or sodium nitrate.

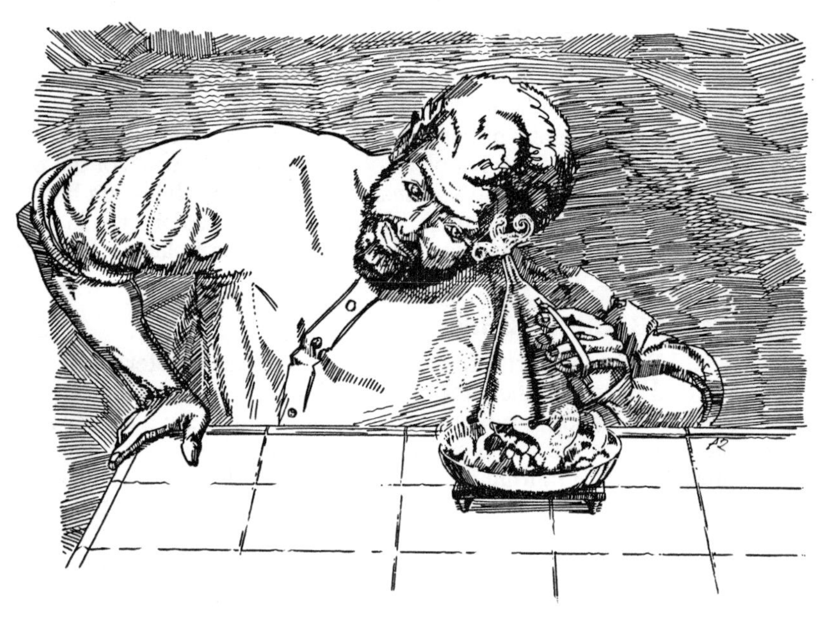

• *Earache Remedy* •

J-K

JARS, COVERING FOR:

A good waterproof paper for covering jars used in preserving, etc., may be made by brushing over the paper with boiled linseed oil, and suspending it over a line until dry.

JARS, TO CLEANSE THE INSIDE OF:

This can be done in a few minutes by filling the jars with hot water (it need not be scalding hot) and then stirring in a tea-spoonful or more of baking-soda. Shake well, then empty the jar at once, and if any of the former odor remains about it fill again with water and soda, shake well, and rinse out in cold water.

JAVELLE WATER, TO MAKE:

Take 2 lbs. washing-soda(1) and 2 lbs. chloride of lime, place them in a hot stone jar, and pour over them 2 gallons of boiling water; then place over it a thick cloth and a board with a stone upon it. Let it stand 24 hours, stirring 2 or 3 times. When quite clear strain it through bed-ticking or thick flannel, rinsing out immediately to save the cloth. Then bottle for future use.

JAVELLE WATER, USES OF:

Javelle water is excellent to remove fruit and vegetable stains, and perhaps some others, but avails nothing with ink and iron-rust. It is intensely alkaline, and therefore it affects acids principally. Half a pint in 3 or 4 pails of boiling water will whiten table-cloths beautifully. Any small article that is to be thoroughly treated should be washed and boiled first, then it may be dipped in the javelle water; let it stand 3 or 4 minutes, watching it very closely, and removing it the moment the stain disappears. If there is yet a faint outline of the stain, that will often come out in the subsequent treatment. Do not let the fabric be in more than 2 minutes, as there is risk of disorganizing it. Then throw it into the hot water, let it stand a few minutes, rinse thoroughly in 2 or 3 waters, and hang to dry in the sun. Do not let a drop of it fall upon colored cloth, and if it falls upon any dry cloth wash out immediately, or it may eat a hole. Do not keep the hands in it longer than half an hour, or it will remove the cuticle.

(1) A crystalline form of sodium carbonate.

JEWELRY, TO CLEAN:

(1) The simplest and best method of cleaning gold jewelry is by washing with tepid water and fine soap, to which a few drops of ammonia has been added. Rinse off with clear water, and lay in fine hardwood shavings, or dry polish with chamois skin.

(2) Wash in soap-suds, rinse in diluted alcohol, and lay in a box of dry sawdust to dry. As simple as this seems, it is the very nicest way possible to clean gold chains or ornaments of any kind.

JINGLING, GAME OF:

This may be considered by some as almost too noisy for an indoor game, but when played in an empty room is proper enough. The players are blindfolded, with the exception of one, who is called the jingler, and who has 2 or 3 little bells fastened to him, which jingle whenever he moves. The object of the blind children is to catch the jingler as he runs to and fro among them, and a line is drawn on the floor beyond which he dare not run in his efforts to evade them. The line is not necessary if the room is a small one. If the jingler can manage to remain uncaught for a certain time he is considered to have won the game. On the other hand, the victory remains with any of the blindfolded children who can catch him before his time probation has expired.

JOCKEY CLUB, TO MAKE:

Spirits of wine, 5 gallons, orange-flower water, 1 gallon; balsam of Peru, 4 ounces; essence of bergamot(1), 8 ounces; essence of cloves, 4 ounces, essence of neroli(2), 2 ounces; mix thoroughly.

KALSOMINE:

Eight pounds of whiting(3) and 1/4 lb. of white glue make the right proportions. Soak the glue over night in cold water, and in the morning heat it until it is perfectly dissolved. Mix the whiting with hot water, stir the two thoroughly together, and have the wash the consistence of thick cream. Apply warm with a kalsomine brush, brushing it well and finishing it as you go on. If warm skim-milk is used instead of water the glue may be omitted. Before the wash is applied all holes and crevices should be stopped with plaster of Paris mixed with water. Colors to tint the walls may be procured at any paint-store.

KEROSENE FIRES:

It ought to be more generally known that wheat flour is probably the best possible article to thrown over a fire caused by the spilling and igniting

(1) Aromatic herb of the mint family.
(2) Oil from orange flowers.
(3) Fine pulverized chalk.

of kerosene. It ought to be known, because flour is always within convenient reach.

KEROSENE STAINS, TO REMOVE:

Cover kerosene stains with Indian meal, and when the oil strikes through remove and put on fresh; repeat this until the oil is removed.

KETTLE, IRON, TO CLEAN:

Some one asks how to cleanse a new iron kettle. Mine was a source of despair to me until I was advised to boil skim-milk in it and then wash in good soap-suds. I had my milk man bring me 6 quarts of skim-milk, which I boiled and simmered in my 8 quart kettle for 24 hours. The kettle was made smooth and clean, and has given me no trouble since.

KETTLES, TO CLEAN:

A good way to clean the inside of pots and pans is to fill them with water in which a few ounces of washing-soda is dissolved, and set them on the fire. Let the water boil until the inside of the pot looks clean.

KEYS, HOW TO FIT INTO LOCKS:

When it is not convenient to take locks apart in the event of keys being lost, stolen, or missing, when you wish to fit a new key, take a lighted match or candle and smoke the new key in the flame, introduce it carefully into the lock, withdraw it, and the indentations in the smoked part of the key will show you exactly where to file.

KID BOOTS, TO CLEAN:

A mixture of oil and ink is good to clean kid boots with; the first softens and the latter blackens them.

KID BOOTS, TO SOFTEN:

Melt 1/4 lb. of tallow, then pour it into a jar, and add to it the same weight of olive-oil; stir and let it stand till cold; apply a small quantity occasionally with a piece of flannel. Should the boots be very dirty, cleanse with warm water. It will soften any leather.

KID GLOVES, HOW TO WASH:

Have ready a little new milk in some saucer and a piece of brown soap in another, and a clean cloth or towel folded 3 or 4 times. On the cloth spread out the glove smooth and neat. Take a piece of flannel, dip it in the milk, then rub off a good quantity of soap to the wetted flannel, and commence to rub the glove downward toward the fingers, holding it firmly with the left hand. Continue this process until the glove, if white, looks of a dingy yellow, though clean; if colored, till it looks dark and spoiled. Lay it to dry, and the old gloves will soon look nearly new. They will be soft, glossy, smooth, shaply, and elastic.

KINDLING, HOW TO MAKE:

To make a handy and cheap kindling, take 1 quart of tar and 3 lbs. of resin; melt them, then cool, and mix as much sawdust, with a little charcoal added, as can be worked in. Spread out on a board, and when cold break up into lumps the size of a large hickory-nut, and you will have enough kindling to last a year. They readily ignite with a match and burn with a strong blaze long enough to kindle any wood that is fit to burn.

KITCHEN, DRESS FOR THE:

The uniform insisted upon for women by those who direct gymnastic exercises is the only one appropriate for housework, so far as the under-garments are concerned. No corsets, loose bands, and the weight of the skirt suspended from the shoulders is the only formula for a comfortable working dress for women. Leaving the matter of under-clothing, the outer garments should certainly be made in one piece. For stout women a wrapper made in Gabrielle or princess fashion is the most becoming, while for slender forms the plain full skirt attached to a spencer or yoke waist is more desirable. For material cotton goods – gingham, seersucker, or calico – are the only suitable fabrics for working dresses. These can be worn the year round by lining with heavy unbleached muslin for winter, and, if necessary, adding an extra under-garment. In these one can always feel and look tidy. Gingham and seersucker are preferable to calico. It takes no longer to make them up, and, although they may cost twice as much, they will wear twice as long. The crinkled seersuckers, too, require no starching, and but little if any ironing. Medium colors are to be preferred, except, perhaps, in mid-winter.

The accessories of a working toilet are as important as those of a ball attire. A white collar is indispensable. As any thing white at the wrists is out of the question, a ruffle of the same material as a dress forms a neat finish for sleeves. Neatly arranged hair is as important an item as the collar. Frizzes(1), while more becoming to most faces than plain bands or pompadours, are not altogether neat for the kitchen. Moreover, steam and perspiration are sworn foes to curls that are not natural.

Kitchen aprons, gloves, and caps to be worn when sweeping, dusting, and attending to fires are essential to cleanliness and soft hands. "O, I can't bother with gloves!" exclaims some one. How much trouble and time are necessary to the slipping on of a pair of loose gloves, kept in a convenient place? And how amply repaid is one for the infinitesimal amount of both involved when she takes up her sewing. Consider, too, how much

(1) Small curls.

more soothing the touch of soft hands to the little ones and invalids than that of hard palms and rough cracked fingers.

Caps should be worn only when necessary, as covering the hair tends to cause baldness. Shoes must not be forgotten. The ankles tire when slippers are worn, and heavy shoes are apt to cause weariness, although useful when the ground is wet. Cloth shoes with moderately thick soles are the most comfortable when working about the house. Be sure to wear shoes sufficiently large or you will reap a bitter harvest of corns, bunions, and tender feet. Overshoes should be kept in a convenient place to be put on when necessary.

KITCHEN, THE:

A neat, well-ordered kitchen will insure not only the comfort, but, in a great degree, the health of the family, and should be the first thing looked to in the household, even if to do so demands a sacrifice of luxury in the parlor and other company apartments. The kitchen should be large and airy, with plenty of light and thorough ventilation, and should be provided with a liberal supply of utensils to simplify and expedite labor.

Then perfect system should be established, for in no department is the old adage more useful—"a place for every thing and every thing in its place"—than in the kitchen. When it is practicable, it is best to have the floor made of hard wood and oiled every 2 or 3 months, as grease will not show and can be easily wiped up. The walls should be kept pure and clean by an occasional coat of whitewash. Two or 3 large, roomy presses with shelves will be found a great convenience, while a safe with drawers in which to keep the small utensils of kitchen use is very necessary. A large lamp should be hung in a kitchen not lighted by gas. Plenty of coarse linen towels and dish-cloths should be furnished the cook, and every housekeeper should see that they are kept clean and free from grease, as indeed every article in the kitchen should be. "Economy counts nowhere so well as in the kitchen," and every wise mistress of the household who has the interests of her family at heart will give her personal supervision to prevent waste in her kitchen, and will know that the watchful eye and frequent suggestions of the mistress are absolutely necessary to keep order and system in the kitchen.

KITCHEN FURNITURE:

Heating New Iron: New iron should be very gradually heated at first. After it has become inured to the heat it is not so likely to crack.

To Prevent Crust in Tea-kettles: Keep an oyster-shell in your tea-kettle. By attracting the stony particles to itself it will prevent the formation of a crust.

To Clean Tea-kettles: Kerosene will make your tea-kettle as bright as new.

Saturate a woolen rag and rub with it. It will also remove stains from clean varnished furniture.

Glass: Glass should be washed in cold water, which gives it a brighter and cleaner look than when cleansed with warm water.

Glass Vessels: Glass vessels and other utensils may be purified and cleansed by rinsing them out with powdered charcoal.

To Clean Coal-oil Cans: After cleansing them as much as possible with wood ashes and hot water, use nitric acid in moderate quantities, which will soon remove the difficulty.

Washing Knives and Forks: Do not let knives be dropped into hot dishwater. It is a good plan to have a large tin pot to wash them in, just high enough to wash the blades without wetting the handles.

To Clean Knives: Cut a small potato in two; dip half in the brick-dust and rub the knives, and rust and stain will disappear like magic from their surfaces.

Scouring Knives: Place a quantity of brick-dust on a board, and having the knife perfectly dry, press it down hard and rub it back and forth crosswise of the blade. When bright, turn and scour the other side. Then wipe off with chamois leather. Knives thus treated will retain their brightness much longer and have a new look after years of usage.

To Extract Stains from Silver: Sal-ammoniac, 1 part; vinegar, 16 parts; mix and use this liquid with a piece of flannel, then wash the plate in clean water.

Silver Soap: For cleaning silver and Britannia 1/2 lb. of soap, 3 table-spoonfuls of spirits of turpentine, and 1/2 tumbler of water; let it boil 10 minutes; add 6 table-spoonfuls of spirits of hartshorn(1). Make a suds and wash silver with it.

To Clean Silver: Cleansing silver is not an easy task; the use of kerosene will greatly facilitate the operation. Wet a flannel cloth in the oil, dip in dry whiting, and thoroughly rub the plated or silver ware; throw it into a dish of scalding soap-suds, wipe with a soft flannel, and polish with a chamois skin.

Cleaning Tinware: An experienced housekeeper says the best thing for cleaning tinware is common soda. She gives the following directions: Dampen a cloth and dip in soda and rub the ware briskly, after which wipe dry. Any blackened ware can be made to look as well as new.

(1) Ammonium carbonate.

To Clean Tin Covers: Get the finest whiting; mix a little of it powdered with the least drop of sweet-oil, rub the covers well with it, and wipe them clean; then dust over them some dry whiting in a muslin bag and rub bright with dry leather. This last is to prevent rust, which the cook must guard against by wiping them dry and putting them by the fire when they come from the dining-room, for if but once hung up damp the inside will rust.

To Polish Tins: First rub them with a damp cloth, then take dry flour and rub it on with the hands; afterward take an old newspaper and rub the flour off, and the tins will shine as well as if half an hour had been spent rubbing them with brick-dust or powder, which spoils the hands.

Papier-maché Articles: Should be washed with a sponge and cold water, without soap, dredged with flour while damp, and polished with a flannel.

Japanned Ware(1): Wet a sponge in warm water and dampen it over, then wipe off with a soft cloth. If a tray becomes spotted, take a bit of woolen cloth and dip into a little sweet-oil and rub it as hard as possible, and the marks, if effaceable, will disappear.

Cleansing Floor-boards: Scrubbing them with a mixture made by dissolving unslaked lime in boiling water will have the desired effect. The proportions are 2 table-spoonfuls to a quart of water. No soap need be used.

To Clean Painted Wood-work: Fuller's earth(2) will be found cheap and useful, and on wood not painted it forms an excellent substitute for soap.

Cleaning Old Brass: The best liquid for cleaning old brass is a solution of oxalic acid.

To Clean a Brass Kettle: Do this before using it for cooking; use salt and vinegar.

To Clean Brasses, Britannia Metals, Tins, Coppers, Etc.: These are cleaned with a mixture of rotten-stone(3), soft-soap, and oil of turpentine, mixed to the consistency of stiff putty. The stone should be powdered very fine and sifted, and a quantity of the mixture may be made sufficient to last for a long while. The articles should first be washed with hot water to remove grease. Then a little of the above mixture, mixed with water, should be rubbed over the metal; then rub off briskly with dry, clean rag or leather, and a beautiful polish will be obtained.

To Keep Iron from Rusting: Kerosene applied by means of a moistened cloth to

(1) Kitchen items with a hard varnish coating.
(2) Absorbent clay.
(3) Siliceous limestone.

stoves will effectually keep them from rusting during the summer. It is also an excellent material to apply to all iron utensils used about the farm. Give plows, cultivators, and the like a coating before they are put away in the fall.

Cleansing Bottles: Many persons clean bottles by putting in some small shot and shaking them around. Water dissolves lead to a certain extent, and a film of this lead attaches itself to the sides of the bottle so closely that the shaking or rinsing with water does not detach it, and it remains to be dissolved by any liquid which has the least sourness in it, and if drank lead poison may be the result. Sometimes a shot becomes wedged in the bottom of a bottle, to be dissolved by wine or cider. Therefore it is better to wash every bottle as soon as emptied with warm water and wood ashes or saleratus, and put the bottle away, mouth open and downward, but be careful to wash again when used, as flies and other insects frequently get into open bottles. Or chop up a large potato very fine and put it into the bottle with some warm water, and shake it rapidly until it is clean.

KNIVES, CARE OF:

To keep knives from rusting, scour bright, wipe thoroughly, dry them by the fire, dust fine wood sashes fresh from the stove plentifully over the knives on both sides, leaving on what adheres to the blades, wrap in a piece of cloth and roll up in a paper, taking care to fold the ends of the paper so that the knives are all covered up. Now you may lay them away for a year, and when you look at them you will not find rusty spots on the steel blades.

KNOCK-KNEES, TO CURE:

An authority says:

"I commenced the practice of placing a small book between my knees, and tying a handkerchief tight around my ankles. This I did 2 or 3 times a day, increasing the substance at every fresh trial, until I could hold a brick with ease breadth-ways. When I first commenced this practice I was as badly knock-kneed as possible, but now I am as straight as any one. I likewise made it a practice of lying on my back in bed, with my legs crossed and my knees fixed tightly together. This I believe did me a great deal of good."

L

LACES, TO CLEAN:

Draw over a bottle a stocking-leg and tie it at each end. On this tack the lace carefully and put in a kettle of cold water with shavings of white soap in it. Raise it to the boiling point, remove, and rinse. If a cream color is desired rinse in cold coffee or saffron-water. Dry and remove from the bottle. Pick out the purling with a pin, and lay between soft papers and under heavy weight.

Lace curtains should be folded and tacked, then washed according to above directions. Rinse in blue water and starch in very thin starch. Then fasten a clean sheet to the carpet or bed-spread, untack the curtains, and pin on the sheet to dry. Put the pins near together, so as to make the edge straight. No laces of any kind should be rubbed or wrung. They may be pressed through a wringer without injury.

Black Lace: When rusty and limp, may be thus restored: Mix with a gill of rain-water in a table-spoonful of borax and one of alcohol; squeeze the lace several times through this; then rinse in a cup of hot water in which a black kid glove has been boiled; pull the lace out carefully till nearly dry, then press 2 or 3 days between sheets of paper under a heavy weight.

LACQUER, JAPANESE:

Japanese lacquer is made as follows: Melt 50 lbs. of Naples asphaltum and 8 lbs of dark gum anime(1); boil for about 2 hours in 12 gallons of linseed oil. Then melt 12 lbs. of dark gum amber, and boil it with 2 gallons of linseed oil; add this to the other, and add dryers. Boil for about 2 hours, or until the mass, when cooled, may be rolled into little pellets. Withdraw the heat, and thin down with 30 gallons of turpentine. During the boiling the mass must be constantly stirred to prevent boiling over.

LADIES' LUNCHES:

These are appropriate entertainments for daylight. The hour is usually 2 P.M. There is a twofold motive for confining the invitations to the fair sex. Gentlemen are seldom at leisure during the day, and as the lunches are sitting-down repasts, it becomes an object to economize num-

(1) A transparent amber resin with an agreeable odor.

bers. The lunches are served in courses, beginning with Blue Point oysters, and extending through soup, fish, meats, and entrées. Wines are usual where there is no temperance proclivity. Coffee concludes the repast, and as each guest makes her adieu she is presented with the cup and saucer she has used, or some other specimen of ceramics.

At ladies' lunches it is not unusual to place the guests in groups of 4 to 8 at small tables. The serving of the courses requires a number of well-trained servants. It is easier to entertain a large than a small party. So greatly has culture increased that the ladies' lunches are by no means dull. Painting is a subject of growing interest. Embroidery is another absorbing topic, and classical costumes are discussed in their application to modern toilets. Ladies are growing learned on scientific subjects, as applied to the improvement and adornment of the home; so that when these are added to the topics ladies are seldom at a loss for interesting conversation. Full dress is not required.

LADY'S MAID, DUTIES OF:

A lady's maid is indispensable to ladies who visit much, but this class of servant is the most difficult to manage. Ladies'-maids must be told, when hired, that they can have no such position in America as they have in England; that they must make their own beds, wash their own clothing, and eat with the other servants. They must be first-rate hair-dressers, good packers of trunks, and understand dress-making and fine starching, and be amiable, willing, and pleasant. A woman who combines these qualifications commands very high wages, and expects as her perquisite her mistress's cast-off dresses. French maids are in demand, as they have a natural taste in all things pertaining to dress and the toilet, but they are apt to be untruthful and treacherous. If a lady can get a girl from some rural district she will find her a most useful and valuable maid after she has been taught.

LAMBREQUINS(1), MANTEL, TO MAKE:

Buy a piece of heaviest burlap (such as is used for floor-mats) half the length of your shelf, divide it through the middle, and sew the ends together; this will form a seam in the center, but when nicely opened and pressed it does not show. Leave about 3 in. of it on the edge to ravel for fringe; above this work the Grecian pattern, or a pretty vine, with Germantown wool, and tie some of the wool in with your fringe. Use a narrow back velvet ribbon to finish the upper edge, and tack to the shelf with gilt-headed tacks.

Mine is worked with shaded red, is very pretty, and inexpensive. Another made of invisible green flannel, lined with cambric, is cut in "picket fence points;" a cluster of bright flowers, cut from satin-finished cretonne cloth, is button-hole stitched on each point, the edges of the points are

(1) A drapery hanging from a mantel.

pinked, and inside of this edge is a row for feather-stitching made with old gold floss on every point on the "picket," and the space between the "pickets" is finished with a tassel or ball of silk or worsted.

LAMP-BURNERS, TO CLEAN:

To clean old lamp-burners wash them in ashes and water, and they will come out bright and new. Many times a burner is condemned because the light is poor, when, having clogged up with sediment, the wick is at fault.

LAMP-CHIMNEYS, TO PREVENT CRACKING:

(1) Place the chimneys in a pot filled with cold water; add a little cooking salt; allow the mixture to boil well over a fire, and then cool slowly; chimneys become very durable by this process, which may also be extended to crockery, stone-ware, porcelain, etc.; the process is simply one of annealing, and the slower the process, especially the cooling portion of it, the more effective will be the work.

(2) If the chimney-glass of a lamp be cut with a diamond on the convex side it will never crack, as the incision affords room for expansion produced by the heat, and the glass, after it is cool, returns to its original shape with only a scratch visible where the cut is made.

LAMPS, REFLECTION FROM:

Never set the lamp upon a red table-cover; if you cannot find time to make a green lamp-mat, put a piece of green card-board under the lamp, and you will find the reflection upon your work much more agreeable to the eyes than that from the red cover.

LAMPS, TO PREVENT SMOKING

Soak the wicks in strong vinegar, and dry them well before using them. No lamp will smoke with wicks so prepared unless they are turned up too high.

LAMPS, WHY THEY EXPLODE:

Many things may occur to cause the flame to pass down the wick-tube and explode the lamp:

(1) A lamp may be standing on a table or mantel, and the slight puff of air from the open window or the sudden opening of a door causes an explosion.

(2) A lamp may be taken quickly from a table or a mantel, and instantly explode.

(3) A lamp is taken into an entry where there is a draught, or out of doors, and an explosion quickly ensues.

(4) A lighted lamp may be taken up a flight of stairs, or is raised quickly

to a place on the mantel, resulting in an explosion. In all these cases the mischief is caused by the air movement—either by suddenly checking the draught or forcing the air down the chimney against the flame.

(5) Blowing down the chimney to extinguish the light is frequently the cause of an explosion.

(6) Lamp explosions have been caused by using a chimney broken off at the top, or one that has a piece broken out, whereby the draft is rendered variable and the flame unsteady.

(7) Sometimes a thoughtless person puts a small-sized wick in a large burner, thus leaving considerable space in the tube along the edges of the wick.

(8) An old burner with its air-draughts clogged up, which rightfully should be thrown away, is sometimes continued in use, and the final result is an explosion.

LAUGHING AND HEALTH:

It is said by good medical authority that there is not the remotest corner or little inlet of the minute blood-vessels of the human body that does not feel some wavelet from the convulsion occasioned by good, hearty laughter, and also that the "central man," or life principle, is shaken to its innermost depths, sending new tides of life and strength to the surface, and thus materially tending to insure good health to the persons who indulge therein. The blood moves more rapidly—probably caused by some chemical or electric modification occasioned by the convulsion—and conveys a different impression to all the organs of the body as it visits them on that particular mystic journey, when the man is laughing, from what it does at other times. For this reason every good, hearty laugh in which a person indulges tends to lengthen his life, conveying as it does new and distinct stimulus to the vital forces.

LAUGHING CURE, THE:

"We doubt not the time will come," says an authority,"when physicians, conceding more importance than they now do to the influence of the mind upon the vital forces of the body, will prescribe to the torpid and melancholy patient a certain number of hearty peals of laughter, to be undergone at stated periods, and believe that they will, in so doing, find the best and most effective method of producing the required effect upon the patient. Our advice to all is, indulge in good, hearty, soulful laughter when the opportunity offers, and if you do not derive material benefit therefrom charge us with uttering false principles of materia medica."

LAUNDRY HINTS:

Washing-fluids shorten labor, but the clothes require such thorough rinsing after their use that only careful hands should be intrusted with the work. To wash flannels so as to leave them soft and pliable instead of hardened into wooden boards requires skill on the part of the washer. Science tells that the oil of perspiration remaining in flannels should be removed before the soap is applied, or a combination is formed with the soap that hardens the flannel instead of softening it. To remove this oil soak them, previous to washing, for at least half an hour in soda-water, moderately strong. After this they are easily washed and remain soft.

Put all the soap used for flannels in the water. Hot water is best for washing and rinsing. They should be well wrung and shaken before they are hung to dry. Always wash flannels by themselves, for if done in the suds used for cotton clothes, the white fluff of the cotton works into the wool and spoils their appearance. Colored flannels are much used now, blue being recommended to wear next to the skin as most healthy. Where white flannels are preferred they can be kept nice and white by an occasional bleaching. This is easily done by fastening ropes across a barrel, near enough to the top to allow the garment to be above it. Put some sulphur into an iron vessel, and after the garments are washed, rinsed, and placed on the ropes, pour some hot coals on the sulphur, and set the barrel down over it, keeping it well covered to retain the flumes. In a half hour or more take them out and hang them to dry.

When starching dark clothes color the starch with coffee, and they will be much improved in appearance, as white spots frequently show on goods where white starch is used. Dark clothes should be turned wrong side out to dry, or hung in the shade so as to prevent fading the colors. To give lawns a fresh look put gum-arabic(1) water into the starch, or use it altogether if the lawn is fine. Gum-arabic is also excellent for stiffening muslins and laces. After using it a few times the quantity liked can easily be found out.

Lace should never be made stiff, however, or it looses its grace and beauty. In washing fine laces do not rub them. Borax or ammonia water cleans them nicely by soaking the soiled parts for several hours. Iron laces very lightly on the wrong side, placing them on a thick, soft cloth first. They may be partially dried, pulled into shape, and then pressed under a light weight. If handkerchiefs used in colds are put to soak in borax-water for a half hour or more the phlegm will be removed, and render the washing easy.

Stockings that are stained or troublesome to clean are improved by being stretched out on a board and scrubbed with a hand-brush. Colored stockings ought to be rinsed quickly and well, and opened by pulling them on the hands on each side, and pinning them by top and side to the line.

(1) Gum obtained from one of several African acacia trees.

Woolen stockings are kept from shrinking if dried on a wooden shape of the right size. These are easily made from shingles or thin boards.

To keep flour-starch from lumping, mix the flour with water first, then remove the boiling water from the fire for a minute before stirring in the mixture or it will cook into lumps before it reaches the bottom. It is well to remember this in making gruel, corn-starch, etc. To set the colors of calico, soak in ox-gall and water, using 1 table-spoonful of ox-gall to 1 gallon of water. A teacup of lye in a bucket of water improves the color of black goods.

To brighten pink or green calicos put vinegar in the rinsing water. Pearl ash answers the same purpose for purple or blue. One tea-spoonful of sugar of lead in 1 quart of water sets blue colors fast. For the latter the articles must be clean. A strong tea made of common hay is said to preserve the tints of gray-colored linen. Before beginning to iron sprinkle the table plentifully with water and lay on the ironing blanket. This will hold it firmly in place and prevent all wrinkling and shoving about. Never try to iron with a blanket having wrinkles or bunches.

LAVENDER-WATER:

Essence of musk, 4 drams; essence of ambergris, 4 drams; oil of cinnamon, 10 drops; English lavender, 6 drams; oil of geranium, 2 drams; spirits of wine, 20 ounces. To be all mixed together.

LAW MAXIMS, COMMON:

- A promise of a debtor to give "satisfactory security" for the payment of a portion of his debt is a sufficient consideration for a release of the residue by his creditor.
- Administrators are liable to account for interest on funds in their hands, although no profit shall have been made upon them, unless the exigencies of the estate rendered it prudent that they should hold the funds thus uninvested.
- Any person who voluntarily becomes an agent for another, and in that capacity obtains information to which as a stranger he could have had no access, is bound, in subsequent dealing with his principal, as purchaser of the property that formed the subject of his agency, to communicate such information.
- When a house is rendered untenantable in consequence of improvements made on the adjoining lot, the owner of such cannot recover damages, because it is presumed he had knowledge of the approaching danger in time to protect himself from it.
- When a merchant-ship is abandoned by order of the master for the purpose of saving life, and a part of the crew

subsequently meet the vessel so abandoned, and bring her safe into port, they will be entitled to salvage.

- A person who has been led to sell goods by means of false pretenses cannot recover them from one who has purchased them in good faith from the fraudulent vendor.
- An agreement by the holder of a note to give the principal debtor time for payment, without depriving himself of the right to sue, does not discharge the surety.
- A seller of goods who accepts, at the time of sale, the note of a third party, not indorsed by the buyer, in payment, cannot, in case the note is not paid, hold the buyer responsible for the value of the goods.
- Common carriers are not liable for extraordinary results of negligence that could not have been foreseen by ordinary skill and foresight.
- A bidder at a sheriff's sale may retract his bid at any time before the property is knocked down to him, whatever may be the conditions of the sale.
- Acknowledgment of a debt to a stranger does not preclude the operation of the statute.
- The fruits and grass on the farm or garden of an intestate descend to the heir.
- A deposit of money in bank by a husband in the name of his wife survives to her.
- Money paid on Sunday contracts may be recovered.
- A debtor may give preference to one creditor over another, unless fraud or special legislation can be proved.
- A court cannot give judgement for a larger sum than that specified in the verdict.
- Imbecility on the part of either the husband or the wife invalidates a marriage.
- An action for malicious prosecution will lie, though nothing further was done than suing out of warrants.
- An agreement not to continue the practice of a profession of business in any specified town, if the party so agreeing has received a consideration for the same, is valid.
- When A. consigns goods to B. to sell on commission, and B. delivers them to C. in payment of his own antecedent debts, A. can recover their value.
- A finder of property is compelled to make diligent inquiry for

the owner thereof, and to restore the same. If, on finding such property, he attempts to conceal such fact, he may be prosecuted for larceny.

- A private person may obtain an injunction to prevent a public mischief by which he is affected in common with others.
- Any person interested may obtain an injunction to restrain the State or a municipal corporation from maintaining a nuisance on its lands.
- A discharge under the insolvent laws of one State will not discharge the insolvent from a contract made with a citizen of another State.
- To prosecute a party with any other motive than to bring him to justice is a malicious prosecution, and actionable as such.
- Ministers of the Gospel, residing in any incorporated town, are not exempt from jury, military, or fire service.
- When a person contracts to build a house, and is prevented by sickness from finishing it, he can recover for the part performed, if such part is beneficial to the other party.
- Permanent erections and fixtures, made by a mortgageor after the execution of the mortgage upon the land conveyed by it become a part of the mortgaged premises.
- When a marriage is denied, and plaintiff has given sufficient evidence to establish it, the defendant cannot examine the wife to disprove the marriage.
- The amount of an express debt cannot be enlarged by application.
- Contracts for advertisements in Sunday newspapers cannot be enforced.
- A seller of goods, chattels, or other property commits no fraud, in law, when he neglects to tell the purchaser of any flaws, defects, or unsoundness in the same.
- In a suit of damages for seduction proof of pregnancy and the birth of a child is not essential. It is sufficient if the illness of the girl, whereby she was unable to labor, was produced by shame for the seduction; and this is such a loss of service as will sustain the action.
- Addressing to a wife a letter containing matter defamatory to the character of her husband is a publication, and renders the writer amendable to damages.
- A parent cannot sustain an action for any wrong done to a

child unless he has incurred some direct pecuniary injury therefrom, in consequence of some loss of service, or expenses necessarily consequent thereupon.

- A master is responsible for an injury resulting from the negligence of his servant while driving his cart or carriage, provided the servant is at the time engaged in his master's business, even though the accident happens in a place to which his master's business does not call him; but if the journey of the servant be solely for the purpose of his own, and undertaken without the knowledge or consent of his master, the latter is not responsible.
- An emigrant depot is not a nuisance in law.
- A railroad track through the streets is not a nuisance in law.
- In an action for libel against a newspaper, extracts from such newspaper may be given to show the circulation and the extent with which the libel has been published. The jury, in estimating the damages, are to look at the character of the libel, and whether the defendant is rich or poor. The plaintiff is entitled in all cases to his actual damages, and should be compensated for the mental sufferings endured, the public disgrace inflicted, and all other actual discomfort produced.
- Delivery of a husband's goods by a wife to her adulterer, he having knowledge that she has taken them without her husband's authority, is sufficient to sustain an indictment for larceny against the adulterer.
- The fact that the insurer was not informed of the existence of impending litigation affecting the premises insured at the time of the insurance was effected does not vitiate the policy.
- The liability of an innkeeper is not confined to personal baggage, but extends to all the property of the guest that he consents to receive.
- When a minor executes a contract, and pays money or delivers property on the same, he cannot afterward disaffirm such contract and recover the money, or property, unless he restores to the other party the consideration received from him for such money or property.
- When a person has, by legal inquisition, been found an habitual drunkard he cannot, even in his sober intervals, make contracts to bind himself or his property until the inquisition is removed.
- Any person dealing with the representative of a deceased

person is presumed, in law, to be fully apprised of the extent of such representative's authority to act in behalf of such estate.

- In an action against a railroad company by a passenger to recover damages for injuries sustained on the road it is not compulsory upon the plaintiff to prove actual negligence in the defendants; but it is obligatory on the part of the latter to prove that the injury was not owing to any fault or negligence of theirs.
- A guest is a competent witness, in an action between himself and an innkeeper, to prove the character and value of lost personal baggage. Money in a trunk, not exceeding the amount reasonably required by the traveler to defray the expenses of the journey which he has undertaken, is a part of his baggage; and in case of its loss while at any inn the plaintiff may prove its amount by his own testimony.
- A married woman can neither sue nor be sued on any contract made by her during her marriage. The action must be commenced either by or against her husband. It is only when an action is brought on a contract made by her before her marriage that she is to be joined as a co-plaintiff or defendant with her husband.
- Any contract made with a person judicially declared a lunatic is void.
- Money paid voluntarily in any transaction, with a knowledge of the fact, cannot be recovered.
- In all cases of special contract for services the plaintiff can recover only the amount stipulated in the contract.
- A wife is a competent witness with her husband to prove the contents of a lost trunk.
- A wife cannot be convicted of receiving stolen goods when she received them of her husband.
- Insurance against fire by lightning or otherwise does not cover loss by lightning when there is no combustion.
- Failure to prove plea of justification in case of slander aggravates the offense.
- It is the agreement of the parties to sell by sample that constitutes a sale by sample, not the mere exhibition of a specimen of the goods.
- Makers of promissory notes given in advance for premiums on pieces of insurance thereafter to be taken are liable thereon.

- An agreement to pay for procuring an appointment to office is void.
- An attorney may plead the statute of limitations when sued by a client for money which he has collected and failed to pay over.
- Testimony given by a deceased witness on first trial is not required to be repeated verbatim on the second.
- A person entitling himself to a reward offered for lost property has a lien upon the property for the reward; but only when a definite reward is offered.
- Confession by a prisoner must be voluntarily made to constitute evidence against him.
- The defendant in a suit must be served with process; but service of such process upon his wife, even in his absence from the State, is not, in the absence of statutory provisions, sufficient.
- The measure of damages in trespass for cutting timber is its value as a chattel on the land where it was felled, and not the market price of the lumber manufactured.
- To support an indictment for malicious mischief in killing an animal, malice toward its owner must be shown, not merely passion excited against the animal itself.
- No action can be maintained against a sheriff for omitting to account for money obtained upon an execution within a reasonable time. He has till the return day to render such account.
- An interest in the profits of an enterprise, as profits, renders the party holding it a partner in the enterprise, and makes him presumptively liable to share any loss.

LAWNS (1) AND THIN MUSLINS, TO WASH:

(1) Boil 2 quarts wheat bran in 6 quarts or more of water half an hour; strain through a coarse towel and mix in the water in which the muslin is to be washed; use no soap and no starch; rinse lightly in fair water. This preparation both cleanses and stiffens the lawn.

(2) Muslin dresses, even the most delicate colors, can be cleaned in 10 or 15 minutes, without losing their color. Melt 1/2 lb. soap in 1 gallon water, empty in a washing tub, place near 2 other large tubs of clear water, and stir into one a quart of bran; put the muslin in the soap, turn it over and knead it for a few minutes, squeeze it out

(1) Lawn linen, a shear cloth used for blouses, curtains, etc.

well, but do not wring it lest it get turned; rinse it about quickly in the bran for a couple of minutes; rinse again well for a couple of minutes in clear water, squeeze out and dry, and hang it between two lines. A clear, dry day should be chosen to wash muslin dresses; half a dozen may be done in this way in half an hour. When the dress is dry make the starch; for a colored muslin, white starch and unboiled, but made with boiling water, is best for muslin dresses; stir the starch with the end of a wax candle; dip the dress; hang it again to dry; when dry rinse it quickly and thoroughly in clear water; hang it to dry again; sprinkle and roll it up; afterward iron it with very hot irons. This rinsing after starching is called clear starching.

LEAF IMPRESSIONS, TO MAKE:

(1) Hold oiled paper in the smoke of a lamp or of pitch until it becomes coated with the smoke; then take a perfect leaf having a pretty outline; after warming it between the hands, lay the leaf upon the smoked side of the paper, with the under side down, press it evenly upon the paper, that every part may come in contact; go over it lightly with a rolling-pin, then remove the leaf with care to a plain piece of white note-paper, and use the rolling-pin again; you will then have a beautiful impression of the delicate veins and outline of the leaf. And this process is so simple that any person, with a little practice to enable him to apply the right quantity of smoke to the oil paper and give the leaf proper pressure, can prepare leaf impressions such as a naturalist would be proud to possess. Specimens can be neatly preserved in book form, interleaving the impressions with tissue-paper.

(2) After warming the leaf between the hands, apply printing ink, by means of a small leather ball containing cotton or some soft substance, or with the end of the finger. The leather ball, (and the finger when used for that purpose), after the ink is applied to it, should be pressed several times on a piece of leather, or some smooth surface, before each application to the leaf, that the ink may be smoothly and evenly applied. After the under surface of the leaf has been sufficiently inked apply it to the paper where you wish the impression, and, after covering it with a slip of paper, use the hand or roller to press upon it, as described in the former process.

LEECHES AND THEIR APPLICATION:

The leech used for medical purposes is called the *Hirudo Medicinalis*, to distinguish it from other varieties, such as the horse-leech and the Lisbon leech. It varies form 2 to 4 inches in length, and is of a blackish brown color, marked on the back with 6 yellow spots, and edged with a yellow line on each side. Formerly leeches were supplied by Sweden, but latterly most of the leeches are procured from France, where they are now becoming scarce.

When leeches are applied to a part it should be thoroughly freed from down or hair by shaving, and all liniments, etc., carefully and effectually cleaned away by washing. If the leech is hungry it will soon bite, but sometimes great difficulty is experienced in getting it to fasten on. When this is the case roll the leech into a little porter, or moisten the surface with a little blood, or milk, or sugar and water.

Leeches may be applied by holding them over the part with a piece of linen cloth or by means of an inverted glass, under which they must be placed. When applied to the gums, care should be taken to use a leech glass, as they are apt to creep down the patient's throat; a large swan's quill will answer the purpose of a leech glass. When leeches are gorged they will drop off themselves; never tear then off from a person, but just dip the point of a moistened finger into some salt and touch them with it.

After leeches have been used they should be placed in water containing 16 per cent, of salt, which facilitates the removal of the blood they contain, and they should afterward be placed one by one in warm water, and the blood forced out by gentle pressure. The leaches should be then thrown into fresh water, which is to be renewed very 24 hours, and they may then be re-applied after an interval of 8 or 10 days. If a leech is accidentally swallowed, or by any means gets into the body, employ an emetic, or enema of salt and water.

LEMONS, MEDICAL QUALITIES OF:

A good deal has been said about the healthfulness of lemons. The latest advice is how to use them so that they will do the most good, as follows: Most people know the benefit of lemonade before breakfast, but few know that it is more than doubled by taking another at night also. The way to get the better of the bilious system without blue pills or quinine is to take the juice of 1, 2, or 3 lemons, as appetite craves, in as much ice-water as makes it pleasant to drink without sugar before going to bed. In the morning, upon rising, at least half an hour before breakfast, take the juice of 1 lemon to a goblet of water. This will clear the system of humor and bile with efficiency without any of the weakening effects of calomel(1) or congress water.

People should not irritate the stomach by eating lemons clear; the powerful acid of the juice, which is always most corrosive, invariably produces inflammation after awhile, but properly diluted, so that it does not burn or draw the throat, it does its medical work without harm, and when the stomach is clear of food has abundant opportunity to work over the system thoroughly, says a medical authority.

(1) Mercurous chloride, generally used as a cathartic.

LEMONS, TO KEEP:

(1) Cover them with buttermilk or sour milk, changing it once a week. Even lemons that are quite dry will seem fresh if kept in this way.

(2) Lemons can be kept sweet and fresh for months by putting them in a clean, tight cask or jar, and covering with cold water. The water must be changed as often as every other day, and the cask kept in a cool place.

LEMON VERBENA:

In Spain the lemon verbena, which we only cultivate as a scented garden-plant, is systematically collected and stored for winter use. With the Spaniards it is said to form one of the finest stomachics and cordials, and is taken either made into a decoction and drank cold with water and sugar as a tonic, or with the morning and evening cup of tea. A sprig of about 5 or 6 leaves of lemon verbena is first put into the cup, and the hot tea poured upon it. By using this Spanish authorities assert "you will never suffer from flatulence, never be made nervous or old maidish, never have cholera, diarrhea, or loss of appetite. Besides, the flavor is simply delicious. No one who has once drank their cup of tea with this addition will ever drink it without a sprig of lemon verbena."

LICE, PLANT:

A tea-spoonful of ammonia to 1 quart of water sprinkled every other day over plants will cause lice to disappear and not injure the plants.

LICE ON CATTLE, TO DESTROY:

Pour kerosene into some shallow dish, to the depth of $^1/_2$ in.; into this dip the teeth of a card(1), then card the animal with it, dipping occasionally while carding.

Another way: Take 1 part lard and 1 part kerosene, warm the lard enough so that the kerosene can be thoroughly and easily incorporated with it, stir until it cools sufficient to prevent separation. Thoroughly anoint the parts where the lice most congregate with the mixture. If the first application does not kill the lice within a few days, make a second.

LICE ON HENS, REMEDY FOR:

A lady who has raised a large number of hens says that after vainly trying recommended remedies for lice she has hit upon the plan of giving them once or twice a week, a large loaf of Graham flour, in which a handful of sulphur has been mixed. The hens like it, and are freed from lice and kept healthy through the season.

(1) Metal comb or wire brush for raising the nap & disentangling fur.

LIGHT:

Daylight exercises considerable influence upon both animal and vegetable life, and also upon a good many inanimate substances. Upon those endowed with life the effects are of the highest importance. The effect upon animal life may not be so apparent, but it should claim our attention. Its hygienic importance should be more studied than it generally is in the building of our houses.

Apartments exposed to the full action of the sun may be less comfortable in hot weather than those from which the sun's rays are excluded, but they are more wholesome. It is the increased intensity of the sunlight in the southern climes, independently of their greater warmth, that makes them so beneficial to many invalids. The little sunlight that finds its way into the narrow courts and alleys of great cities is partly the cause of the stunted growth and pale faces of children living there.

When the outer skin is tanned the sympathetic influence is felt also by the connecting mucous membranes lining every part of the body and stomach, and bowel derangements are less liable to occur. The inner as well as the outer skin is toughened. This shows the beneficial influence of light and fresh air in the summer complaints of children.

LIGHT FOR THE TABLE:

At night a dining- or sitting-room should be illumined either by a drop-light or by one of the fine lamps that, under the names of the Rochester, the Climax, the Fireside Electric, and other titles, are rapidly crowding the Argand gas-burners(1) out of the way. Easily managed and kept clean, they pay for themselves in a short time by saving the consumption of gas.

The brass lamps are very pretty, but the nickel-plated ones require much less work to keep bright, and do not tarnish readily. A low light is an absolute essential to the comfort and safety of the eyes that must superintend finger-work in the evening.

Half a dozen of the most brilliant gas-jets in a chandelier of ordinary height will not do as much service as one good lamp placed on a table. About this the family may gather with their various employments.

LIMBS, FROZEN, TREATMENT OF:

Frozen limbs should be thawed out slowly. The patient should be placed in a cold room and the limb bathed in ice-water or cloths wrung out in ice-water. When the limb begins to tingle the bathing must be stopped and the temperature of the room gradually raised.

LIME FOR BLASTING:

Every one who has slowly added water to a lump of quicklime to

(1) Gas or oil burner with a cylindrical wick to enable air to flow inside & outside the flame.

slake it has noticed that in combining with water the lime swells up and becomes much larger than before. This expansion of quicklime when in contact with water is a force exercised through a short distance, but, like the expansion of water in freezing, is almost irresistible. The force has lately been used in the coal-mines of England to throw down the coal.

To prepare quicklime for use in blasting it is first reduced to powder, and then forced into cartridges or cylinders by means of an hydraulic press. A mold 2 in. across and 7 in. long is filled with powdered lime, and compressed by an hydraulic press of 40-ton power into a solid mass of about 4 in. long. When these cylinders or cartridges have lengthwise grooves cut in them to admit water they are ready for use. Holes are drilled as for blasting with powder, a cylinder of compressed lime is placed in each and tamped. A tube is provided for in the tamping, and water, by means of a force-pump, is forced through the tube and brought in contact with the lime cartridge. In slaking the swelling of the lime throws down the coal without any smoke or the liberation of unwholesome gases, and there is no loss of time in getting rid of these. This method of blasting will, no doubt, find a wider application than for coal-mines.

LIME IN THE EYE, TO REMOVE:

Bathe the eye with a little vinegar and water, and carefully remove any little pieces of lime which may be seen, with a feather. If any lime has got entangled in the eyelashes, carefully clear it away with a bit of soft linen soaked in vinegar and water. Violent inflammation is sure to follow; a smart purge must therefore be administered, and in all probability a blister must be applied on the temple, behind the ear, or on the nape of the neck.

LIME-WATER, TO MAKE:

To $^1/_2$ lb. of unslaked lime add three fourths of a pint of water; put the lime into an earthen pot, and pour a little of the water upon it, and as the lime slakes pour the water on by little and little, and stir up with a stick. The water must be added very slowly, otherwise the lime will fly about in all directions, and may bread the vessel. In 3 or 4 hours' time, when the slaked lime has sunk to the bottom, pour the clear fluid off, and put it in stoppered bottles away from the light.

LIME-WATER, USE OF:

If good milk disagrees with a child or grown person lime-water at the rate of 3 or 4 table-spoonfuls to the pint, mixed with the milk or taken after it, will usually help digestion and prevent flatulence. Lime-water is a simple ant-acid, and is a little tonic. It often counteracts pain from acid fruits, from "wind in the stomach," and from acids produced by eating candies and other sweets; also "stomach-ache" (indigestion) from over-eating of any kind.

A table-spoonful for a child of 2 yrs. old, to a gill or more for an adult, is an ordinary dose, while considerable more will produce no serious injury.

A pint of cold water dissolves less than 10 grains of lime, and warm water still less. Pure lime-water, even though pretty closely corked, soon deteriorates by carbonic acid in the air, which unites with the lime and settles as an insoluble carbonate.

To have it always ready and good, and at no cost, put into a tall pint or quart glass bottle of any kind a gill or so of good lime just slaked with water. Then fill the bottle nearly full of rain or other pure water, and let it stand quietly, corking well. The lime will settle, leaving clear lime-water at the top. Pour off gently as wanted, adding more water as needed. Some carbonic acid will enter, but the carbonate will settle, often upon the sides of the bottle, and freshly saturated water remain. The lime should be removed and a new supply put in once a year or so, unless kept very tightly corked.

LINEN CLOSET, THE:

In the linen closet skill in assortment is needed. The cotton and linen sheets must be in separate piles, as must cotton and linen pillow-cases and bolster-slips. Those of different sizes must also be divided. Great confusion is saved by this simple method. No one who has unfolded one sheet and pillow-case after another, vainly seeking those devoted to some particular bed, will fail to see the necessity of keeping unlike pieces in separate piles.

LINIMENT FOR SPRAINS AND BRUISES:

For strain, sprain, bruise, or broken bone in either man or beast dissolve gum camphor in sweet-oil and rub on 3 times a day with flannel or woolen cloth, wrapping up the wound with the cloth after rubbing it in. I have tried the above and know its value.

LIPS, CARE OF THE:

There is no art potent enough to give the beauty of symmetry which nature may have refused to the lips. If they become unnaturally pale, more or less rouge mixed with beeswax will give them a deceitful and temporary gloss of nature. To this daubing our fashionable dames are constantly obliged to resort, for their exhausting lives of dissipation impoverish and decolorize the blood, and the effect is apparent at once in the blanched lip. A frequent use, however, of the lip salve, as it is ingeniously called, but which is merely a red pigment in disguise, so inflames, thickens, roughens, and gives such a peculiar tint to the mouth, that it has the look of the shriveled, purplish one of a sick Negress.

The habit of biting the lips soon destroys any grace of form they may have originally possessed. Mme. De Pompadour, while lamenting the decay of her charms, confessed that she first began to spoil at the mouth. She had early acquired the habit of biting her lips in order to conceal her emotion.

"at 30 years," says an historian," her mouth had lost all its striking brilliancy."

LIP SALVE:

(1) Oil of almonds, 3 ounces; alkanet(1), 1/2 ounce. Let them stand together in a warm place until the oil is colored, then strain. Melt 1 1/2 ounces of white-wax, and 1/2 ounce of spermaceti with the oil, stir till it begins to thicken, and add 12 drops of attar of roses.

(2) White wax, 1 ounce; almond oil, 2 ounces; alkanet, 1 dram. Digest in a warm place till sufficiently colored, strain, and stir in 6 drops of attar of roses.

LOBSTERS, HOW TO SELECT:

Lobsters recently caught have always some remains of muscular action in the claws, which may be excited by pressing the eyes with the finger; when this cannot be produced the lobster must have been too long kept. When boiled the tail preserves its elasticity if fresh, but loses it as soon as it becomes stale. The heaviest lobsters are the best; when light they are watery and poor. Hen-lobsters may generally be known by the spawn or by the breadth of the "flap."

LOCK-JAW, OR TETANUS:

There are two varieties of this disease, the traumatic and idiopathic. Traumatic lock-jaw is a very dangerous malady, and is usually caused by wounds, the irritation of splintered bones, and sometimes follows amputations. Idiopathic lock-jaw proceeds from constitutional causes, and is far less dangerous than the former. It may arise from debility of the nervous system, and from affections of the brain.

The disease commences with stiffness and pain in the neck and jaws as if from a cold; the voice is husky; there is difficulty in protruding the tongue, and in articulating; the muscles of the jaws and throat become rigid, with great difficulty in swallowing; a pain at the pit of the stomach succeeds these, shooting to the back, with difficulty of breathing; as the disease advances the paroxysms become more frequent., the jaws locked, and breathing obstructed, and the patient dies from exhaustion or suffocation.

Treatment: All wounds made by nails and other sharp instruments, especially in the bottom of the foot or in the palm of the hand, should not be allowed to heal up too quickly; such wounds should be thoroughly cleansed with a solution of chlorinated soda, tea-spoonful to 6 of water, and compresses, wet with same, bound to the parts. When there is a foreign body in the wound, as dirt, rust, a splinter, or a piece of bone, it should at once be cut out.

(1) (Henna) The root of a flowering plant used to give a red color to oils (Alkanna tinctoria).

LOCK-JAW, REMEDIES FOR:

(1) *The following is said to be a positive cure:* Let any one who has an attack of lock-jaw take a small quantity of spirits of turpentine, warm it, and pour it on the wound, no matter where the wound is or what is its nature. Relief will follow in less than 1 minute. Turpentine is also a sovereign remedy for croup. Saturate a piece of flannel with it and place on to the throat and chest, and in severe cases 3 to 5 drops on a lump of sugar may be taken internally.

(2) If any person is threatened with lock-jaw from injuries to the arms, legs, or feet, do not wait for a doctor, but put the part injured in the following preparation: Put hot wood-ashes into water as warm as can be borne; if the injured part cannot be put into water, then wet thick-folded cloths in the water and apply them to the part as soon as possible, and at the same time bathe the back-bone from the neck down with some laxative stimulant—say cayenne pepper and water, or mustard and water, (good vinegar is better than water); it should be as hot as the patient can bear it. Don't hesitate; go to work and do it, and don't stop until the jaws will come open. No person need die of lock-jaw if these directions are followed.

(3) Take a red-hot coal from the fire and pour sweet-oil (olive-oil) on it; then hold the wounded part over the thick smoke, as near as possible without burning. It will be necessary to repeat the operation 2 or 3 times a day. This remedy has been known to cure after jaws had commenced to get stiff.

LOO, GAME OF:

Loo, or lue, is subdivided into limited and unlimited loo, and is a game the complete knowledge of which can easily be acquired; it is played two ways, both with 5 and 3 cards, though most commonly with 5, dealt from a whole pack, either first 3 and then 2, or by 1 at a time. Several persons may play together, but the greatest number can be admitted when with 3 cards only. After 5 cards have been given to each player another is turned up for trump; the knave of the clubs generally, or sometimes the knave of the trump suit, as agreed upon, is the highest card, and is styled pam; the ace of trumps is next in value, and the rest in succession as at whist. Each player has the liberty of changing for others, from the pack, all or any of the 5 cards dealt, or of throwing up the hand, in order to escape being looed.

Those who play their cards, either with or without changing, and do not gain a trick, are looed; as is likewise the case with all who have stood the game, when a flush or flushes occur and each, excepting any player holding pam, of an inferior flush, is required to deposit a stake to be given to the person who sweeps the board, or divided among the winners at the ensuing deal, according to the tricks which may then be made. For instance, if every one at dealing stakes half a dollar, the tricks are entitled to 6 cents a piece, and whoever is looed must put down half a dollar, exclusive of the deal; sometimes it is settled that each person looed shall pay a sum equal to what happens to be on the table at the time. Five cards of a suit or 4 with pam compose a flush, which sweeps the board and yields only to a superior flush, or the elder hand.

When the ace of trumps is led it is usual to say, "Pam, be civil"; the holder of which last mentioned card is then expected to let the ace pass. When Loo is played with 3 cards they are dealt one at a time, pam is omitted, and the cards are not exchanged, nor permitted to be thrown up.

LOOKING-GLASS, TO CLEAN:

(1) Remove with a damp sponge fly-stains and other soils, (the sponge may be dampened with water or spirits of wine). After this dust the surface with the finest sifted whiting or powder-blue, and polish it with a silk handkerchief or soft cloth. Snuff of candle, if quite free from grease, is an excellent polish for a looking-glass.

(2) Remove all fly-stains and dirt by breathing on them, and rubbing with a soft rag; then tie up some powder-blue in a piece of thick flannel, and with this carefully polish the whole surface.

LOTIONS:

Lotions are usually applied to the parts required by means of a piece of linen rag wetted with them, or by wetting the bandage itself.

Emollient: Use decoction of marsh-mallow or linseed.

Elder flowers: Add 2½ drams of elder flowers to 1 quart of boiling water; infuse for 1 hour and strain. Use as a discutient.

Sedative: Dissolve 1 dram of extract of henbane(1) in 24 drams of water.

Opium: Mix 2 drams of bruised opium with ½ pint of boiling water, allow it to grow cold, and use for painful ulcers, bruises, etc.

Stimulant: Dissolve 1 dram of caustic potash in 1 pint of water, and then gradually pour it upon 24 grains of camphor and 1 dram of sugar, previously bruised together in a mortar. Use as in fungold(2) and flabby ulcers.

Ordinary: Mix 1 dram of salt with 8 ounces of water. Used for foul ulcers and flabby wounds.

(1) Medicine from a smelly poisonous plant of the nightshade family.
(2) Resembling a fungus.

Cold Evaporating: Add 2 drams of Sulard's extract *(Liquor plumbi diacetatis)* and the same quantity of sweet spirit of niter *(Spiritus etheris nitrici)* to a pint of cold water. Use as a lotion for contusions, sprains, inflamed parts, etc.

Hydrochlorate of Ammonia: Dissolve 1/2 ounce of sal ammoniac *(Ammonia hydrochloras)* in 6 ounces of water, then add 1 ounce of distilled vinegar and the same quantity of rectified spirit. Use as a refrigerant.

Black Wash: Add 1/2 dram of calomel to 4 ounces of lime-water, or 8 grains to an ounce of lime-water, shake well. Use as a detergent.

Acetate of Lead with Opium: Take 10 grains of acetate of lead, and then a dram of powdered opium, mix, and add an ounce of vinegar and 4 ounces of warm water, set aside for 1 hour, then filter. Use as an astringent.

Creasote: Add 1 dram of creasote to a pint of water, and mix by shaking. Use as an application in tinca capitis, or other cutaneous diseases.

Galls(1): Boil 1 dram of bruised galls in 12 ounces of water until only 1/2 pint remains, then strain and add 1 ounce of laudanum. Use as an astringent.

LOUNGE COVER:

A lovely lounge-cover or coverlet for an invalid can be made of cast-off neckties, old bonnet-pieces, and scraps of silk. Cut the pattern of a hexagon, 5 in. from the center to the outer edge. Put a center of black silk on velvet about 2 in. in diameter, and piece around this in log-cabin style, preserving the form throughout. Twelve will make a very good-sized coverlet. Put together with squares of black silk or velvet, and lined with bright flannel pinked on the edges so that it projects a little on the right side. Wool pieces make a very pretty one, too.

LUNCHEON, THE:

To mention the work luncheon is to call up a picture of rest and quiet and homelike peace. Once more the busy wheels of life cease to whirr, and its golden grain or worthless chaff remains undisturbed. The carpenter beside the idle plane, the mason with his brick and mortar, the farmer by his patient horse, the needle-woman raising a weary face from her interminable work, all pause for the grateful hour of luncheon. Within the home where peace and order reign the cloth is neatly spread and the dishes tidily arranged for even a morsel of toast and a cup of tea.

Perhaps a cloth of yellow or pink or crimson is provided for this meal, with napkins to match. In that case the dishes ought to be white. American wares now vie in every respect with the imported and are less ex-

(1) Gall nut; a tumor-like growth following a puncture by a Cynip in a stem or leaf of various trees..

pensive. Stamped patterns of the wild rose or daisy, or grass, or of conventional forms, on ware of a good quality, can be purchased very reasonably, with the comforting certainty that any thing broken can be readily duplicated. As for nicked dishes—those horrors for a sensitive eye—a fine piece of china had better be broken and thrown away than be degraded to kitchen service. The fitness of things forbids such desecration.

No other meal so well shows the care and thrift of the housekeeper as the family luncheon. A little forethought provides a savory stew or soup from the bones and remnants of meats and gravies, and stewed fruit and patties, or the old-fashioned baked turnovers served warm on a cold winter's day when the children rush in from school asking for something savory. This is the case where, unfortunately, circumstances compel a late dinner, if the father or other members find it impossible to be home at the midday meal.

Let the table be ever so perfect, the success of a luncheon depends on the congeniality of the guests. It is essentially a woman's repast. Those who know each other too well are bored in being brought together in a very formal way. Generally some one whom it is designated to honor becomes the cause of a conventional lunch party, and no more charming way can be found to introduce a friend into a social circle.

M

MACKEREL, HOW TO SELECT:

Mackerel must be perfectly fresh or it is a very indifferent fish; it will neither bear carriage nor being kept many hours out of the water. The firmness of the flesh and the clearness of the eyes must be the criterion of fresh mackerel, as they are of all other fish.

MAD ANIMALS, BITE OF:

Tie a string tightly over the part, cut out the bite, and cauterize the wound with a red-hot poker or lunar caustic. Then apply a piece of "sponglo-piline,"(1) give a purgative, and plenty of warm drink. Get a physician instantly.

MAGAZINES, TO BIND:

With an awl, needle, and shoe-thread (waxed) tack them firmly together, paste a piece of muslin over the backs, and have it extend an inch on either cover. Then over this paste covers of brown paper, (that of which flour-sacks are made is best), and on the cover, also on the back, write the name and date. Thus bound, magazines are conveniently handled, and are not likely to be mislaid or injured. Three or four of the size of Harper's may thus be bound together with a slight expense, and with no charge of the book-binder.

MAGIC HATS, GAME OF:

Though the following trick cannot exactly be designated a round game, it may be performed by one of the company with great success during an interval of rest from playing. The performer begins by placing his own hat, along with another which he has borrowed, on the table, crown upward. He then requests that the sugar basin may be produced, from which, on its arrival, a lump is selected and given to him. Taking it in his fingers, he promises, by some wonderful process, that he will swallow the sugar, and then, within a very short time, will let its position be under one of the two hats on the table, the company deciding which hat it shall be. It is generally suspected that a second lump of sugar will be taken from the basin, if it can be done without observation, consequently all eyes are fixed upon it. Instead of that, after swallowing the sugar the performer places the selected hat up on his own head, thus, of course, fulfilling his undertaking.

(1) A substitute for a poultice made from sponge and fibre with Indian rubber backing.

MAGIC MUSIC, GAME OF:

This is a game in which music is made to take a prominent part. On one of the company volunteering to leave the room, some particular article agreed upon is hidden. On being recalled, the person, ignorant of the hiding-place, must commence a diligent search, taking the piano as his guide. The loud tones will mean that he is very near the object of his search, and the soft tones that he is far from it. Another method of playing the same game is for the person who has been out of the room to try to discover on his return what the remainder of the company desire him to do. It may be to pick up something from the floor, to take off his coat, to look at himself in the glass, or anything else as absurd. The only clew afforded him of solving the riddle must be the loud or soft tones of the music.

MANTEL ORNAMENTS:

A very pretty mantel ornament may be obtained by suspending an acorn, by a piece of thread tied around it, within 1/2 in. of the surface of some water contained in a vase, tumbler, or saucer, and allowing it to remain undisturbed for several weeks. It will soon burst open, and small roots will seek the water; a straight and tapering stem, with beautiful, glossy green leaves, will shoot upward, and present a very pleasing appearance. Chestnut trees may be grown in this manner, but their leaves are not as beautiful as those of the oak. The water should be changed once a month, taking care to supply water of the same warmth; bits of charcoal added to it will prevent water from souring. If the leaves turn yellow add one drop of ammonia into the utensil which holds the water, and it will renew their luxuriance.

Take a saucer and fill it with fresh green moss. Place it in the center of a pine cone, large size, having first watered it thoroughly. Then sprinkle it thoroughly with grass seed. The moisture will close the cone partially, and in a day or two the tiny grass spires will appear in the interstices, and in a week you will have a perfect cone of beautiful verdure. Keep secure from the frost, and give it plenty of water, and you will have a "thing of beauty" all the winter.

MARBLE, TO CLEAN:

(1) It is said that marble may be cleaned by mixing up a quantity of the strongest soap lye with quick-lime to the consistency of milk, and laying it on the marble for 24 hours. Clean it afterward with soap and water. Or else use the following: Take 2 parts of common soda, 1 part of pumice-stone, and 1 part of powdered chalk; sift through a very fine sieve, and mix with water; then rub it well all over the marble, and the stains will be removed; then wash with soap and water, as before, and it will be as clean as it was at first.

(2) Brush the dust of the dish to be cleaned, then apply with a brush a

good coat of gum arabic, about the consistency of a thick office mucilage, expose it to the sun or dry wind, or both. In a short time it will crack and peel off; wash it with clean water and clean cloth. Of course, if the first application does not have the desired effect, it should be applied again.

(3) Make a paste with soft-soap and whiting. Wash the marble first with it, and then leave a coat of the paste upon it for 2 or 3 days. Afterward wash off with warm (not hot) water and soap.

(4) Chalk, in fine powder, 1 part; pumice, 1 part; common soda, 2 parts; mix; wash the spots with this powder, mixed with a little water; then clean the whole of the stone and wash off with soap and water.

MARBLE, TO REMOVE DIRT AND STAINS FROM:

A solution of gum arabic will remove dirt and stains from marble. Let it remain until it dries, when it will peel off or can be washed off.

MARBLE AND GLASS, TO POLISH:

Marble of any kind, alabaster, and hard stone or glass may be repolished by rubbing it with a linen cloth dressed with oxide of tin, (sold under the name of putty powder). For this purpose a couple or more folds of linen should be fastened tight over a piece of wood, flat or otherwise, according to the form of the stone. To repolish a mantel-piece it should be first perfectly clean. This is best done by making a paste of lime soda, and water, wetting well the marble, and applying the paste. Then let it remain for a day or so, keeping it moist during the interval. When this paste has been removed the polishing may begin. Chips in the marble should be rubbed out first with emery and water. At every stage of polishing the linen and putty powder must be kept constantly wet. Glass, such as jewelers' show counter-cases, which become scratched, may be polished in the same way.

MAT, FOOT, TO MAKE:

Cut woolen and flannel pieces of cloth into strips 3 in. long and 1/2 in. wide. Get a pair of very coarse steel knitting-needles and some jute twine—no other will answer—the same that is used in making gunny sacks, and can always be obtained where they are made, if not at the shops. Set up 15 stitches on the needles, and knit once across; knit the first stitch on the second row, and between the needles put a piece of the cloth at right angles with the stitch, and knit another stitch; then turn the end of the cloth that points toward you out between the needles, so that the ends will be even, and so on clear across, 2 stitches to every piece of cloth; then knit across again plain to get back to the side where you began.

The ends of the cloth must always point from you as you knit them in. They are very warm for the feet and are very pretty, and it is a good way to use up discarded coats, vests, and pants. The cloth must not be too thick. Broad cloth, waterproof, ladies' cloth, etc., are the best for the purpose.

MATS, HUSK, TO MAKE:

A good, respectable-looking husk mat is not an unsightly-looking object. One bushel basket and a boiler full of husks is sufficient to braid a large mat. If you have boys or girls, it will be fun for them to braid one in the evening; but if, like myself, you have neither, it would pay you to take the time and do it yourself. Have ready a tea-kettle full of hot water and turn into the boiler of husks.

Begin a common 3-strand braid, and as you bring over a strand place about 3 husks on; leave the large ends of the husks up. When enough is braided for a mat, sew firmly with twine in any shape you choose—long, round, or oval. Then sprinkle warm water on the upper side. Run a fork through the husks, splintering the ends into a mass of little curly fibers. Then, with the shears, trim off evenly. This can all be done in one evening by a good worker.

MEALS, NUMBER OF:

In regard to the number of meals stomachs differ, of course, according to their ability to digest with rapidity. A serpent may take a meal once a month. Some people feed their dogs one meal a day. There are many men who get on best with two meals a day. But for the average healthy man who is working, three meals are best. One key to enduring health will be the religious observances of rest after dinner. Let the evening be for relaxation, not only for the sake of rest to the mind, but out of fair treatment of the stomach, when, if the dinner be at night, it is doing its hardest work.

MEALY BUG:

This species is reddish and strewed with white dust. At the sides of the 12 segments of the body it is provided with small tubercles. The male is slender and gnat-like, with two rather broad wings and two long, brush-shaped tail filaments. It attacks a number of species of plants, and can only be diminished in number by brushing it off carefully with soft brushes and crushing it.

MEASLES, TREATMENT:

Measles are an acute inflammation of the skin, internal and external, combined with an infectious fever.

Symptoms: Chills, succeeded by great heat, languor, and drowsiness, pains in the head, back and limbs, quick pulse, soreness of throat, thirst, nausea, and vomiting, a dry cough, and high-colored urine. These symptoms increase in violence for 4 days. The eyes are inflamed and weak and the nose pours forth a watery secretion, with frequent sneezing. There is considerable inflammation in the larynx, windpipe, and bronchial tubes, with soreness of the breast and hoarseness. About the fourth day the skin is covered with a breaking out which produces heat and itching, and is red in spots, upon the face first, gradually spreading over the whole body.

It goes off in the same way, from the face first and then from the body, and the hoarseness and other symptoms decline with it; at last the outside skin peels off in scales.

Treatment: In a mild form nothing is required but a light diet, slightly acid drinks, and flaxseed or slippery elm tea. Warm herb teas and frequent sponge baths with tepid water serve to allay the fever; care should be taken not to let the patient take cold. If the fever is very high, and prevents the rash coming out, a slight dose of salts, or a nauseating dose of ipecac(1), lobelia(2), or hive syrup should be given, and followed by tea-spoonful doses of compound tincture of Virginia snake-root(3) until the fever is allayed. If the patient from any derangement takes on a low typhoid type of fever and the rash does not come out until the seventh day, and is then of a dark and livid color, tonics and stimulants must be given, and the expectoration promoted by some suitable remedy.

The room should be kept dark to protect the inflamed eyes. As long as the fever remains the patient should be kept in bed. Exposure may cause pneumonia, which, in other words, is acute inflammation of the lungs. Keep in the room as long as the cough lasts. There is always danger of the lungs being left in an inflamed state after the measles unless the greatest possible care is taken not to suffer the patient to take cold. If, however, there should be much pain and a severe cough, this must be treated as a separate disease, with other remedies.

MEDICAL HINTS, SHORT AND SAFE:

- In health and disease endeavor always to live on the sunny side. Sir James Wyle, late physician to the Emperor of Russia, remarked during long observation in the hospitals of that country that cases of death occurring in rooms averted from the light of the sun were four times more numerous than the fatal cases in the rooms exposed to the direct action of the solar rays.
- When poison is swallowed a good off-hand remedy is to mix salt and mustard, 1 heaped tea-spoonful of each in a glass of water, and drink immediately. It is quick in its operation. Then give the whites of 2 eggs in a cup of coffee, or the eggs

(1) From the dried roots of a plant of the madder family.
(2) An expectorant and diaphoretic.
(3) Senega, rattlesnake-root, an expectorant and diuretic.

alone if coffee cannot be had. For acid poisons give acids. In cases of opium poisoning give strong coffee and keep moving.

- For light burns or scalds dip the part in cold water or in flour; if the skin is destroyed cover with varnish.
- If you fall into the water float on the back, with the nose and mouth projecting.
- For apoplexy, raise the head and body; for fainting, lay the person flat.
- Suck poisonous wounds, unless your mouth is sore. Enlarge the wound, or, better, cut out the part without delay, cauterize it with caustic, the end of a cigar, or a hot coal.
- If an artery is cut, compress above the wound; if a vein is cut, compress below.
- If choked, get upon all fours and cough.
- Before passing through smoke take a full breath, stoop low, then go ahead; but if you fear carbonic acid gas, walk erect and be careful. Smother a fire with blankets or carpets; water tends to spread boiling oil and increase the danger.
- Remove dust from the eyes by dashing water into them, and avoid rubbing. Remove cinders, etc., with a soft, smooth wooden point.
- Preserve health and avoid catching cold by regular diet, healthy food, and cleanliness. Sir Astley Cooper said: "The methods by which I have preserved my own health are temperance, early rising, and sponging the body every morning with cold water immediately after getting out of bed, a practice which I have adopted for 30 yrs. without ever catching cold."
- Water diluted with 2 per cent. of carbolic acid will disinfect any room or building if liberally used as a sprinkle.
- Diphtheria can be cured by a gargle of lemon-juice, swallowing a little so as to reach all the affected parts.
- To avert cold from the feet wear 2 pairs of stockings made from different fabrics, one pair of cotton or silk, the other of wool, and the natural heat of the feet will be preserved if the feet are kept clean.
- In arranging sleeping-rooms the soundest and most refreshing slumber will be enjoyed when the head is toward the north.
- Late hours and anxious pursuits exhaust vitality, producing disease and premature death; therefore the hours of labor and study should be short.

- Take abundant exercise and recreation.
- Be moderate in eating and drinking, using simple and plain diet, avoiding strong drink, tobacco, snuff, opium, and every excess.
- Keep the body warm, the temper calm, serene, and placid; shun idleness; if your hands cannot be usefully employed, attend to the cultivation of your minds.
- For pure, health-giving fresh air, go the country. Dr. Stockton Hough asserts that if all the inhabitants of the world were living in cities of the magnitude of London the human race would become extinct in a century or two. The mean average of human life in the United States is 39 1/2 yrs., while in New York and Philadelphia it is only 23 yrs., about 50 per cent. of the deaths in these cities being of children under 5 yrs. of age. A great percentage of this excessive mortality is caused by bad air and bad food.

MICA, TO CLEAN:

Mica in stoves, (often wrongly called "isinglass"(1)), when smoked, is readily cleaned by taking it out and thoroughly washing with vinegar a little diluted. If the black does not come off at once, let it soak a little.

MICE IN CORN-STACKS, TO PREVENT RAVAGES OF:

Sprinkle from 4 to 6 bushels of dry white sand upon the root of the stack before the thatch is put on. The sand is no detriment to the corn, and stacks thus dressed have remained without injury. So very effective is the remedy that nests of dead young mice have been found where the sand has been used, but not a live mouse could be seen.

MILDEW:

To prevent mildew on roses and other plants syringe with the following: Mix 1 lb. of flower of sulphur and 1 lb. of fresh lime in 5 quarts of water; repeatedly shake the mixture; and after settling put it into well-corked bottles. For using, 1 gill of this mixture is put in 3 gallons of water.

MILDEW, TO REMOVE FROM CLOTH:

The most effectual method is one which has never failed with us, but which needs to be used with care. It worked to a charm in one case where a careless laundress left a basket of clothes, including the fine clothing of 2 little children, to stand in hot weather till every article was mildewed. Despairing, we put them in the hands of a woman noted for her wisdom in all household ways, and she brought them back in perfect condition.

(1) Dried swimming bladder of the Acipenser. Gelatinous tissue, which on boiling yields gelatin.

Dissolve 2 ounces of chloride of lime in 1 quart of boiling water, then add 3 quarts of cold water. Strain this through cloth, lest any tiny lumps remain, and soak the mildewed spots in the liquid for 5 or 6 hours, and then thoroughly rinse in clean water. This is effectual. The dangers to be avoided are the use of too strong a solution, soaking too long, and insufficient rinsing, the natural result of which would be a weakening of the fiber of the cloth itself.

MILDEW, TO REMOVE FROM LINEN:

Remove mildew from linen by wetting the spot, rubbing on chalk, and exposing it to the air. Diluted hartshorn(1) will take out mildew from woolen stuffs. A weak solution of chloride of lime can be applied to almost any fabric, but must be used with care, especially on some colors.

MILK:

Milk is an article of diet which all persons may use under nearly all conditions. A person who is sick may take milk with the greatest possible advantage, because it contains, in the form of assimilation, all the elements essential for maintaining nutrition. It should be taken slowly in mouthfuls, never in draughts like other fluids. It should not be taken after other food, as it will be almost sure to burden the stomach. Milk is theoretically a perfect food, combining every element necessary to nutrition. Yet some say they cannot drink it. It makes them bilious. If this be the fact it probably is to be attributed to the fat contained in the cream. Drink skimmed milk merely, then, and you will get on well.

Some persons are adverse to milk because they find it indigestible. A frequent reason for such consequences is that milk is drunk as if it were so much water. Where digestion is not strong it only agrees when leisurely sipped and bread eaten with it, or else cooked with suitable solids. Milk, moreover, particularly the large supplies of it given to cities, is full of germs which may produce a bad effect upon some systems. In that case it should be sterilized, as it is called, and that can be done by heating it, not to the boiling point, but as high as 170 degrees. It will be found that milk in that condition can be taken by almost every one. For kindred reasons cold milk must be pronounced undesirable.

MILK, HEALTHFULNESS OF:

If any one wishes to grow fleshy a pint of milk on retiring at night will soon cover the scrawniest bones. Although we see a good many fleshy persons nowadays, there are a great many lean and lank ones, who sigh for the fashionable measure of plumpness, and who would be vastly improved in health and appearance could their flesh be rounded with good, solid flesh. Nothing is more coveted by a thin woman than a full figure, and noth-

(1) Ammonium carbonate.

ing will so raise the ire and provoke the scandal of the "clipper-build" as the consciousness of plumpness in a rival. In a case of fever and summer complaint milk is now given with excellent results. The idea that milk is feverish has exploded, and it is now the physician's great reliance in bringing through typhoid patients, or those in too low a state to be nourished by solid food. It is a mistake to scrimp the milk-pitcher. Take more milk and buy less meat.

MILK, HOW TO TEST THE QUALITY OF:

Procure any long glass vessel—a cologne bottle or long phial. Take a narrow strip of paper just the length from the neck to the bottom of the phial, and mark it off with 100 lines at equal distances, or into 50 lines, and count each as 2, and paste it upon the phial, so as to divide its length into 100 equal parts. Fill it to the highest part with milk fresh from the cow and allow it to stand in a perpendicular position 24 hours. The number of spaces occupied by the cream will give you the exact percentage in the milk without any guess-work.

MILK, TO PRESERVE:

Provide bottles, which must be perfectly clean, sweet, and dry; draw the milk from the cow into the bottles, and as they are filled immediately cork them well up, and fasten the corks with pack-thread or wire. Then spread a little straw at the bottom of a boiler, on which place bottles with straw between them until the boiler contains a sufficient quantity. Fill it up with cold water; heat the water, and as soon as it begins to boil draw the bottles and pack them in sawdust in hampers, and stow them in the coolest part of the house. Milk preserved in this manner and allowed to remain even 18 months in the bottles will be as sweet as when first milked from the cow.

MINERAL WATERS, USE AND ABUSE OF:

Their indiscriminate use is harmful. They put too much salts in the blood, and this has to go off through the kidneys, stimulating them altogether too much. Mineral waters are useful at times, and the less frequently used the more beneficial they are. If indulged in they had better be the saline waters, such as apollinaris and seltzers, rather than the alkaline like vichy.

MIRRORS, TO TAKE CARE:

The strong light of the sun should never be allowed to fall directly upon a mirror. The amalgam or union of tin-foil and mercury which is spread on glass to form a looking-glass is easily ruined by the direct continued exposure to the solar rays, causing the glass to look misty.

MIRRORS, TO CLEAN:

Cleaning mirrors is an easy operation when rightly understood. The greatest care should be taken in cleaning to use only the softest articles, lest the glass should be scratched. It should first be dusted with a feather brush, then washed over with a sponge dipped in spirits to remove the fly spots; after this it should be dusted with the powder blue in a thin muslin bag, and finally polished with an old silk handkerchief.

MIRRORS, TO REPAIR:

To repair a damaged mirror pour upon a sheet of tin-foil about 3 drams of quicksilver to the square foot of foil. Rub smartly with a piece of buckskin until the foil becomes brilliant. Lay the glass upon a flat table, face downward; place the foil upon the damaged portion of the glass, lay a sheet of paper over the foil, and place upon it a block of wood or a piece of marble with perfectly flat surface; put upon it sufficient weight to press it down tight; let it remain in this position a few hours. The foil will adhere to the glass.

MITES IN CHEESE, TO DESTROY:

(1) These are at all times better avoided than destroyed, for when they have become very numerous they do a great deal of damage in a short time. To avoid mites the best plan seems to be to leave the cheese exposed to the air, and to brush it occasionally; some prefer wrapping the cheese in a buttered paper, but the former plan, we think, is the best. When mites have become very numerous they may be killed by suspending the cheese by a piece of wire or string and dipping it for a moment into a pail of boiling water. The boiling water will kill all the mites and do no harm to the cheese unless it is left in too long.

(2) Cheese kept in a cool larder or cellar, with a cloth rung out of clean cold water constantly upon it, will never have mites in it, or if it has, this will soon destroy them and also greatly improve the cheese, keeping it always moist.

MITTENS, SILK, FOR GENTLEMEN:

Four No. 18 needles, $3^1/_2$-ounce balls of knitting silk. Cast on 78 stitches; knit 2 and purl 2 round the needles till there is about $1^1/_2$ in. of webbing; then knit plain once around, knit to the middle of the needle, seam 1, make 1, knit 1, make 1, seam 1. Knit plain, always seaming the seam stitch, and every sixth or seventh row make a stitch inside the seam stitch as directed, until there are as many stitches between the seams as there are in the other needles, (26.) Slip these stitches on a thread; tie the ends. Cast on 8 or 10 stitches between the seams and knit around plain till the mitten reaches the nail of the third rows, narrow and knit 2 rows plain, narrow and knit 1 row, then narrow every time till all of the stitches but 2 are knit.

Draw the end of the silk through these stitches and fasten securely; a fine darning-needle is the best thing to do it with. For the thumb take the stitches off the thread and take up the 8 or 10 stitches made between the seams. Knit once around plain, then knit 2 together of the made stitches every time around till they are all taken up. Then knit round and round till the thumb is long enough. Narrow it off by knitting 2 together at the beginning of each needle till it can be finished as the hand. These directions are equally good for yarn mittens, changing the size of the needles and the number of stitches according to the size of the yarn used.

MITTENS, TO KNIT:

For the hand cast on 60 stitches, and widen at one end every time you knit across until you have widened 12 stitches; knit plain 4 times across; narrow down 12 stitches; widen 12 stitches; narrow 12, and you have the heap of the mitten. Bind off and sew it off, leaving a space for the thumb to be sewed in.

For the thumb cast on 18 stitches and widen at both ends; at the top widen 5 stitches, knit 2 plain, then narrow 5, but at the other end of the needle widen continuously, as this is the gore that runs toward the wrist. When half of the thumb has been knitted begin to narrow at this end, while you repeat the widening and narrowing at the top. When the thumb is knitted bind off all but 6 stitches, knit a little square with them for a gore between the thumb and hand. Sew up and then sew into the space left in the hand.

The wrist may be finished as long as wanted, either by knitting or crocheting. This number of stitches makes a medium-sized mitten in Saxony yarn, and, of course, is to be varied according to the size of the yarn used.

MIXED-UP POETRY, GAME OF:

A great amount of fun may be obtained from this game of mixing up poetry, which is nothing more than selecting lines from different authors and arranging them so as to make rhyme. The specimens below will illustrate our meaning:

There was a sound of revelry by night, Away down south where I was born; Let dogs delight to bark and bite Cows in the meadow and sheep in the corn.

A chieftain to the Highlands bound, His father's hope, his mother's joy, Found something smooth and hard and round, John Brown's little Indian boy.

Man wants but little here below, Oats, peas, beans, and barley; This world is all a fleeting show Over the water to Charley.

There is a calm for those who weep In famous London town; Little Bo Peep she lost her sheep— The bark that held a prince went down.

John Gilpin was a citizen From India's coral strand; Far from the busy haunts of men There is a happy land.

Hark! from the tombs a doleful sound; Dear, dear, what can the matter be? Shake the forum round and round, Come to the sunset tree.

MIXTURES:

Aromatic: Mix 2 drams of aromatic confection with 2 drams of compound tincture of cardamoms and 8 ounces of peppermint water. Dose, from 1 to 1 1/2 ounces.

Cathartic: Dissolve 1 ounce of Epsom salts in 4 ounces of compound infusion of senna, then add 3 ounces of peppermint water. Dose, from 1 1/2 to 2 ounces. Use as a warm stomachic(1) and cathartic.

Diuretic: Add 1/2 ounce of sweet spirit of niter, 2 drams of tincture of squills, and 2 ounces of liquid acetate of ammonia, to 6 ounces of decoction of broom(2). Dose, 1 ounce every 2 hours. Use in dropsies.

Cough: Dissolve 3 grains of tartar emetic and 15 grains of opium to 1 pint of boiling water, then add 4 ounces of treacle, 2 ounces of vinegar, and 1 pint more of boiling water. Dose, from 2 drams to 1 ounce.

Cough, for Children: Mix 2 drams of ipecacuanha wine with 1/2 ounce of oxymel of squills and the same quantity of mucilage, and 2 ounces of water. Dose, 1 tea-spoonful for children under 1 yr., 2 tea-spoonfuls from 1 to 5 yrs., and a table-spoonful from 5 yrs. every time the cough is troublesome.

Antispasmodic: Dissolve 50 grains of camphor in 2 drams of chloroform, and then add 2 drams tincture of lavender, 6 drams of mucilage of gum arabic, 8 ounces of aniseed, cinnamon, or some other aromatic water, and 2 ounces of water; mix well. Dose, 1 table-spoonful every 1/2 hour if necessary. Use in cholera in the cold stage when cramps are severe or exhaustion very great; as a general antispasmodic in doses of 1 dessert-spoonful when the spasms are severe.

Tonic and Stimulant: Dissolve 1 dram of extract of bark and 1/2 dram of powdered gum arabic in 6 ounces of water, and then add 1 ounce of syrup of marsh-mallow and the same quantity of syrup of tolu. Dose, 1 table-spoonful every 3 hours. Use after fevers and catarrhs.

(1) A digestive tonic.
(2) Diuretic concoctions either of scoparine and water or sparteia juice and rectified spirit.

Stomachic: Take 20 grains of powdered rhubarb and dissolve it in $3^1/2$ ounces of peppermint water, then add sal volatile and compound tincture of gentian, each $1^1/2$ drams; mix. Dose, from 1 to $1^1/2$ ounces. Use as a tonic, stimulant, and stomachic.

MOLES:

(1) To destroy moles take caster beans, and where they have recently been passing along to their underground passages make a small hole in the passage with the finger or some other way, drop in a couple of beans, and cover up the hole with dirt carefully, so as to disturb their track as little as possible. This course persevered in for a few weeks will exterminate them. The striped leaf variety that bears a speckled bean is best.

(2) Make a stiff dough of corn meal, mixing with it a small quantity of arsenic; make a hole with a finger in the runways, drop in a lump of dough about the size of a marble, and then cover over with a lump of earth to exclude the light. After the first rain go over the field again and deposit in all freshly made roads.

(3) Sink a glass or stone-ware jug into the ground under the mole-runs. The moles while running along fall into the jar, and the vertical, slippery sides of the jar prevent their escape.

MOLES, TO REMOVE:

The common mole is situated in the middle layer of the skin; the coloring matter is probably some chemical combination of iron. They are often elevated above the surface, and then the natural down of the skin over them is changed into a tuft of hair. The less they are trifled with the better, and avoid particularly the use of depilatories to remove the hair from them, as it often causes a fetid, suppurating wound. When slight they may be removed by touching them every day with a little concentrated acetic acid, by means of an hair pencil, observing due care to prevent the application from spreading to the surrounding parts. The application of lunar caustic is also effective, but it turns the spot temporarily black. When other means fail the hair may be safely removed by surgical means. They can also be removed with a sun-glass. Seat the patient in a clear, strong sunlight; bring the concentrated rays of the sun to bear on the excrescence 5 to 10 minutes. In 3 or 4 weeks the mole will scale off and a new skin form.

MONARCHS OF ENGLAND, RULE FOR MEMORIZING:

First William the Norman,
Then William his son;
Henry, Stephen, and Henry,
Then Richard and John.

Next Henry the Third,
Edwards one, two, and three,
And again, after Richard,
Three Henrys we see,

Two Edwards, third Richard,
If rightly I guess;
Two Henrys, sixth Edward,
Queen Mary, Queen Bess.

Next Jamie, the Scotsman,
And Charles whom they slew;
Yet received after Cromwell
Another Charles, too.

Next James the Second
Ascended the throne,
And good William and Mary
Together came on;

Then Anne, Georges four,
And fourth William all past,
God sent us Victoria—
May she long be the last!

MOSQUITOES, TO GET RID OF:

Mosquitoes, says some-body, love beef-blood better than they do any that flows in the veins of human kind. Just put a couple of generous pieces on plates near your bed at night, and you will sleep untroubled by these pests. In the morning you will find them full and stupid with the beef-blood and the meat sucked as dry as a cork.

MOSQUITOES, TO PROTECT FROM:

Quassia(1) is used in medicine as a powerful tonic, and the chips are sold by chemists at 15 to 25 cents per pound. The tree is indigenous to the West Indies and to South America. A young friend of mine, severely bitten by mosquitoes, and unwilling to be seen so disfigured, sent for quassia chips, and had boiling water poured upon them. At night, after washing, she dipped her hands into the quassia-water and left it to dry on her face. This was a perfect protection, and continued to be so whenever applied.

At the approach of winter, when flies and gnats get into houses and sometimes bite venomously, a grandchild of mine, 18 months old, was thus attacked. I gave the nurse some of my weak solution of quassia to be let dry on his face, and he was not bitten again. It is innocuous to children, and it may be a protection also against bed insects, which I have not had the opportunity of trying. When the solution of the quassia is strong it is well known to be an active fly poison, and is mixed with sugar to attract flies, but this is not strong enough to kill at once.

(1) A bitter drug extracted from the roots of the quassia plant.

MOSQUITO REMEDY:

To clear a sleeping-room of mosquitoes take a piece of paper rolled around a lead-pencil to form a case, and fill this with very dry pyrethrum powder, (Persian insect powder), putting in a little at a time and pressing it down with the pencil. This cartridge, or cigarette, may be set in a cup of sand to hold it erect. An hour before going to bed the room is to be closed and one of these cartridges burned. A single cartridge will answer for a small room, but for a large one two are required. Those who have tried this find that it effectually disposes of the mosquitoes.

MOTHER-OF-PEARL, TO CLEAN:

Mother-of-pearl may be polished with finely powdered pumice-stone which has been washed to separate the impurities and dirt, and then finished with putty powder and water applied by a rubber, which will produce a fine gloss.

MOTHER-OF-PEARL WORK:

This delicate substance requires great care in its workmanship, but it may be cut by the use of saws, files, and drills, with the aid of muriatic or sulphuric acid, and it is polished by colcothar(1), or the brown-red oxide of iron left after the distillation of the acid from sulphate of iron. In all ornamental work, where pearl is said to be used for flat surfaces, such as inlaying, mosaic work, etc., it is not real pearl, but mother-or-pearl that is used.

MOTH FROM THE FACE, TO REMOVE:

The principal causes of moth-spots are biliousness and a torpid liver. A distinguished and successful physician prescribes this remedy: "Put 10 drops of elixir of vitriol(2) into half a tumbler of water, and drink the whole dilution twice daily." Pimples about the face are extremely common and very annoying. Eating in moderate quantities nourishing and simple food, keeping the bowels regular, exercising and sleeping wisely; in brief, observing the laws of health, elevating and purifying the system, is the only cure. The skin must be thoroughly bathed with soap and water every night on going to bed, or every morning, as may be more convenient.

MOTHS, PROTECTION AGAINST:

(1) Steep 1/4 lb. of Cayenne pepper in 1 gallon of water; add 2 drams of strychnia powder; strain and pour this tea into a shallow vessel. Before unrolling a new carpet set the roll on each end alternately in this poisoned tea for 10 minutes, or long enough to wet its edges for at least an inch. After beating an old carpet, roll and treat all its seams and edges to the same bath; let the carpet dry thoroughly

(1) Red oxide of iron.
(2) Probably refers to sulphuric acid.

before tacking it to the floor, in order to avoid the accidental poisoning of the tacker's fingers by the liquid. If preserved for future use carefully label, "Poison." This preparation will not stain or disfigure carpets, nor corrode metals in contact with the carpet.

(2) One pound of quassia chips, 1/4 lb. of Cayenne pepper steeped in 2 gallons of water; strain and use as above.

(3) Little black carpet moths can be effectually destroyed by a free use of benzine or naphtha; poured around the edge of carpet it leaves no stain; the odor soon disappears and so do the moths. All use of either must be attended with care, and applied in the day-time and not near an open fire.

(4) Wring a cloth out of hot water; lay it over the bindings and edges, and iron with as hot an iron as can be used without scorching. This will destroy both the moths and their eggs.

(5) If fine-cut tobacco be sprinkled under the edges of the carpets, and under places where bureaus, book-cases, and the like make it dark, the moths will be prevented from laying their eggs in them, as it will drive them away.

MOUSE-TRAP, CHEAP AND GOOD:

Take the bowl of a clean clay pipe and fill it with cheese; put it under the edge of a tumbler in such a manner that a slight touch will cause the tumbler to slip off—the bait and mouse of course underneath. This arrangement will catch more mice than any trap, at the cost of 1 cent.

MOUTH, INFLAMMATION OF, OR STOMATITIS:

It begins with small red elevations, with minute, white, pearly points or vesicles on them, which soon break out and allow serum to escape, leaving little rounded ulcers of grayish color, with more or less thickened edges, and surrounded with redness; they appear first on the inner surface of the lips and gums, and then on the cheeks, edges of the tongue, and soft palate; in severe cases there is often fever, thirst, nausea and vomiting, offensive breath, and high-colored urine, with constipated bowels or diarrhea; in the milder attacks some or all of these may exist in a mild degree; it may last but a few days or continue for weeks.

Treatment: In mild attacks all that may be required is to regulate the diet, and gargle or wash the mouth with infusions of elm-bark, flaxseed, marsh-mallow(1), or quince-seeds, to which 1 dram to the pint of chlorate of potash solution is added, and touching the ulcers occasionally with a mixture of 1 part borax to 2 of honey; or prepared chalk rubbed up in a glycerine to the consistence of a thin paste. If the bowels are costive 1/2

(1) A confection from the root of the marsh mallow (altheae).

ounce of Epsom or Rochelle salts may be given, or 10 grains of rhubarb, with twice as much magnesia.

MOUTH, MUST BE KEPT CLOSED:

The peculiar arrangement of the narrowed and branched and delicately furnished nasal passages are specially suited to strain the air and to warm it before it enters the lungs. The foul air and sickening effluvia which one meets in a day's travel through the crowded city are breathed with greater impunity through the nose than through the mouth. Raw air, inhaled through the mouth, induces hoarseness, coughs, etc. No one who has been snoring through the night feels properly refreshed in the morning. Keep the mouth shut when reading silently, when writing, when listening, when in pain, when walking or riding, when angry, and when asleep.

MOUTH WASH:

Proof spirits(1), 1 quart; borax and honey, of each 1 ounce; gum myrrh, 1 ounce; red sanders wood, 1 ounce. Rub the honey and borax well together in a mortar, then gradually add the spirit, the myrrh, and sanders wood, and macerate 14 days.

MUFFS FOR THE FEET:

A nice present for any one who has got to get out of bed at night in order to tend to small children or an invalid is a pair of foot-muffs. They are of clouded zephyr, knit on wooden needles, garter fashion. Forty stitches are set up, and the knitting proceeds back and forth across the needles until the strip is about 10 in. long. Bind it off and double it together and make it into a gag, whole at the bottom and with a seam at each side. The seams are crocheted together, or may be loosely sewed with zephyr, like that used in knitting. With a coarse crochet-needle make loops around the top of the bag, crocheting a long stitch into every third stitch around the bag, and joining these together by chain-stitch. These loops are for a rubber tape about 10 in. long. Crochet scallops around the top, as ornamental as you like. This bag does not look much like boot, shoe, or slipper, but put it on your foot and it answers nicely for a foot-warmer. The number of stitches required would depend upon the size of the needles. The knitting would be loose and elastic.

MUMPS:

This disease, most common among children, begins with soreness and stiffness in the side of the neck. Soon a swelling of the paratoid gland takes place, which is painful and continues to increase for 4 or 5 days, sometimes making it difficult to swallow or open the mouth. The swelling sometimes comes on one side at a time, but commonly upon both. There is often

(1) Water and alcohol.

heat and sometimes fever, with a dry skin, quick pulse, furred tongue, constipated bowels, and scanty and high-colored urine. The disease is contagious.

Treatment: Keep the face and neck warm, and avoid taking cold. Drink warm herb teas, and if the symptoms are severe, 4 to 6 grains of Dover's powder; or if there is costiveness, a slight physic(1), and observe a very simple diet. If the disease is aggravated by taking cold and is very severe, or is translated to other glands, physic must be used freely, leeches applied to the swelling, or cooling poultices. Sweating must be resorted to in this case.

MUSH:

Farinaceous(2) food, such as mush and farina, are carbonaceous. It may be called slow "burning," but if it can have a steady supply of oxygen it will burn well and do good service. If a man is engaged in mechanical labor which requires activity and muscular exercise, let him eat of mush and oatmeal. He will do well. Then it burns and is consumed, and enters into the system easily and slowly and with advantage. It may be better than meat. But for men of sedentary habits it is to be used with care. It is by no means the all agreeing and faultless food that it was once thought to be. As a general rule it must be pronounced not the best food. More concentrated sustenance for men engaged in intellectual occupations without exercise is better, such as meat and eggs. If a man is confined to an office he does not get the oxygen necessary, nor indulge in the steady bodily movements which make carbonaceous food agree well with the stomach. Oatmeal in the morning, as a rule the coarser the better, serves sometimes as an aperient, but generally its disadvantages for a business man are greater than its advantages.

MUSHROOMS, INDICATIONS OF WHOLESOME:

When a fungus is pleasant in flavor and odor it may be considered wholesome; if, on the contrary, it have an offensive smell, a bitter, astringent, or styptic taste, or even if it leave an unpleasant flavor in the mouth, it should not be considered fit for food. The color, figure, and texture of these vegetables do not afford any characters on which we can safely rely; yet it may be remarked that in color the pure yellow, gold color, bluish pale, dark or luster brown, wine-red, or the violet belong to many that are esculent(3); while the pale or sulphur yellow, bright or blood-red, and the greenish belong to few but the poisonous. The same kinds have most frequently a compact, brittle texture; the flesh is white; they grow more readily in open places, such as dry pastures and waste lands, than in places humid or shaded by wood. In general those should be suspected which grow in

(1) Laxative.
(2) Cooked cereal made from grains of wheat, potato, nuts, etc.
(3) Edible, fit or good for food.

caverns and subterranean passages, on animal matter undergoing putrefaction, as well as those whose flesh is soft or watery.

Mushrooms vs. Poisonous Fungi:

(1) Sprinkle a little salt on the spongy part or gills of the sample to be tried. If they turn yellow they are poisonous; if black, they are wholesome. Allow the salt to act before you decide on the question.

(2) False mushrooms have a warty cap, or else fragments of membrane, adhering to the upper surface, are heavy, and emerge from a vulva or bag; they grow in tufts or clusters in woods, on the stumps of trees, etc., whereas the true mushrooms grow in pastures.

(3) False mushrooms have an astringent, styptic, and disagreeable taste.

(4) When cut they turn blue.

(5) They are moist on the surface, and generally;

(6) of a rose or orange color.

(7) The gills of the true mushroom are of a pinky red, changing to a live color.

(8) The flesh is white.

(9) The stem is white, solid, and cylindrical.

MUSTY FLOORS, TO SWEETEN:

Scrub the floor as clean as soap-suds and the scrubbing-brush will make it. Then make a strong hot solution of chloride of lime and scrub it into the floor with a broom. Make a second application of lime if necessary.

CHOOSE A PHYSICIAN OF CLEAN LIPS:

"No one of impure speech, of reckless or even careless words, or hints bordering on the obscene or immodest or vulgar, should find a place even professionally in any home."

N

NAILS, CARE OF THE:

Persons who possess well-filled purses can indulge in the luxury of a manicure's services, and thus relieve themselves of all responsibility as to their digits, but with the majority personal care and attention are necessary. If one aims only at the simplest possible method of caring for the nails he will find that very few utensils are required—a chamois-covered polisher, a little file for paring, and a powder for polishing, all of which can be bought of any apothecary.

An almond-shaped nail is very desirable and to secure it the skin which tends to grow over its base should be pushed down daily. This may be done with advantage every time the hands are bathed, for then the skin is soft and pliable. One may use for the purpose a finger of the other hand covered by the towel, or the blunted ivory end of the little instrument connected with the file. A manicure is able skillfully to cut away the superfluous border of the skin, but an unprofessional person is likely to do it bunglingly, with the result of hangnails.

The nails should be filed away at each side to insure their oval shape. Their length must depend upon the taste of the wearer, although the pianist finds his fashion prescribed by necessity, and is obliged literally to "cut his claws." In cleaning them it is best to use a brush or an ivory point, as scraping with a sharp knife tends to harden them. Polishing is done by placing a small quantity of powder on the chamois pad, and rubbing the nails back and forth.

To Whiten the Nails: Diluted sulphuric acid, 2 drams; tincture of myrrh, 1 dram; spring water, 4 ounces; mix. First cleanse with white soap, and then dip the fingers into the mixture. A good hand is one of the chief points of beauty, and these applications are really effective.

NAPERY(1):

Every housekeeper feels the need of at least one set of handsome table-linen that shall always be ready for company occasions. Fringed and embroidered damask table-cloths are very expensive, but I have seen a table-cloth in a mountain farm-house that was pretty without being costly. The material was good linen sheeting with a fringe raveled out and tied by the daughter of the owner. Above the fringe was a running pattern, not exactly

(1) Household linen.

a vine, but closely set groups of leaves and small fruits of various kinds, done very sketchily in outline work, which is simply long back-stitching in colored thread, crewel, or silk.

The work I refer to was indelible cotton of various shades. In the center was a large June apple with leaves. From the same linen, which, as it was bought, was of course too wide for a table-cover, small square napkins had been cut off and finished with a narrow fringe. In the center of each was worked patterns of fruit; a bunch of grapes on one, a pear on another, and berries of different kinds on others. The designs were all taken with the help of transfer-paper from agricultural papers and seed catalogues, and the outlining is such rapid work that 2 or 3 napkins could be embroidered in an afternoon. Kate Greenaway patterns, copied from Under the Window and other children's books, or even from advertising cards, would be as pretty as fruit designs, and easy to execute. If they are used the patterns on the table-cloth should correspond.

NAPKIN-RING, TO CROCHET:

Use cotton twine of a quality between the common wrapping twine and macrame thread. It is smoother and harder twisted than the common white twine, yet not so stiff as the macrame. Use a small steel needle and crochet rather tight and firm.

(1) Make a chain of 40 stitches. Join the ends.

(2) One chain. (Draw thread through the 2 upper threads of first stitch at first row, then through the 2 stitches on the needle, thus making a single crochet). Finish the row in single crochet.

(3) Like the second row.

(4) Five chain, 1 double crochet into the fourth stitch of third row, (3 chain, 1 double crochet into the fourth stitch of third row from the last double crochet). Repeat between parentheses until you have finished the row, but at the end, instead of 1 double crochet catch it into the second stitch of fine chain.

(5) Same as second row.

(6) Same as second row.

(7) Two chain, 3 double crochet into the first stitch of sixth row, (skip 3 stitches in sixth row and 4 double crochet into the next stitch). Repeat between parentheses until you finish the row.

(8) (Five double crochet into the middle of 4 double crochet in seventh row). Repeat between parentheses until the row is finished, then break off the thread.

(9) Tie the thread on to the end where you first began, and make 2 rows on this edge like the seventh and eighth rows. Make some very thick

flour starch and starch your ring, rubbing well into the twine, then pull into the shape of an hour-glass and dry. Repeat the starching 2 or 3 times until it is perfectly stiff. When thoroughly dry give it a coat of unbleached shellac. Weave ribbon into the open meshes in the middle, and finish with a knot.

NAUSEA, TO RELIEVE:

The following drink for relieving sickness of the stomach is said to be very palatable and agreeable:

Beat up 1 egg very well, say for about 20 minutes, then add fresh milk, 1 pint; water, 1 pint; sugar to make it palatable; boil, and get it cool. Do not drink until cold. If it becomes curds and whey it is useless.

NECK, THE:

The usual means for keeping the neck warm are by very light goods, with large meshes like woven worsted, which best serve the purpose. But covering is not desirable if it can be avoided.

Many wise men, whose faces illumine the milder seasons with the bright aspects of clean shaven cheeks and chin, prudently put a shield over the most valuable portion of the neck, if not of the entire body, the throat, by growing a winter beard. Probably every one can count among his friends some who, by letting their beards grow, hardly ever have a sore throat in winter. It will be seen by this illustration what is meant by goods that hold air and provide warmth without overheating.

The beard is like one of those light fabrics spoken of above. It is loosely put together, holds a great deal of air, and keeps the skin warm without making it perspire, which is the secret of sensible protection. There is a great deal of protection, not considering beauty, in a winter beard. Somewhat the same result is produced by putting on a high collar. For men of delicate throats the high collar is as desirable an article of winter dress as the flannel shirt is to others in summer. And no man should hesitate from so protecting himself through dread of being identified as a dude. Dudedom is as dudedom does.

NERVOUSNESS:

This unhealthy state of system depends upon general debility. It is often inherited from birth, and as often brought on by excess of sedentary occupation, overstrained employment of the brain, mental emotion, dissipation, and excess. The nerves consist of a structure of fibers or cords passing through the entire body, branching off from and having a connection with each other, and finally centering on the brain. They are the organs of feeling and sensation of every kind, and through them the mind operates upon the body. It is obvious, therefore, that what is termed the "nervous system" plays an important part in the bodily functions, and upon them not only much of the health but happiness depends.

Treatment: The cure of nervous complaints lies rather in moral than in medical treatment. For although much good may be effected by tonics, such as bark, quinine, etc., there is far more benefit to be derived from attention to diet and regimen. In such cases solid food should preponderate over liquid, and the indulgence in warm and relaxing fluids should be especially avoided; plain and nourishing meat, as beef or mutton, a steak or chop, together with 1/2 pint of bitter ale or stout, forming the best dinner. Cocoa is preferable to tea; vegetables should be but sparingly eaten. Sedentary pursuits should be cast aside as much as possible, but where they are compulsory every spare moment should be devoted to outdoor employment and brisk exercise.

Early bed-time and early rising will prove beneficial, and the use of the cold shower-bath is excellent. Gymnastic exercises, fencing, horse-riding, rowing, dancing, and other pursuits which call forth the energies serve also to brace and invigorate the nervous system. It will also be as well to mingle with society, frequent public assemblies, and amusements, and thus dispel that morbid desire for seclusion and quietude which, if indulged in to excess, renders a person unfitted for intercourse with mankind, and materially interferes with advancement in life.

NEURALGIA, TEMPORARY RELIEF FOR:

(1) *A New Hampshire gentleman says:* "Take 2 large table-spoonfuls of cologne and 2 tea-spoonfuls of fine salt; mix them together in a small bottle; every time you have any acute affection of the facial nerves, or neuralgia, simply breathe the fumes into your nose from the bottle, and you will be immediately relieved."

(2) Prepare horse-radish by grating and mixing in vinegar, and same as for the table, and apply to the temple when the face or head is affected, or to the wrist when the pain is in the arm or shoulder.

NICKEL ORNAMENTS, TO POLISH:

Nickel ornaments on stoves, etc., may be kept bright by using ammonia and whiting. Mix together in a bottle and apply with a cloth. A very little polishing gives a fine luster. It is good for silver-plated ware as well. We use pumice powder to polish tin pans when we use any thing.

NICKEL-PLATING, TO POLISH:

Take the finest of coal ashes—you will find deposits as fine as flour in your stove—and sift through muslin. Dip a soft cloth in kerosene, then in the ash-dust, and rub vigorously on the plating. Dry and polish with a woolen cloth.

NIGHT-DRESS, THE:

The old-fashioned night-shirt is being rapidly supplanted by pajamas, and this is a very sensible revolution. The sudden change from complete street or house dress to a thin sheet of linen or of cotton or silk was productive not only of colds, but of rheumatism and often of pneumonia. Draught strikes the legs of a person who wears a night-shirt, and the legs are very sensitive, because they are at other times heavily clothed. Then, again, such is the flighty nature of an old-fashioned night-gown on a restless sleeper that it is always apt to work up above his stomach and expose it to sudden chilling, and that is often fraught with serious results.

If you will wear the old-fogy night-shirt, wear a flannel band about the waist. Athletes do in training, when the system becomes especially sensitive. The pajama not only insures a covering for the legs the night through, but it guards the bowels, too. And it is incomparably better in case the sleeper should be called suddenly to get out of bed. In a suit of pajamas a man may always be called "clothed," to a certain extent. In a night-gown he is always an old womanish-looking fright, and uncompromisingly unpresentable. Physicians do not think that it matters much to a healthy person whether pajamas are made of silk or flannel or linen. But those who are in poor health or advanced in years would doubtless do well to wear none but flannel.

NIGHTMARE:

The symptoms are generally well understood, and they are caused by the effects of too hearty or indigestible suppers eaten too short a while before going to bed.

Treatment: This must be mainly preventive. The diet should be simple and well regulated, and the supper light, and the evening spent in some pleasant recreation or amusement; avoid sleeping on the back or in constrained, uneasy positions; the bowels should be kept regular by mild laxatives when required, and as much outdoor exercise as possible taken.

NIGHT-SWEATS:

(1) The cure for night-sweats depends entirely on the cause. Malaria gives rise to them, and then the cure is quinine and arsenic. Debility may cause them. In that case tonics and good nutritious food should be used. Consumption causes them and the remedy is sulphuric acid, 10 to 20 drops in water each hour.

(2) Drink freely cold sage tea, which is said to be a certain remedy; or take elixir of vitriol in a little sweetened water. Dose, from 20 to 30 drops.

NIPPLES, SORE:

Excoriations and cracks of the nipples not only cause great pain and inconvenience in suckling, but are a frequent cause of acute inflammation of the breast. The tannin lotion, made of 1/2 dram of tannin, 1 fluid dram of alcohol, and 4 fluid ounces of water, mixed together, should be used.

The nipple may be defended from the clothes and the child's mouth by a metallic shield or rubber band. Women who are subject to the affection should frequently wash the parts with salt and water, or solution of alum; or should apply every night a liniment composed of equal parts of rectified spirit and olive-oil.

Ointment for Sore Nipples:

(1) Take of tincture of tolu(1), 2 drams; spermaceti ointment, 1/2 ounce; powdered gum, 2 drams; mix, make an ointment.

(2) The white of an egg mixed with brandy is the best application for sore nipples; the person should at the same time use a nipple-shield.

(3) Glycerine and tannin(2), equal weights, rubbed together, is very highly recommended, as is also mutton tallow.

NOSE, CARE OF THE:

The Sense of Smell: The nostrils open at the back into the pharynx, and are lined by a continuation of the mucous membrane of the throat. The olfactory nerves enter through a sieve-like bony plate at the roof of the nose, and are distributed over the inner surface of the two olfactory chambers. The purpose of the sense of smell is to warn us of the presence of cold air, and to aid us in the selection of food.

Foreign Substances in the Nose: Beans, cherry-pits, peas etc., often cause considerable but not serious inconvenience among children. The simplest way of getting rid of the intruder is to close the opposite nostril, and blow forcibly into the patient's mouth. Sometimes sneezing, caused by snuff introduced into the nostril, will dislodge the object. In place of this a stream of water carried into the nostril by means of a nasal douche may wash out the material. When simple measures fail, a physician must be called, and the forceps resorted to.

Bleeding from the Nose: The causes which commonly produce bleeding from the nose are those which send the blood too strongly to the head, such as strong coffee, too full living, exposure to heat, excess in drinking, and violent mental excitement, constipation, etc. It is also caused by tight

(1) A stimulant and expectorant from the balsam of Tolu (Myrospermum Toluiferum).
(2) Tannic acid.

lacing, tight neck-cloths, blows on the nose, etc. In the majority of cases it is beneficial, but may be so persistent as to endanger life.

Treatment of Nose-bleed: The patient should be exposed to cool air. The head should not hang over a basin, but be kept raised. Find which nostril the blood escapes from, and on that side raise the arm perpendicularly, and hold the nose firmly with the finger and thumb. At the same time a towel wet with ice-water may be laid on the forehead. A piece of ice, a snowball, or cold water compress applied to the back of the neck will often stop the bleeding. The popular remedy of placing a cold key between the clothes and the back should not be forgotten. A more powerful remedy, one which seldom fails, is that of blowing, by means of a quill, powdered gum arabic into the nostrils. When clotted blood forms in the nostrils it should be disturbed as little as possible.

To Arrest Bleeding of the Nose: Introduce by means of a probe a small piece of lint or soft cotton, previously dipped into some mild styptic, and a solution of alum, white vitriol, creasote, or even cold water. This will generally succeed; but should it not, cold water may be snuffed up the nostrils. Should the bleeding be very profuse, medical advice should be procured.

Catarrh: This disease is not usually painful, but it is yet in many cases intensely harassing. It is universal, for neither sex and no age is free from liability to acute attacks of it. The one great cause of it is exposure to cold, but sitting in draughts, wetting the feet, and all circumstances that conspire to close the pores of the skin may bring on a severe attack in a few hours. The chief predisposing causes are confinement in over-heated rooms, and the eating and drinking of hot substances.

Treatment of Nasal Catarrh: No two cases can be treated exactly alike. The special remedy to be used and the strength of the solution must be determined by the progress of the case. In almost all cases a weak solution of chlorate of potash, applied by means of a syringe, will prove beneficial. Carbolic acid, nitric acid, Lugol's solution, iodine and glycerine, tannin and glycerine, are also beneficial, and are to be applied in the same manner, or, in the absence of a syringe, be snuffed into the nostrils.

NOSE, THE:

There seems to be no absolute standard of nasal beauty. The Romans were proud of their stern and portentous aquilines, and the Israelites would probably not be content to lose the smallest tip of their redundant beaks. The Tartars, having no noses to speak of, affect to consider the deficiency a beauty. The wife of Genghis Khan was esteemed the most charming woman in all Tartary because she only had two holes where her nose should have been.

The peculiar form of the nose seems in fact to have but little influence upon our likes and dislikes. Mirabeau, who had a nose as wide-spread as that of a Hottentot, and Gibbon and Wilkes, whose noses were reduced to barely perceptible snubs, were very successful suitors of the female sex. The turn-up nose cannot be justified by any principle of taste, and yet the *nez retrouss*, by which French appellation we are fond of dignifying the pug, is so far from diminishing, that it seems to increase the admiration of man for the woman who possesses it.

NURSE, THE:

Where there are children the nurse is of course a most important part of the household, and often gives more trouble than any of the other servants, for she is usually an elderly person, impatient of control and "set in her ways." The mistress must make her obey at once.

Nurses are only human, and can be made to conform to the rules by which humanity is governed. Ladies have adopted for their nurses the French style of dress—dark stuff gowns, white aprons, and caps. French nurses are, indeed, very much the fashion, as it is deemed all-important that children should learn to speak French as soon as they can articulate. But it is so difficult to find a French nurse who will speak the truth that many mothers have renounced the accomplished Gaul and hired the Anglo-Saxon, who is often not more veracious.

NURSERY:

Food and drink are matters of great importance to an invalid, especially to one who is confined to the sick-room for some time. They should always be given according to the doctor's orders, both as regards the nature of the food, the quantity, and the time of eating. The least disobedience here has sometimes produced fatal consequences, particularly in cases of typhoid fever.

In dealing with a sick person who is impatient and unwilling to obey the physician a nurse, even though she be young and inexperienced, should try to be firm, and do nothing against the doctor's commands. It is better to endure the complaints of an invalid than the remorse and reproaches that would follow an indulgence that proved fatal to the one who asked for it.

Whether the nurse prepares the food herself or has it made at her request, she should be very careful to see that it is exactly right before serving. No half-done or slovenly cooking will answer here. Hot food and drinks should be served hot, not lukewarm; cold food or drinks should be refreshingly cold. Above all, there should be no suspicion of grease in broth or soup; no lumps on gruel; no burnt toast or soggy bread; no milk half turned sour; no doubtful meat or vegetables admitted to the invalid's tray. Such seasoning as is allowed should be used in moderation while cooking, and more added afterward if the patient's taste is not suited. It is always possible to put in more, but not to take any out.

Dainty china and glass add much to a well-cooked meal, and sick persons are often tempted by the inviting appearance of food, when they would not touch it if served carelessly. A spray of fresh flowers laid beside the plate is very pretty, but be sure there are no spiders or bugs on them to creep out and spoil one's appetite.

Avoid handling bread or fruit or similar articles in the sight of the sick, if intended for them to eat, and remember never to be offended if the most carefully and daintily prepared food is reduced, because an invalid's appetite is the most capricious thing in the world. Study the different recipes for the sick-room in reliable cook-books, prepare unexpected dishes in small quantities, after asking the doctor's advice, and never ask patients what they would like to eat. Cook such food as the physician orders, and take it to them at the proper time; but if they do express preferences, spare no pains to get the desired article, provided it is allowable.

NURSERY GOVERNESS, THE:

The nursery governess is much oftener employed now in this country than in former years. This position is often filled by well-mannered and well-educated young women, who are the daughters of poor men, and obliged to earn their own living. These young women, if they are good and amiable, are invaluable to their mistresses. They perform the duties of a nurse, wash and dress the children, eat with them, and teach them, the nursery-maid doing the coarse, rough work of the nursery. If a good nursery governess can be found, she is worth her weight in gold to her employer. She should not eat with the servants; there should be a separate table for her and her charges. This meal is prepared by the kitchen-maid, who is a very important functionary, almost an under-cook, as the cook in "grand houses" is absorbed in the composition of the dishes and dinners.

NIGHTMARE:

"The symptoms, are generally well understood, and they are caused by the efects of too hearty or indigestible suppers eaten too short a while before going to bed."

O

OIL-CLOTH, TO POLISH:

Wash it clean in lukewarm water, using a scrubbing-brush, then rub it with a woolen cloth wrung out of skim-milk.

OIL LINIMENTS:

(1) In cases of whooping-cough and some chronic bronchitic affections the following liniment may be advantageously rubbed into the chest and along the spine. Spirits of camphor, 2 parts; laudanum, 1/2 part; spirits of turpentine, 1 part; castile soap in powder finely divided, 1/2 ounce; alcohol, 3 parts; digest the whole together for 3 days, and strain through linen. This liniment should be gently warmed before using.

(2) *A powerful liniment for all rheumatic pains, especially when affecting the loins, is the following:*

Camphorated-oil and spirits of turpentine, of each 2 parts; water of hartshorn, 1 part; laudanum, 1 part; to be well shaken together.

(3) *Another very efficient liniment or embrocation, serviceable in chronic painful affections, may be conveniently and easily made as follows:*

Take of camphor, 1 ounce; Cayenne pepper, in powder, 2 teaspoonfuls; alcohol, 1 pint. The whole to be digested with moderate heat for 10 days, and filtered. It is an active rubificant(1); and after a slight friction with it produces a grateful thrilling sensation of heat in the pained part, which is rapidly relieved.

OIL-PAINTINGS, TO CLEAN:

Oil-paintings on canvas or panel are best cleaned by washing with soap and soft water just warm. When wiped dry with a soft cloth they should be rubbed with a warm silk handkerchief before the fire. An immediate brightness may be given to any very dull oil-paintings by gently wiping the surface over with a fresh-cut onion.

OIL-PAINTINGS, TO RENEW:

The blackened lights of old pictures may be instantly restored to their original hue by touching them with deutoxide of hydrogen diluted with

(1) A reddening agent.

6 or 8 times its weight of water. The part must be afterward washed with a clean sponge and water.

OINTMENTS:

Ointments are used as topical applications to parts, generally ulcers, and are usually spread upon linen or other materials.

Camphorated: Mix 1/2 ounce of camphor with 1 ounce of lard, having, of course, previously powdered the camphor. Use as a discutient and stimulant in idolent tumors.

Chalk: Mix as much prepared chalk as you can into some lard so as to form a thick ointment. Use as an application to burns and scalds.

For Itch: Mix 4 drams of sublimated sulphur, 2 ounces of lard, and 2 drams of sulphuric acid together. This is to be rubbed into the body.

For Scrofulous Ulcerations: Mix 1 dram of ioduret of zinc and 1 ounce of lard together. Use twice a day in the ulcerations.

Catechu: Mix 1 ounce of powdered catechu, 2 1/2 drams of olive-oil together. Use to apply to flabby and indolent ulcerations.

Tartar Emetic: Mix 20 grains of tartar emetic and 10 grains of white sugar with 1 1/2 drams of lard. Use as a counter irritant in white swellings, etc.

For Old Sores: Red precipitate(1), 1/2 ounce; sugar of lead, 1/2 ounce; burnt alum, 1 ounce; white vitriol, 1/4 ounce, or a little less; all to be very finely pulverized; have mutton tallow made warm, 1/2 lb.; stir all in, and stir until cool.

OLD CLOTHES:

It is a mystery to many people how scourers of old clothes can make them look almost as good as new. Take, for instance, a shiny old coat, vest, or pair of pants of broadcloth, cassimere, or diagonal. The scourer makes a strong, warm soap-suds and plunges the garment in it, souses it up and down, rubs the dirty places, if necessary puts it through a second suds, then rinses it through several waters and hangs it to dry. When nearly dry he takes it in, rolls it up for an hour or two, and then presses it. An old cotton cloth is laid on the outside of the coat and the iron passed over that until all the wrinkles are out; but the iron is removed before steam ceases to rise from the goods, else they will be shiny. Wrinkles that are obstinate are removed by laying a wet cloth over them and passing the iron over that.

If any shiny places are seen they are treated as the wrinkles are; the

(1) Red oxide of mercury.

iron is lifted while the full cloud of steam rises and brings the nap up with it. Cloth should always have a suds made specially for it, for if washed in that which has been used for white cotton or woolen clothes lint will be left in the water and cling to the cloth. In this manner we have known the same coat and pantaloons to be renewed time and again, and have all the look and feel of new garments. Good broadcloth and its fellow clothes will bear many washings and look better every time because of them.

ONIONS, HEALTHFUL PROPERTIES OF:

Lung and liver complaints are certainly benefited, often cured, by a free consumption of onions, either cooked or raw. Colds yield to them like magic. Don't be afraid of them. Taken at night all offense will be wanting by morning, and the good effects will amply compensate for the trifling annoyance. Taken regularly they greatly promote the health of the lungs and the digestive organs. An extract made by boiling down the juice of onions to a syrup and taken as a medicine answers the purpose very well, but fried, roasted, or boiled onions are better. Onions are very cheap medicine, within every body's reach, and they are not by any means as "bad to take" as the costly nostrums a neglect of their use may necessitate.

ONIONS, MEDICINAL QUALITIES OF:

The free use of onions for the table has always been considered by most people a healthy and desirable vegetable, and but for their odor, which is objectionable to many, they would be found more generally on our dining tables. For a cold on the chest there is no better specific for most persons than well boiled or roasted onions. They may not agree with every one, but to persons with good digestion they will not only be found to be most excellent remedy for a cough, and the clogging of the bronchial tubes, which is usually the cause of the cough, but if eaten freely at the outset of a cold they will usually break up what promised, from the severity of the attack, to have been a serious one.

A writer in one of our medical journals recently recommended the giving of young raw onions to children 3 or 4 times a week, and when they get too large and strong to be eaten raw, then boil and roast them, but not abandon their free use. Another writer advocating their use says; "During unhealthy seasons, when diphtheria and like contagious diseases prevail, onions ought to be eaten in the spring of the year at least once a week. Onions are invigorating and prophylactic beyond description. Further, I challenge the medical fraternity or any mother to point out a place where children have died from diphtheria or scarlatina anginosa, etc., where onions were freely used."

ONIONS, TO PEEL:

To many persons peeling onions is a most disagreeable operation, and causes the greatest pain in the eyes. All this inconvenience may be avoided, and as many onions as you please be peeled with impunity, merely by taking a needle or any small piece of polished steel between the teeth during the operation. The steel will attract the acid juice of the onion and save the eyes.

OPIUM HABIT:

Opium holds its victims with a power well-nigh resistless. No other drug can compare with it in this respect, and no other has yet been discovered to take its place.

Treatment: Where this habit has existed for a comparatively brief period, and patients are young and strong, the best plan is to stop it at once, and sustain the strength with food and tonics until recovery; where the habit has been existing several years, and the patients are old and weak, such a course would be highly dangerous and might prove fatal. These should adopt a gradual and systematic reduction of the opiate dose, supplying its place as much as possible with a tonic prescribed by a physician.

ORANGES AND LEMONS, GAME OF:

Oranges and Lemons, or "London Bells," is a game that will often cause considerable sport for a party of young people. Two of the tallest players are chosen, who join hands and hold them up to form an arch. The rest of the company take hold of each other's dresses or coats, and march, one after the other, beneath the arch, singing in chorus, "Oranges and lemons, say the bells of St. Clemet's. You owe me 5 farthings, say the bells of St. Martin's. When will you pay me? say the bells of Old Bailey. When I grow rich, say the bells of Shoreditch. When will that be? say the bells of Stepney. I do not know, says the great bell of Bow. Here comes a candle to light you to bed; and here comes a chopper to chop off the last, last, last man's head."

The last one in the line being cut off by the descent of the arms forming the arch, is asked whether oranges or lemons are preferred, and according to the answer is sent to the right or left side of the room. This is repeated until all heads are off, when the oranges and lemons have a tug of war. The contestants clasp each other around the waist, the foremost players of each party grasp hands, and all pull with might and main. The party wins which brings the other over to their side of the room. The war tug may well be confined to the boys in the party, the girls looking on and cheering their respective sides. This play is also best adapted to uncarpeted floors.

ORATOR, GAME OF:

A manager is elected, who invites the guests to come and hear Mr. Gladstone, Mr. Evarts, or some other distinguished orator. It requires two to deliver the oration. The one who is to speak puts his arms behind his back; a shorter friend (well concealed by the window curtains) passes his arms around the speaker's waist, and supplies with his own the latter's want of hands. He is then to gesticulate to this friend's words, and the fun of the performance consists in the singular inappropriateness of the action to the speech, the invisible gesticulator making the orator absurd by his gestures. A table placed before the speaker and a good arrangement of the curtains makes the illusion very perfect. The speaker must be able to keep his countenance, as his gravity is likely to be severely taxed by his friend's pantomimical illustration of his speech.

ORCHARDS, TO RENEW:

(1) It is very well known that the reason why peach, apple, quince, and pear orchards gradually grow poorer and poorer, until they cease to produce at all, is because the potash is exhausted from the soil by the plant. This potash must be restored, and the most effective way to do it is to use the following compound, discovered by a distinguished German chemist: 30 parts sulphate of potash, 15 parts sulphate of magnesia, 35 parts salt, 15 parts gypsum, (plaster of Paris), 5 parts chloride of magnesia. This should be roughly powdered and mixed and then mingled with barn-yard manure, or dug in about the roots of the trees. From 10 to 20 lbs. to a tree are quite enough.

(2) Early in the spring plow the entire orchard and enrich the whole soil with a good dressing of compost of manure, swamp-muck, and lime, and scrape off the old bark with a deck-scraper or a sharp hoe; apply 1/2 bushel of lime, and soap of strong soap-suds on the trunks and limbs, as high as a man can reach. When the trees are in full bloom throw over them a good proportion of the fine slaked lime, and you will reap abundant fruits from your labors.

OSTRICH FEATHERS, TO CLEAN:

(1) Four ounces of white soap cut small, dissolved in 4 pints of water, rather hot, in a large basin; make the solution into a lather by beating it with birch rods or wires. Introduce the feathers and rub well with the hands for 5 or 6 minutes. After this soaping wash in clean water as hot as the hand can bear. Shake until dry.

(2) White or light tinted ones can be laid on a plate and scrubbed gently with a tooth-brush in warm soap-suds, then well shaken out and well dried either by the hot sun or a good fire. At first the feather will have a most discouraging appearance, and a novice is apt to think it perfectly spoiled. But after it is perfectly dry it should be carefully curled with a penknife or scissors blade, and it will recover all its former plumy softness.

OTTOMAN, TO MAKE:

A neat and useful ottoman may be made by taking a box in which fine-cut tobacco is packed and covering it with cretonne. The top may be taken off and put on without difficulty, if, after covering, a narrow ruffle to fall over the edge is tacked on. An ottoman of this sort is convenient in the bedroom, where it may serve as a receptacle for stockings. If one does not care to buy cretonne, bits of carpet may be used for the covering.

OVEN-HOLDERS, TO MAKE:

Oven-holders for taking out bread, meat, etc., are made $2^1/_2$ ft. long by 1 ft. wide, or coffee-sacking, first boiling it in ashes to soften and then washing it, or of 3 or 4 thicknesses of old cotton cloth. They are a great necessity. Have 3 or 4 of them, or better half a dozen, so part can be washed each week. Keep those in use on nails beside the stove, and it is handy to have a smaller one with a loop; and tied with a tape to the apron-binding of the cook.

P

PAIN EXTRACTOR:

Spirits of ammonia, 1 ounce; laudanum, 1 ounce; oil of origanum(1), 1 ounce; mutton tallow, 1/2 lb.; combine the articles with the tallow when it is nearly cool.

PAIN IN THE FEET, TO CURE:

If your feet become painful from walking or standing too long, put them into warm salt and water mixed in the proportion of large handfuls of salt to a gallon of water. Sea-water made warm is still better. Keep your feet and ankles in the water until they begin to feel cool, rubbing them well with your hands. Then wipe them dry and rub them long and hard with a coarse towel. Where the feet are tender and easily fatigued it is an excellent thing to go through this practice regularly every night; also on coming home from a walk. With perserverance this has cured neuralgia in the feet.

PAINT, MIXTURE FOR CLEANING:

Dissolve 2 ounces of soda in a quart of hot water, which will make a ready and useful solution for cleaning old painted work preparatory to re-painting. The mixture in the above proportions should be used when warm, and the wood-work afterward washed with water to remove the remains of the soda.

PAINT, OLD, TO REMOVE:

Cover with a wash of 3 parts quick stone lime slaked in water, to which 1 part pearlash is added. Allow the coating to remain 16 hours, when the paint may be easily scraped off.

PAINT, TO REMOVE FROM A WALL:

If you intend papering a painted wall you must first get off the paint, otherwise the paper will not stick. To do this, mix in a bucket with warm water a sufficient quantity of pearlash or potash, so as to make a strong solution. Dip a brush into this and with it scour off all the paint, finishing with cold water and a flannel.

PAINT, TO REMOVE FROM WINDOWS:

To remove paint from windows take strong bicarbonate of soda and

(1) In 1800's, margoram; today may refer to oregano.

dissolve it in hot water. Wash the glass, and in 20 minutes or 1/2 hour rub thoroughly with a dry cloth. Paint, varnish, or Japan may be softened or easily removed from old surfaces with a solution of caustic soda.

PAINT-CLEANER:

Provide a plate with some of the best whiting to be had, and have ready some clean warm water and a piece of flannel, which dip into the water and squeeze nearly dry; then take as much whiting as will adhere to it, apply it to the painted surface, when a little rubbing will instantly remove any dirt or grease. After which wash the part well with clean water, rubbing it dry with a soft chamois. Paint thus cleaned looks as well as when first laid on, without any injury to the most delicate colors. It is far better than using soap, and does not require more than half the time and labor.

PAINT FOR BARNS, ANY COLOR:

Mix water lime and skim-milk to a proper consistence to apply with a brush, and it is ready to use. It will adhere well to wood, whether smooth or rough, to brick, mortar, or stone, where oil has not been used, (in which case it cleaves to some extent), and forms a very hard substance, as durable as the best oil paint. It is too cheap to estimate, and any one can put it on who can use a brush. Any color may be given to it by using colors of the tinge desired. If a red is preferred, mix Venetian red with milk, not using any lime. It looks well for 15 yrs.

PAINT FOR MAGIC-LANTERN SLIDES:

Transparent colors only are used for this work, such as lakes, sap-green, ultra-marine, verdigris(1), gamboge(2), asphaltum, etc., mixed in oil, and tempered with light-colored varnish, (white Demar). Draw on the paper the design desired, and stick it to the glass with water or gum; then with a fine pencil put the outlines on the opposite side of the glass with the proper colors; then shade or fill up with black Vandyke brown(3), as you find best.

PAINTING BANNERS:

Lay out the letters very accurately with charcoal or crayon, then saturate the cloth with water to render the painting easy. On large work a stencil will be found useful. Take a piece of tin, lay the straight edge to the mark, brush over with a wash tool, and by this means you will make a very clean-edged letter. Use stiff bristle pencils in painting on canvas.

PAINTING HOUSES, BEST SEASON FOR:

The outside of buildings should be painted during autumn or winter.

(1) The green encrustation found on brass or copper, originally in France, from the action of grape refuse on copper pans.
(2) A gum resin from a tree of the Saint Johnswort family used as a yellow pigment.
(3) Pigment obtained from a kind of peat or bog earth.

Hot weather injures the paint by drying in the oil too quickly; then the paint will easily rub off. But when the paint is laid on during the cold weather, it hardens in drying and is firmly set.

PAINTING WALLS:

Before paint or kalsomine is applied to walls every crevice should be filled with plaster or cement. For the kalsomine put 1/4 lb. of white glue in cold water over night, and heat gradually in the morning until dissolved. Mix 8 lbs. of whiting with hot water, add the dissolved glue and stir together, adding warm water until about the consistency of thick cream. Use a kalsomine brush, and finish as you go along. If skim-milk is used instead of water the glue may be omitted.

PAINT ODORS, TO GET RID OF:

Place a vessel full of lighted charcoal in the middle of the room and throw on it 2 or 3 handfuls of juniper-berries; shut the windows, the chimney, and the door close; 24 hours afterward the room may be opened; then it will be found that the sickly unwholesome smell will be entirely gone. The smoke of the juniper-berry possesses this advantage, that should any thing be left in the room, such as tapestry, etc., none of it will be spoiled.

PAPER, TO FUMIGATE:

Dip light paper in a solution of alum; strength of alum, 1 ounce; water, 1 pint. Dry thoroughly, and on one side spread a mixture of equal parts of gum benzoin, galbanum(1), or Peruvian balsam; melt the gums in an earthenware dish and spread with a hot spatula; slips of the paper are held over a light, when the odorous matter will be evaporated, the alum preventing the paper from igniting.

PAPER, WALL, HOW TO CLEAN:

To clean wall-paper take off the dust with a soft cloth. With a little flour and water make a lump of stiff dough and rub the wall gently downward, taking the length of the arm each stroke, and in this way go around the whole room. As the dough becomes dirty, cut the soiled parts off. In the second round commence the stroke a little above where the last one ended, and be very careful not to cross the paper or to go up again. Ordinary papers cleaned in this way will look fresh and bright, and almost as good as new. Some papers, however, and these the most expensive ones, will not clean nicely; and in order to ascertain whether a paper can be cleaned nicely it is best to try it in some obscure corner where it will not be noticed if the result is unsatisfactory. If there be any broken places in the wall, fill them up with a mixture of equal parts of plaster of Paris and silver

(1) A gum resin from the Ferula Galbaniflua, found in India and Persia.

sand, made into a paste with a little water, then cover the place with a piece of paper like the rest, if it can be had.

PAPERING AND PAINTING:

Papering and painting are best done in cold weather, especially the latter, for the wood absorbs the oil of paint in warm weather, while in cold weather the oil hardens on the outside, making a coat which will protect the wood instead of soaking into it.

PARING AND BURNING OF THE SOIL:

Pare off the turf to a depth of 2 or 3 in., generally by a breast plow worked by hand or by a turf-paring plow drawn by a horse; allow it to dry and then burn in heaps. The result is a mixture of burned earth, charred vegetable fiber, the ashes of that part which is entirely consumed thus producing a powerful manure. Insects are also killed by the process.

To ascertain whether a soil will be improved by paring and burning, a few sods may be taken and exposed to heat in a closely covered iron pot; the heat should not be so intense as to produce light, but should be kept up for a considerable time till the sods are consumed. If the ashes are red, and the whole is a fine powder with particles of charcoal in it, the soil from which it was taken may be safely pared and burned; especially if it forms a mud with water, and the earth is not readily through, and soon settles when mixed with it, burning will not be advantageous.

PARLOR MAGIC:

The Tobacco Pipe Cannon: Take of saltpeter, 1 ounce; cream of tartar, 1 ounce; sulphur, $^1/_2$ ounce; heat them to powder separately, then mix them together. Put a grain into a pipe of tobacco, and when it is lighted it will give the report of a musket without breaking the pipe. By putting as much as may lie on your nail in a piece of paper and setting fire to it, a tremendous report will be the result.

The Erratic Egg: Have 2 wine-glasses. Transfer the egg from one wine-glass to the other and back again to its original position without touching the egg or glasses, or allowing any person any thing to touch them. To perform this trick all you have to do is to blow smartly on one side of the egg, and it will hop into the next glass, repeat this and it will hop back again.

To Melt Lead in a Paper: Wrap up a very smooth ball of lead in a piece of paper, taking care that there be no wrinkles in it, and that it be every-where in contact with the ball. If it be held in this state over the flame of a taper the lead will be melted without the paper being burned. The lead, indeed, when once fused, will not fail in a short time to pierce the paper, and, of course, runs through.

PASTES AND CEMENTS:

These include all substances employed for the purpose of causing the adhesion of two or more bodies, whether originally separate or divided by an accidental fracture. As the substances that are required to be connected together are exceedingly variable and differ very much in their properties as to texture, and as the conditions under which they are placed, with regard to heat and moisture, are also exceedingly variable, a number of articles possessed of very different properties are required; for an adhesive substance that answers admirably under one set of circumstances may be perfectly useless in others. We give a variety sufficient for all needs.

Rice-flour Cement: This cement, much used in china and Japan, is made by mixing fine rice-flour with cold water, and simmering over a slow fire until a thick paste is formed. This is superior to any other paste, either for parlor or workshop purposes. When made of the consistence of plaster, clay models, busts, bass-reliefs, etc., may be formed of it, and the articles when dry are susceptible of high polish and very durable.

Compound Glue: Take very fine flour, mix it with white of eggs, isinglass, and a little yeast; mingle the materials; heat them well together; spread them, the batter being made thin with gum-water, or even tin-plates; tinge the paste with Brazil or vermilion for red; indigo or verditer(1), etc., for blue; saffron, turmeric, or gamboge for yellow.

Cement for Iron and Stone: Glycerine and litharge stirred to a paste hardens rapidly and makes a suitable cement for iron upon iron, for two stone surfaces, and especially for fastening iron to stone. The cement is insoluble and is not attacked by strong acids.

Cement for Metal and Glass: The following cement will firmly attach any metallic substances to glass or porcelain: Mix 2 ounces of a thick solution of glue with 1 ounce of linseed-oil varnish, or three-fourths ounce of Venice turpentine; boil them together, stirring them until they mix as thoroughly as possible. The pieces cemented should be tied together for 2 or 3 days.

Glue for Uniting Card-board, etc.: For uniting card-board, paper, and small articles of fancy work the best glue dissolved with about one third its weight of coarse brown sugar in the smallest quantity of boiling water is very good. When this is in a liquid state it may be dropped in a thin cake upon a plate and allowed to dry; when required for use, one end of the cake may be moistened by the mouth and rubbed on the substances to be joined.

Cement for Crockery: To make a good cement for crockery take 1 lb. of white shellac pulverized, 2 ounces of clean gum-mastic, put these into a bottle,

(1) A blue pigment prepared by adding chalk to a solution of copper in nitric acid.

and then add $^1/_2$ lb. pure sulphuric ether. Let it stand half an hour, and then add $^1/_2$ gallon 90 per cent. alcohol and shake occasionally until it is dissolved. Heat the edges of the article to be mended, and apply the cement with a pencil-brush; hold the article firmly together till the cement cools.

Diamond Cement: Soak isinglass in water till it is soft, then dissolve it in the smallest possible quantity of proof spirit by the aid of a gentle heat; in 2 ounces of this mixture dissolve 10 grains of ammoniacum, and while still liquid add $^1/_2$ dram of mastic dissolved in 3 drams of rectified spirit; stir well together, and put into small bottles for sale.

Directions for Use:

Liquefy the cement by standing the bottle in hot water and use it directly. The cement improves the oftener the bottle is thus armed, and resists the action of water and moisture perfectly.

Mouth Glue: A very useful preparation is sold by many of the law stationers under this title; it is merely a thin cake of soluble glue, (4 in. by $1^1/_2$), which, when moistened by the tongue, furnishes a ready means of fastening papers, etc., together. It is made by dissolving 1 lb. of brown sugar, and boiling the whole until it is sufficiently thick to become solid on cooling; it is then poured into molds or on a slab slightly greased, and cut into the required shape when cool.

Liquid Glue: Dissolve 1 ounce of borax in a pint of boiling water, add 2 ounces of shellac, and boil in a covered vessel until the lac is dissolved. This forms a very useful and cheap cement; it answers well for pasting labels on tin, and withstands damp much better than the common glue. The liquid glue made by dissolving shellac in naphtha is dearer, soon dries up, and has an unpleasant smell.

Paste for Wall-paper: Moisten common laundry starch with cold water to the consistency of paste, pour on boiling water until it is quite thin, stirring briskly till it is smooth, let it boil up once, and remove from the fire; then dissolve a small piece of glue, $^1/_2$ ounce to a gallon of starch in boiling water, and add it to the starch just before removing it from the fire.

PASTILS:

Dry compounds for perfuming or correcting the breath.

(1) Extract of liquorice, 3 ounces; oil of cloves, $1^1/_2$ drams; oil of cinnamon, 15 drops; mix and divide into 1 grain pills, and silver them.

(2) Chocolate powder and ground coffee, of each $1^1/_2$ ounces; prepared charcoal, 1 ounce; sugar, 1 ounce; vanilla, (pulverized with the

sugar), 1 ounce; enough mucilage. Make into lozenges of any form, of which 6 or 8 may be used daily to disinfect the breath.

(3) **Bolonga Catechu:** Extract of liquorice, 3 ounces; water, 3 ounces; dissolve by heat in a water bath and add catechu, 1 ounce; gum arabic, 1/2 ounce. Evaporate to the consistence of an extract, and add (in powder) 1/2 dram each mastic, cascarilla(1), charcoal, and orris; remove from the fire and add oil of peppermint, 1/2 dram; essence of ambergris and essence of musk, each 5 drops; roll it flat on an oiled marble slab, and cut into small lozenges. Used by smokers.

(4) Catechu, 7 drams; orris powder, 40 grains; ;sugar, 3 ounces; oil of rosemary, (or of peppermint, cloves or cinnamon), 4 drops. Make as before.

PATENT MEDICINES:

The popular habit of self-doctoring with patent medicines is one of the most peculiar developments of our times. Men form the habit of prescribing for themselves with a distinct formula that, taken in toto, rivals the pharmacopoeia. After too heavy or frequent drinking they dose themselves with aromatic spirits of ammonia or acid phosphate; a tinge of rheumatism sends them to a druggist's for St. Somebody's oil; a tired feeling too prolonged suggests to them a course of tincture of iron; for coughs and colds every one seems to have his own patent remedy, so numerous are they; patent preparations of pepsin, patent after-dinner pills, mineral waters, and a veritable host of compounds, pellets, and draughts are resorted to against dyspepsia. Both sexes victimize themselves with all sorts of powerful sedatives, like choral and sulphonal; and less harmful salts, like bromide of potassium. The craze is more than foolish, it is wicked.

The drugs that are used bring relief only for the time being, and in the end leave the nervous system shattered, if not wrecked. The best nerve-medicines are plenty of sleep, regular habits, a free movement of the bowels, a clear conscience, and a fixed intention to drop business after business hours. The patent medicines that are of most good are those which come from some scientific or expert doctor's prescription. But, as a rule, patent medicines do a world of harm. They do this not because they are all essentially harmful in themselves, but because they prevent the persons who use them from appreciating the causes of their illnesses.

What cures they effect are at the best only temporary. They serve precisely the end that a man gains by tearing off the top of a weed in his garden. The root is left, and the weed reappears. A man who goes to a doctor finds out how and why he is out of order; often the "why" is most important. Without knowing the cause of one's illness it is impossible to treat

(1) An aromatic bitter tonic from the bark of the Croton Eleuteria; when burnt it emits a fragrant smell.

one's self intelligently, to know what to do besides the mere taking of medicine—what to leave off and what to modify. It is not alone necessary to hinder the symptoms of an illness, which is all that patent medicines can do; it is equally desirable to know what it is that is making us sick.

PATTERNS, TO STAMP ON CLOTH:

A very good way to stamp any patterns on muslin, canvas, or paper is to procure from the stationery store a sheet of blue tracing-paper. Place a piece of tracing-paper over the goods on which you want the pattern, now put your pattern on the tracing-paper with the pattern up, and trace every line with a pencil or any thing sharp. Do not move the pattern after you have begun to trace until you have finished, then take up both pattern and paper, and your stamping is completed.

PEACHES, TO DRY:

Let the peaches get mellow enough to be in good eating condition; put them in boiling water for a moment or two, and the skins will come off like a charm; let them be in the water long enough, but no longer.

PEACHES, TO KEEP:

Peaches can be kept several weeks beyond the usual time if carefully gathered when hard, and each peach at once wrapped in thin paper such as is used for keeping oranges, and then packing in stone jars, and storing in a cool, dry place, where the temperature does not rise above 60 degrees.

PEARL WATER FOR THE COMPLEXION:

Castile soap, 1 lb.; water, 1 gallon; dissolve; then add alcohol, 1 quart; oil of rosemary and oil of lavender, each 2 drams; mix well.

PEARS, HINTS ON MARKETING:

Pears, whether early or late, should never remain on the tree until they become mellow. Whenever they have made their growth they should be gathered. It is easy to tell the proper condition by observing the ease with which the stem parts from the tree. If, on taking hold of the pear and lifting it, the stem readily breaks away from the spur to which it is attached, the fruit has received all the nourishment it can get from the tree, and the sooner it is gathered the better.

Pears are sent to market in crates and half-barrels; especially fine specimens are sent in shallow boxes, only deep enough for a single layer of fruit, and each pear is wrapped in thin white paper. Extra specimens of any of the standard kinds will bring enough more to pay for this extra care in packing. The early varieties mature quicker after gathering than the later kinds, but all should reach the market in a firm and hard condition. As with all other fruits, it will pay to carefully assort pears. Make lots, firsts and seconds for market, and thirds for keeping at home, for the pigs, if need be; there is positively no sale for poor pears.

PEARS, TO KEEP:

Summer pears gathered a few days before fully ripe and wrapped in thin paper and kept in a cool place away from the changes of light and air may be kept in good condition for several weeks.

PEAR-TREES, TO PROTECT FROM BLIGHT:

One method of preserving pear-trees from blight is winding a rope of straw around the trunks so as to completely cover them from the ground to the limbs, keeping it on moderately tight through the season. The theory is that the blight is caused by the rays of the hot sun coming in contact with the body of the tree, heating the sap and causing it to dry up and the bark to grow to the wood of the tree.

PEAS, GREEN, TO KEEP:

When full-grown pick and shell; lay them on dishes or tins in a cool oven or before a bright fire; do not heap the peas on the dishes, but merely cover them; stir them frequently and let them dry very gradually. When hard let them cool, then pack in stone jars, cover close, and keep in a very dry place. When required for use soak them for some hours in cold water till they look plump before boiling; they are excellent for soup.

PEAS, TO DRY:

Look the peas over and remove any that are bad, then place them in the sun until they are dried.

PENCIL-MARKS, TO MAKE INDELIBLE:

To fix pencil-marks so they will not rub out, take skimmed milk and dilute with an equal bulk of water. Wash the pencil-marks (whether writing or drawing) with this liquid, using a soft flat camel's-hair brush, and avoiding all rubbing. Place upon a flat board to dry.

PEPPERS, PICKLED:

Cut out the stems of bell-peppers or cut a slit in the side and remove the seeds. Soak them 24 hours in brine strong enough to bear up an egg. Chop cabbage fine, sprinkle salt on it, and let it stand 24 hours. Drain the peppers from the brine, strain the brine from the cabbage through a colander, fill the peppers with cabbage, tie them up, and put in a jar. Pour over them scalding vinegar. Next day scald the vinegar again, and the following day repeat the scalding of the vinegar and pour it over the peppers. Nasturtium pods, tiny cucumbers, and little onions are preferred by some to cabbage for stuffing. Only the very best vinegar should be used.

PERFUMES:

Bouquet de la Rhine: Take 1 ounce of essence of bergamot, 3 drams of English oil of lavender, $\frac{1}{2}$ dram of oil of cloves, $\frac{1}{2}$ dram of aromatic vinegar, 6 grains of musk, and $1\frac{1}{2}$ pints of rectified spirits of wine; distill.

Jockey Club: Spirits of wine, 5 gallons; orange-flower water, 1 gallon; balsam of Peru, 4 ounces; essence of bergamot, 8 ounces; essence of musk, 8 ounces; essence of cloves, 4 ounces; essence of neroli(1), 2 ounces.

Kiss Me Quick: Spirit, 1 gallon; essence of thyme, $\frac{1}{4}$ ounce; essence of orange flowers, 2 ounces; essence of neroli, $\frac{1}{2}$ ounce; attar of roses, 30 drops; essence of jasmine, 1 ounce; essence of balm mint, $\frac{1}{2}$ ounce; petals of roses, 4 ounces; oil of lemon, 20 drops; *calorus aromaticus*, $\frac{1}{2}$ ounce; essence of neroli, $\frac{1}{4}$ ounce; mix and strain.

Upper Ten: Spirits of wine, 4 quarts; essence of cedrat(2), 2 drams; essence of violets, $\frac{1}{4}$ ounce; essence of neroli, $\frac{1}{2}$ ounce; attar of roses, 20 drops; oils bergamot and neroli, each $\frac{1}{2}$ ounce.

Ladies' Own: Spirits of wine, 1 gallon; attar of roses, 20 drops; essence of thyme, $\frac{1}{2}$ ounce; essence of neroli, $\frac{1}{4}$ ounce; essence of vanilla, $\frac{1}{2}$ ounce; essence of bergamot, $\frac{1}{4}$ ounce; orange-flower water, 6 ounces.

PERFUMES, GARDEN:

Simple garden perfumes are charming in linen when put away in trunks or drawers. To handkerchiefs the perfume is more delicate and much more desirable than the stronger odors so freely used. Always preserve the trimmings of rose-geraniums in envelopes for such purposes, and lay in plenty of sweet clover when in blossom.

PERFUMES, TO EXTRACT:

The perfumes of different flowers may be extracted by a very simple process, and without any apparatus. Gather the flowers the perfume of which you desire to obtain with as little stalk as possible, and place them in a jar three parts filled with olive or almond oil. After 24 hours turn them out in a coarse cloth and squeeze all the oil from them. Throw away the old flowers and repeat the process with fresh-gathered flowers 3 or 4 times, according to the strength of the perfume desired. The oil being thoroughly impregnated with the volatile particles of the flowers, is then to be mixed with an equal quantity of pure rectified spirit, and shaken every day for a fortnight. It may then be poured off, when it will be found beautifully scented and fit for use.

(1) Oil distilled from orange flowers.
(2) From a variety of citron tree (Citrus Medica).

PERSPIRATION, TO REMOVE ODOR OF:

The unpleasant odor produced by perspiration is frequently the source of vexation to persons who are subject to it. Nothing is simpler than to remove this odor much more effectually than by the application of such costly unguents and perfumes as are in use. It is only necessary to procure some compound spirits of ammonia and place about 2 table-spoonfuls in a basin of water. Washing the face, hands, and arms with this leaves the skin as clean and sweet as one could wish. The wash is perfectly harmless and very cheap. It is recommended on the authority of an experienced physician.

PERSPIRING FEET:

Persons troubled with feet that perspire or smell offensively may perhaps effect a cure by bathing them every night or oftener in a strong solution of borax. Two or 3 weeks of this treatment will probably be found sufficient.

PERSPIRING HANDS:

The only effective method of preventing excessive perspiration in the hands is to mix club moss in the water when washing them. They should be washed 2 or 3 times a day in tepid water with the club moss, which need only be used fresh every morning.

PHYSICIAN, CHOOSING A:

Select the Physician Early: Choose him, if possible, before he is needed. There is then time for greater care in the selection. There come emergencies in every home. If no selection has then been made the messenger may rush from door to door, seeking help from the first one met. There may then be no time for discrimination, and the practitioner may be one of doubtful excellence. The questions involved may be too important for such hurry.

Select a Physician of Integrity: No amount of medical or surgical skill can compensate for the lack of good morals and a scrupulous conscience. The relation is too intimate and sacred for the admission of any one of doubtful habits or reputation. Shun the physician of bad habits as you would a person bearing the infection of yellow fever or the plague.

Choose a Physician of Clean Lips: No one of impure speech, of reckless or even careless words, or hints bordering on the obscene or immodest or vulgar, should find a place even professionally in any home.

Give Him your Confidence: A good physician will repay in thoroughness and zeal what is awarded him in ready and unmistaken confidence. However strong in his own convictions and rigidly earnest in his professional work, he is sensitive almost to a fault. A word or a look of mistrust disheartens him in his work, while a word or look of unreserved trust becomes an inspiration to an intense zeal for the patient.

Be Considerate of his Time and Rest: His season for sleep and for recreation should be respected. In case of necessity it may be appropriately disturbed, but "before doing it," says a well-known medical writer, "one should think twice." "It is his trade," is a harsh expression and unworthy of considerate and devoted patients. Consider carefully your physician's hours for repose, for meals, and for church, and then care for him as you would have him care for you. Such appreciative care on your part will be reciprocated by him a hundred-fold.

The Physician Should be Reverential: If that profound naturalist, Agassiz, surrounded by his pupils in his laboratory, where the fossils representing the past ages of life, would not enter upon his work without first uncovering his head in silent prayer to God, how should a physician feel on entering the mysterious chamber where disease and health, life and death, time and eternity, are brought into juxtaposition. If we speak of responsibility in connection with other professions, how immeasurably greater is the responsibility connected with the medical profession.

Qualities of a Good Doctor: Here is a very suggestive summary of hints covering the question of choosing a physician. It has the authority of an experienced and able member of the profession. Read and ponder:

- Avoid the mean man, for you may be sure he will be a mean doctor, just as certainly as he would make a mean husband.
- Avoid a dishonest man; he will not be honest with you as your physician. Shun the doctor that you can buy to help you out of a scrape; a good doctor cannot be bought.
- Avoid the untidy, coarse, blundering fellow, though he may bear the parchments of a medical college.
- Avoid the doctor who flatters you, and humors your lusts and appetites.
- Avoid the man who puts on an extra amount of airs; be assured that it is done to cover his ignorance.
- Avoid the empty blow-horn who boasts of his numerous cases, and tells you of his seeing 40 to 50 patients a day, while he spends 2 hours to convince you of the fact. Put him down for a fool.
- To be a doctor one must be a man in the true sense of the word. He should be a moral man, honest in his dealings. He must have good sense or he cannot be a good doctor.

- He should be strictly temperate. No one should trust his life in the hands of an intemperate doctor.
- He must have some mechanical genius, or it is impossible for him to be a good surgeon.
- It is a good sign if he tells you how to keep well.
- It is a good sign if the members of his own family respect him.
- It is a good sign if the children like him.
- It is a good sign if he is neat and handy at making pills and folding powder.
- It is a good sign if he is still a good student, and keeps posted in all the latest improvements known to the profession for alleviating human suffering.

PILES, OR HEMORRHOIDS, OINTMENT FOR:

Take of hog's lard, 4 ounces; camphor, 2 drams; powdered galls, 1 ounce; laudanum, 1/2 ounce. Mix; make an ointment to be applied every night at bed-time.

PILLS:

Strong Purgative: Take of powdered aloes, scammony(1), and gamboge(2), each 15 grains; mix, and add sufficient Venice turpentine to make into a mass, then divide into 12 pills. Dose, 1 or 2 occasionally.

Milder Purgative: Take 4 grains of powdered scammony, the same quantity of compound extract of colocynth(3), and 2 grains of calomel; mix well, and add a few drops of oil of cloves or thin gum-water, to enable the ingredients to combine properly; divide into 2 pills. Dose, 1 or 2 when necessary.

Common Purgative: Take of powdered jalap(4) and compound extract of colocynth, each 4 grains; of calomel, 2 grains; mix as usual, and divide into 2 pills. Dose, 1 or 2 occasionally.

Tonic: Mix 24 grains of extract gentian and the same of green vitriol together, and divide into 12 pills. Dose, 1 or 2 when necessary. Use in debility.

Cough: Mix 1 dram of compound powder of ipecacuanha(5) with 1 scruple of gum ammoniacum and dried squill(6) bulb, and make into a mass with mucilage, then divide into 20 pills. Dose, 1 three times a day.

(1) A climbing Asian plant with thick roots used for medicines.
(2) A gum resin of the Saint Johnwort family used as a cathartic and as a yellow pigment.
(3) From the dried fruits of a vine belonging to the gourd family.
(4) A resin obtained from the dried root of a Mexican vine.
(5) Ipecac, the dried roots of which yield a vomit inducing drug.
(6) Scilla Maritima, increases bronchial mucus membrane secretions; is an expectorant and a diuretic.

Astringent: Mix 16 grains of acetate of lead with 4 grains of opium, and make into a mass with syrup so as to make 8 pills. Dose, from 1 to 2. Use as an astringent in obstinate diarrhea, dysentery, and cholera.

PIP, TO CURE:

This is a troublesome and somewhat fatal complaint to which all domestic poultry are liable; it is also a very common one. Some writers say it is the result of cold; others, that it is prompted by the use of bad water. But, whatever the cause, the disease is easily detected. There is a thickening of the membrane of the tongue, particularly at the tip; also a difficulty in breathing; the beak is frequently held open, the tongue dry, the feathers of the head ruffled, and the bird falls off its food, and, if neglected, dies. The mode of cure which, if put in practice in time, is generally successful, is to remove the thickened membrane from the tongue with the nails of the forefinger and thumb. The process is not difficult, for the membrane is not adhesive.

Then take a lump of butter, mix into it some strong Scotch snuff, and put 2 or 3 pills of this down the fowl's throat. Keep it from cold and damp and it will soon recover. It may perhaps be necessary to repeat the snuff-balls. Some writers recommend a mixture of butter, pepper, garlic, and scraped horse-radish; but we believe the Scotch snuff to be the safest, as it is the most simple.

PITTING, TO PREVENT:

The following treatment has been found very successful in preventing those fearful marks which small-pox and other like diseases so often leave behind: With a camel's-hair brush apply to each spot or pustule on all exposed surfaces of the face and person a little *acetum cantharidis*, or any vesicating fluid. As soon as blistering is evident by the whitening of the skin in the parts subjected to the application, the fluid producing it must be washed off with warm water or very thin arrow-root. The pain of this application is very slight and very transient, the benefit of it immense and permanent.

PLANTS, HOUSE, FERTILIZER FOR:

When plants are in a growing state they may be stimulated by the use of guano water. A small tea-cupful of Peruvian guano dissolved in a pailful of rainwater is strong enough; water the soil with this once, or at most twice a week. The water of ammonia (hartshorn) is about as good.

PLANTS, SPECIMENS FOR PRESERVATION:

The plants you wish to preserve should be gathered when the weather is dry; and after placing the ends in water let them remain in a cool place till the next day. When about to be submitted to the process of drying, place each plant between several sheets of blotting-paper, and iron it with a large smooth heater, pretty strongly warmed, till all the moisture is dissipated. Colors may thus be fixed which otherwise become pale or nearly white. Some plants require more moderate heat than others, and herein consists the nicety of the experiment; but I have generally found that if the iron be not too hot, and is passed rapidly yet carefully over the surface of the blotting-paper, it answers the purpose equally well with plants of almost every variety of hue and thickness.

In compound flowers, with those also of a stubborn and solid form, as the centaurea(1), some little art is required in cutting away the under part, by which means the profile and forms of the flowers will be more distinctly exhibited. This is especially necessary when the method employed by Maj. Velley is adapted, viz., to fix the flowers and fructification down with gum upon the paper previous to ironing, by which means they become almost incorporated with the surface. When this very delicate process is attempted, blotting-paper should be laid under every part excepting the blossoms, in order to prevent staining the white paper. Great care must be taken to keep preserved specimens in a dry place.

PLANTS, TO RE-POT:

Shake the old earth from the plants after they commence to grow in spring, then pot them into smaller pots than those just occupied, as the plants make fresh growth, and fill these pots with roots, re-pot into those of a size larger, and so on until the plants are in their flowering pots. By adopting this plan the plants are supplied with fresh soil from time to time, and not kept growing on from year to year in the same soil, which soon becomes exhausted. The above remarks apply more particularly to such plants as fuchsias, perlargoniums, etc.

PLASTERS, MUSTARD:

By using syrup or molasses for mustard-plasters they will keep soft and flexible, and not dry up and become hard, as when mixed with water. A thin paper or fine cloth should come between the plaster and the skin. The strength of the plaster may be varied by the addition of more or less flour.

PLATE, TO CLEAN:

Hartshorn is one of the best possible ingredients for plate-powder in daily use. It leaves on the silver a deep polish and is less hurtful than any other article. To wash plate carefully first remove all the grease from it, and this can be done with the use of warm water and soap. The water should be as nearly hot as the hand can bear it. Then mix as much hartshorn powder as will be required into a thick paste with cold water.

(1) A plant with funnel shaped scaly leaves and variously colored flowers.

Smear this lightly over the plate with a piece of soft rag and leave it for some little time to dry. When perfectly dry brush it off quite clean with a soft plate-brush and polish the plate with a dry leather. If the plate be very dirty or much tarnished, spirits of wine will be found to answer better than the water for mixing the paste.

POINTER'S BLUFF, GAME OF:

A little girl is blinded carefully with a handkerchief, and a wand or stick is put into her hand. The rest take hands and skip round her. When she waves her wand they stop; she touches the one nearest to her with it, and says, "Who is this?" The little girl touched answers, in a voice as unlike her own as possible, "It is I." If the blindfolded child guesses rightly by the voice who it is the two exchange places. The little girl who is caught then becomes "blind," and the player in the center resigns her wand and joins the circle.

POISON IVY, HOW TO DETECT:

The poison ivy and the innocuous kind differ in one particular, which is too easy of remembrance to be overlooked by any one who is interested enough in the brilliant-hued leaves in autumn to care for gathering them:

The leaves of the former grow in clusters of threes and those of the latter in fives. As some body has suggested in a juvenile story-book, every child should be taught to associate the 5 leaves to the cluster with the fingers on the human hand, and given to understand that when these numbers agree they can be brought into contact with perfect safety.

POLISH:

For Brass Ornaments Inlaid in Wood: If the brass-work is very dull, file it with a small, smooth file; then polish it with a piece of soft felt dipped in Tripoli powder(1) mixed with linseed oil until the desired effect is obtained.

For Boots and Shoes: Mix together 2 pints of the best vinegar and 1 pint of water; stir into 1/4 lb. of glue, broken up, 1/2 lb. of logwood chips, 1/4 ounce of isinglass; put the mixture over the fire and let it boil 10 or 15 minutes; then strain the liquid and bottle and cork it.

For Furniture: Fill a pint bottle with equal parts of boiled linseed oil and kerosene oil; shake together well, apply with a soft piece of flannel, rubbing dry with a second piece of flannel. This will remove all scratches and white stains. Burn up the rags when through with them.

(1) A finely divided polishing powder from weathered chert or siliceous limestone.

For Leather: Mix intimately together 3 or 4 lbs. of lamp-black and 1/2 lb. of burned bones with 5 lbs. of syrup. Then gently warm 2 and three-quarter ounces of gutta-percha(1) in an iron or copper kettle until it flows easily; add 10 ounces of olive-oil, and when completely dissolved, 1 ounce of stearine. This solution while still warm is poured into the former and well mixed. Then add 5 ounces of gum senegal dissolved in 1 1/2 lbs. of water, and 1/2 ounce of lavender or other oils to flavor it. For use it is diluted with 3 or 4 parts of water. It gives a fine polish, is free from acid, and the glycerine keeps the leather soft and pliable.

For Woods: Mahogany, walnut, and some other woods may be polished by the use of the following mixture: Dissolve by heat so much beeswax in spirits of turpentine that the mixture, when cold, shall be of about the thickness of honey. This may be applied to furniture or to work running in the lathe by means of a piece of clean cloth, and as much as possible should be rubbed off by using a clean flannel or other cloth.

For Mahogany: *Ingredients:* 1/4 lb. of beeswax, 1 ounce of colophony(2), 2 ounces of oil of turpentine.

Cut the wax into thin pieces, pound the colophony, and melt them together in a pipkin; then warm the oil of turpentine and stir it gradually into the pipkin. When thoroughly mixed the polish may be put into a jar and tied over till required. It should be well rubbed into the mahogany by means of a smooth piece of woolen cloth. This is an excellent polish for general furniture.

For Stoves: If stove-polish is mixed with very strong soap-suds the luster appears immediately, and the dust of the polish does not fly around as it usually does.

For Patent-Leather Goods: Take 1/2 lb. of molasses or sugar, 1 ounce of gum arabic, and 2 lbs. of ivory black; boil them well together, then let the vessel stand until quite cooled and the contents are settled, after which bottle off. This is an excellent reviver, and may be used as a blacking in the ordinary way, no brushes for polishing being required.

POLISH, STARCH:

White wax, 1 ounce; spermaceti, 2 ounces; melt them together with a gentle heat. When you have prepared a sufficient amount of starch in the usual way for a dozen pieces put into it a piece of the polish about the size of a large pea, more or less, according to large or small washings. Thick

(1) A rubber-like gum from trees of the sapodilla family.
(2) The resinous substance remaining after turpentine has been heated, removing water & volitile oils.

gum solution, (made by pouring boiling water upon gum arabic), 1 teaspoonful to a pint of starch, also gives clothes a beautiful gloss.

POLISHING POWDER FOR GOLD AND SILVER:

Rock alum burned and finely powdered, 5 parts; levigated chalk, 1 part; mix; apply with a dry brush.

POLISHING TORTOISE-SHELL:

Rub the tortoise shell with a linen rag dipped in rouge powder; afterward polish with the hand. Tortoise-shell combs should always be rubbed with the hand after they are removed from the hair; they will not then lose their polish.

POPE JOAN, GAME OF:

Pope, a game somewhat similar to that of matrimony, is played by a number of people, who generally use a board painted for this purpose, which may be purchased at most turners' or toy-shops. The eight of diamonds must first be taken from the pack, and after settling the deal, shuffling, etc., the dealer dresses the board by putting fish-counters or other stakes, 1 each to ace, king, queen, knave, and the game; 2 to matrimony, 2 to intrigue, and 6 to the nine of diamonds, styled pope. This dressing is, in some companies, at the individual expense of the dealer, though in others the players contribute 2 stakes apiece toward the same.

The cards are next to be dealt round equally to every player, 1 turned up for the trump, and about 6 or 8 left in the stock to form stops; as, for example, if the ten of spades be turned up the nine consequently becomes a stop; the 4 kings and the seven of diamonds are always fixed stops, and the dealer is the only person permitted in the course of the game to refer to the stock for information as to what other cards are stops in their respective deals. If either ace, king, queen, or knave happen to be the turned-up trump, the dealer may take whatever is deposited on that head; but when pope be turned up the dealer is entitled both to that and the game, besides a stake for every card dealt to each player.

Unless the game be determined by pope being turned up, the oldest hand must begin by playing out as many cards as possible; first the stops, then pope, if he has it, and afterward the lowest card of his longest suit, particularly an ace, for that never can be led through; the other players are to follow, when they can, in sequence of the same suit till a stop occurs, and the party having the stop thereby becomes eldest hand and is to lead accordingly; and so on until some person part with all his cards, by which he wins the pool, (game), and becomes entitled besides to a stake for every card not played by the others, except from any one holding pope, which excuses him from paying; but if pope has been played, then the party having held it is not excused.

King and queen form what is denominated matrimony, queen and knave make intrigue when in the same hand; but neither these, no ace, king, queen, knave, nor pope, entitle the holder to the stakes deposited thereon unless played out, and no claim can be allowed after the board be dressed for the succeeding deal, but in all such cases the stakes are to remain for future determination. This game only requires a little attention to recollect what stops have been made in the course of the play; as, for instance, if a player begin by laying down the eight of clubs, then the seven in another hand forms a stop, whenever that suit be led for any lower card; or the elder, when eldest, may safely lay it down in order to clear his hand.

PORCELAIN, TO CLEAN:

Porcelain or chinaware stained with iron can be cleaned with muriatic acid, but it must not be used on marble, as it dissolves it with great rapidity and the polish is lost.

Oxalic acid is purchased in white crystals, and for use a saturated solution is made. As one part of it dissolves only in several parts of water, it is well to keep an excess of crystals in the bottle. It is poisonous and should not be left about in solid form within reach of careless people. A small bottle of the liquid can, however, be kept with other laundry articles.

This acid is particularly useful in removing shoe-leather stains from white stockings. It will also remove most fruit stains on napkins and from the fingers after preserving; for the latter purpose tartaric acid is also good. Oxalic acid is invaluable to the housekeeper as a means of removing black iron-stains. It is more powerful than acetic acid, and must be carefully rinsed from the cloth in water and then in water with a little ammonia in it. Oxalic acid is very efficient in cleaning brass, and it is even softer to use than the acetic, as the compound of the latter with copper salts is one of the most dangerous of the copper compounds.

Sulphurous acid gas is obtained by burning sulphur, and is the well-known agent for bleaching. It will remove spots which nothing else will touch. The cloth or substance should be moistened and held over a bit of burning sulphur; as the agent is an acid, the same precautions must be obtained as in the case of the other acid as to the removal of the corrosive substance.

PORTABLE VAPOR BATH:

Make a small circular boiler of copper or tin and fit the same into an upright tin stand, in which, directly under the boiler, leave an aperture to contain a small spirit lamp. The boiler lid must fit tightly and be provided with 3 small tubes pointing upward. The boiler being filled with water and the lamp lighted, as soon as the steam gets up it rushes through these tubes, and the patient, seated on a cane chair, with his or her feet in a pan of warm water, with a suitable cloak tightly fastened around the neck, is speedily enveloped in a cloud of steam.

Ten minutes is the time for the duration of the first few baths. It may be afterward increased, but not beyond half an hour. In getting out of the cloak plunge into a cool bath for a few minutes, then rub the skin till it is quite dry and glowing with a coarse towel and a pair of good hair gloves. Persons in health or disease will experience a wonderful recuperative power in the frequent use of this bath, and all will find it incomparably superior to the use of drugs in any form whatever.

POSTS, TO PRESERVE:

Experience proves that wood which is exposed to the action of water or put into the ground should first be subjected to charring, and then, before it has entirely cooled, be treated with tar until the wood is impregnated in the most thorough manner. Proceeding in this manner the acetic acid and the oils contained in the tar are evaporated by the heat and only the resin left behind, which penetrates the pores of the wood and forms an air-tight and waterproof envelope, It is found important that the posts be impregnated somewhat above the line of exposure, as it is here that the action of decay affects the wood first.

POTATOES, TO DRY:

The potatoes are to be washed clean, placed in trays, and thrust into a steam box. At the end of 35 minutes they are removed and the skins stripped off by hand. Great care is necessary that the potatoes are not too much cooked, or they are worthless for drying. After peeling they are placed in a press with a tight-fitting plunger and a perforated bottom, and pressed through upon trays, which move on a tramway so as to secure an equal distribution. They are then ready for the dryer, and after being dried hard are placed in a grinder and coarsely pulverized. They can then be cooked in 15 minutes in a little boiling water.

POTATOES, TO KEEP:

A cave dug in the side of a hill, or a pit in a sand-bank, affords an excellent place for storing potatoes. If piled on top of the ground and covered with straw and earth, care should be taken not to leave them exposed to the light. A dark cellar is preferable to a light one for keeping potatoes.

POT-POURRI PERFUME, TO MAKE:

One-half pound of common salt, $^1/_4$ lb. of saltpeter, $^1/_4$ ounce of storax, 6 cloves, a handful of dried bay-leaves, a handful of dried lavender-flowers. Mix these well together to form the basis of the pot-pourri. It will last for years. Rose-leaves and the leaves of any other fragrant flowers gathered on dry days may be added from time to time. If approved, powdered benzoin, chips of sandal-wood, cinnamon, orris-root—indeed, any aromatic plant dried—may be mixed in.

OTTERY, TO DECORATE:

In this work, wood, glass, or tin can be used, and two or more articles of different material may be cemented with white paint prepared as follows:

Mix two-thirds of No. 1 coach varnish and one-third Japan dryer; use paints to color; if desired to paint brown, pour a little of the above in a dish and mix in with a paint-brush burnt umber to give the right shade; do not get it too thick; for scarlet use a little of the best vermilion by mixing what you need in another dish; decorate with embossed pictures or any fancy pictures, gilt bands, etc.; then varnish with the prepared varnish, clear, not too thick.

If light tints are desired, procure white zinc ground in varnish, and for pale pink mix a very little vermilion in some of the zinc; pale blue, use ultra-marine blue; pale green, use some of the zinc; use chrome green, or Paris green will do; mix these colors for pale tints with the white zinc, and always finish with a coat of demar varnish.

OULTICES AND THEIR APPLICATION:

The use of poultices is to promote warmth and moisture, hence those which keep warm and moist the longer are the best. They are employed in the treatment of abscesses, suppurating wounds, inflammation, and pain. In making them the attendant should have them smooth, light, and as hot as they can be made without burning in their application.

(1) *Bread Poultice:* Cold, light wheat bread soaked in sweet milk makes a good one.

(2) *Beet Poultice:* A beet fresh from the garden and pounded fine makes an excellent poultice.

(3) *Linseed Meal Poultice:* In preparing this the basin should be scalded in which it is made. Pour in boiling water, according to the size of the poultice required. Add gradually sufficient linseed meal to form a thick paste, stirring it one way until it is of the proper consistency and smoothness; then spread it on linen or muslin and apply it.

(4) *Charcoal Poultice:* Take 2 ounces of bread in crumbs, soak for 10 minutes in boiling water—say 10 ounces; then mix and add gradually 1/2 ounce of pulverized charcoal and 1/2 ounce of linseed meal, well stirred together; spread as above and apply.

(5) *Chlorinated Soda Poultice*: Made like linseed meal poultice; consisting of 2 parts of linseed meal poultice to 1 of chlorinated soda, mixed with boiling water.

(6) *Yeast Poultice:* Made by mixing 1 lb. of flour or linseed meal with 1/2 pint of yeast; heat and stir it carefully. All poultices are made with boiling water, except yeast, and with this the temperature should not be over 100 degrees.

(7) *Mustard Poultice:* Take a sufficient quantity of powdered mustard to make a thin paste of the required size. It should be mixed with boiling water, with a small quantity of vinegar added, if a very strong poultice is required. Spread it on brown paper or linen, with a piece of thin muslin over it. It should be kept on from 10 to 20 minutes. If the skin is very irritable afterward, a little flour should be sprinkled over it. By mixing the mustard with the white of an egg the poultice will not cause a blister.

POULTRY RAISING:

In raising poultry or stock of any kind it should be the aim of every one to keep it healthy and improve it. You can do it very easily by adapting some systematic rules. These may be summed up in brief as follows:

(1) Construct your house good and warm, avoid damp floors, and afford a flood of sunlight. Sunshine is better than medicine.

(2) Provide a dusting and scratching place where you can bury wheat and corn, and thus induce the fowls to take the needful exercise.

(3) Provide yourself with some good, healthy chickens, none to be over 3 or 4 yrs. old, giving 1 cock to every 12 hens.

(4) Give plenty of fresh air at all times, especially in summer.

(5) Give plenty of fresh air daily and never allow the fowls to go thirsty.

(6) Feed them systematically 2 or 3 times a day; scatter the food so they can't eat too fast or without proper exercise. Do not feed more than they will eat up clean, or they will get tired of that kind of food.

(7) Give them a variety of both dry and cooked feed; a mixture of cooked meat and vegetables is an excellent thing for their morning meal.

(8) Give soft feed in the morning and the whole grain at night, with a little wheat or cracked corn placed in the scratching-places to give them exercise during the day.

(9) Above all things keep the hen-house clean and well ventilated.

(10) Do not crowd too many in one house. If you do, look out for disease.

(11) Use carbolic powder occasionally in the dusting bins to destroy lice.

(12) Wash your roosts and bottom of laying nests, and whitewash once a week in summer and once a month in winter.

(13) Let the old and young have as large a range as possible—the larger the better.

(14) Don't breed too many kinds of fowls at the same time unless you are going into the business. Three or 4 will give you your hands full.

(15) Introduce new blood into your stock every year or so by either buying a cockerel or sittings of eggs from some reliable breeder.

(16) In buying birds or eggs go to some reliable breeder who has his reputation at stake.

(17) Save the best birds for next year's breeding, and send the others to market. In shipping fancy poultry to market send it dressed.

(18) For very young chicks we make the clabbered milk into "Dutch cheese," and use the whey to mix feed for older fowls and chickens. From the time they are a week old till sent to market for broilers our early chicks have all the milk, sweet or sour, or butter-milk, that they can drink. If the home supply of milk falls short of the demand we buy skim-milk at 2 cents a quart, and consider it cheap at that.

(19) For laying hens in winter there is nothing better than a liberal supply of milk. A pan of warm milk with a dash of pepper in it every morning will do more toward inducing hens to lay in cold weather than all the egg-food in creation.

(20) For fattening fowls we find that boiled vegetables mixed with milk and barley or corn-meal will put on flesh at an astonishing rate.

(21) The best way to prevent or cure gapes in chickens is to commence feeding them whole grains of corn as soon as they are old enough to swallow them—say 2 or 3 weeks old. The effort made by the chick to swallow the whole grain will kill the little red worms in the throat which are the cause of the gapes, and it is easier and safer to kill the worms in that way than to attempt to take them from the throat with a bent horse-hair, as is sometimes done.

(22) Sunflower seeds fed in small quantities impart a fine glow to the plumage of poultry.

(23) A good way to make a cheap and simple chicken nest is to take a common box about 2 ft. high, 1 ft. wide, and 1 ft. deep; have the back to work on hinges, for which 2 strips of leather will do; nail on to the front a board half the height of the box, put 2 screw-eyes in the top to hang it up.

(24) If one has several broods of chickens they ought to have the shelter of some glass roofing. They need not be confined under the glass all the time, but should have easy access to outdoor exercise if it is not too cold. A small building or shed after the style of a greenhouse will be found very convenient and useful in rearing early broods.

(25) The nest of a setting hen should be nearly flat at the bottom, so that the eggs will move easily when the hen puts her feet among them. If too rounding, the eggs will crowd together, and when the biddy puts her foot down with the characteristic force of her sex something has to give way, and usually it is the shells of the eggs.

(26) The coops for young broods should have broad bottoms and these should be separated from the coop. On clear days let the hen and her brood out, turn up the coop, clean off the bottom thoroughly, let it dry, and sprinkle on a layer of dry earth.

(27) A lath fence made in sections of 8 ft. and wired to light posts makes a good temporary fence for a poultry yard. It is cheap and will last for several years. It will confine the heavier breeds.

(28) Feed setting hens on corn. It digests slowly, is of an oily and heating nature, and much better than any other food for the purpose.

(29) Little chickens need no feed until they are 24 hours old. Some of the brood may be late in hatching. In this case take the older ones and feed them by themselves. When all are hatched, and when they have been dried and vitalized by the hen, remove to a nice, roomy, clean, warm coop. Feed the hen as much corn as she wants to eat and give her water. Feed the little things some bread-crumbs and corn-meal, or crushed wheat slightly moistened with sweet milk. Coarsely ground or broken corn scalded is a good food for the broods. The morning feed should always be warm. Feed the little things apart from the hen, or she will get more than her share. Give but little water. Keep the hen in the coop and allow the chicks to run about in its vicinity. When they get cold they will return to be hovered and warmed. Keep things clean and neat in and about the coop, and close it up carefully every night. Visit it early in the morning with a nice warm breakfast for the chickens, though care and regularity are necessary to success.

(30) The best remedy for gapes ever tried is caustic lime in a dry, powdered state. It may be either air or water slaked. Hold the chicken in the left hand, open its mouth by the thumb and forefinger, and with the other hand drop a pinch of lime into it. Hold in this position a few seconds, until it is obliged to breathe, when it will inhale some of the lime; then let it go. One application of the lime in this manner has cured every case of the gapes, some of them in the last stages.

(31) Old nails, etc., laid in the drinking-fountain will do no harm, but sometimes good, as iron is a tonic for poultry. Old rusty iron may not dissolve in water, but if the rust is fine and mingles with the water,

iron is sometimes taken into the system that way. A solution of copperas, however, is better, as copperas is sulphate of iron.

POWDERS:

Compound Soda: Mix 1 dram of calomel, 5 drams of sesquicarbonate of soda, and 10 drams of compound chalk powder together. Dose, 5 grains. Use as a mild purgative for children during teething.

Tonic: Mix 1 dram of powdered rhubarb with the same quantity of dried carbonate of soda, then add 2 drams of powdered calumba root. Dose, from 10 to 20 grains as a tonic after fevers, in all cases of debility, and dyspepsia attended with acidity.

Rhubarb and Magnesia: Mix 1 dram of powdered rhubarb with 2 drams of carbonate of magnesia and 1/2 dram of ginger. Dose, from 15 grains to 1 dram. Use as a purgative for children.

Sulphur and Potash: Mix 1 dram of sulphur with 4 scruples of niter. Dose, from 1/2 dram to 1 dram. Use as a purgative, diuretic, and refrigerant.

Anti-diarrheal: Mix 1 grain of powdered ipecacuanha and 1 grain of powdered opium with the same quantity of camphor. Dose, 1 of these powders to be given in jam, treacle, etc., 5 or 6 times a day if necessary.

Antispasmodic: Mix 4 grains of subnitrate of bismuth, 48 grains of carbonate of magnesia, and the same quantity of white sugar, and then divide in 4 equal parts. Dose, one fourth part. Use in obstinate pain in the stomach; with cramps unattended by inflammation.

Antipertussal, or against Whooping-cough: Mix 1 dram of powdered belladonna root and 5 drams of white sugar together. Dose, 6 grains morning and evening for children under 1 yr., 12 grains for those under 2 and 3 yrs. of age, 24 grains for those between 5 and 10, and 48 grains for adults.

Caution: This should be prepared by a chemist, as the belladonna is a poison, and occasional doses of castor oil should be given while it is being taken.

Purgative, (common): Mix 10 grains of calomel with 1 dram of powdered jalap and 20 grains of sugar. Dose, 50 grains for adults.

Sudorific: Mix 6 grains of compound antimonial powder and 2 grains of sugar together. Dose, as mixed, to be taken at bed-time. Use in catarrh and fever.

PRINTS, TO TAKE IMPRESSIONS FROM:

The print is soaked first in a solution of potash, and then in one of tartaric acid. This produces a perfect diffusion of crystals in bi-tartrate of potash, through the texture of the unprinted part of the paper. As this salt repels the oil, the ink-roller may now be passed over the surface without transferring any of its contents to the paper, except in those parts to which the ink has been originally applied. The ink of the print prevents the saline matter from penetrating wherever it is present, and wherever there is no saline matter present the ink adheres; so that many impressions may be taken, as in lithography.

PRUNES, TO DRY:

Prunes are mostly imported from France, where several varieties are raised especially for drying, among which are German prune, St. Catherine, Brignolles, and others. The fruit is not gathered until the sun has dried off the dew; it is then picked by hand and spread in shallow baskets, which are kept in a cool and dry place. When they have become soft they are shut up close in spent ovens and left for 24 hours; they are then taken out and replaced after the ovens have been slightly re-heated. On the next day they are taken out and turned by slightly shaking the sieves on which they have been laid; the ovens are heated again, and they are put in a third time. After remaining 24 hours they are taken out and left to get quite cold; after some manipulations they are submitted to oven heat twice more, and then packed in boxes and jars for sale.

PUMPKINS, TO DRY:

Take ripe pumpkins, pare, cut into small pieces, stew soft, mash, and strain through a colander, as if for making pies; spread this pulp on plates in layers about 1/2 in. thick; dry it in a stove oven, which should be kept at so low a temperature as not to scorch it; in about a day it will become dry and crisp. The sheets thus made can be stowed away in a dry place and are always ready for use, either for pies or stewing. The quick drying after cooking prevents the souring, which is almost always the case when the uncooked pieces are dried, while the flavor is much better preserved.

Q

QUINSY(1), OR ULCERATED SORE THROAT:

Those who suffer from these distressing maladies will find relief from an onion poultice made as follows:

Bake or roast till quite soft 3 or 4 large onions, peel them quickly, and beat them quite flat with a rolling-pin; put them into a muslin bag that

(1) Inflammatory sore throat.

will reach from ear to ear and about 3 in. deep. Apply this bag to the throat as hot as possible. Keep it on night and day, using fresh ones as the strength of the onions becomes exhausted. The throat must be protected from cold when the poultices are removed.

QUINSY, RELIEF FOR:

(1) A tea-cupful of red sage leaves to 1 quart of water, boil 10 minutes, add 4 table-spoonfuls of vinegar, and sweeten with honey. In the first stage of the disease it might be used as a gargle, and then to rinse the mouth; it should be used warm. It will be found invaluable.

(2) Tar spread on the throat and quite up under the ears. Cover with a cloth and go to sleep and wake up well. Only a brown stain will remain, which is easily washed off with castile soap. It is a sure relief. It is our opinion that in cases of insipient scarlet fever or diphtheria this is the remedy. It looks reasonable if it brings sure relief in quinsy which it does.

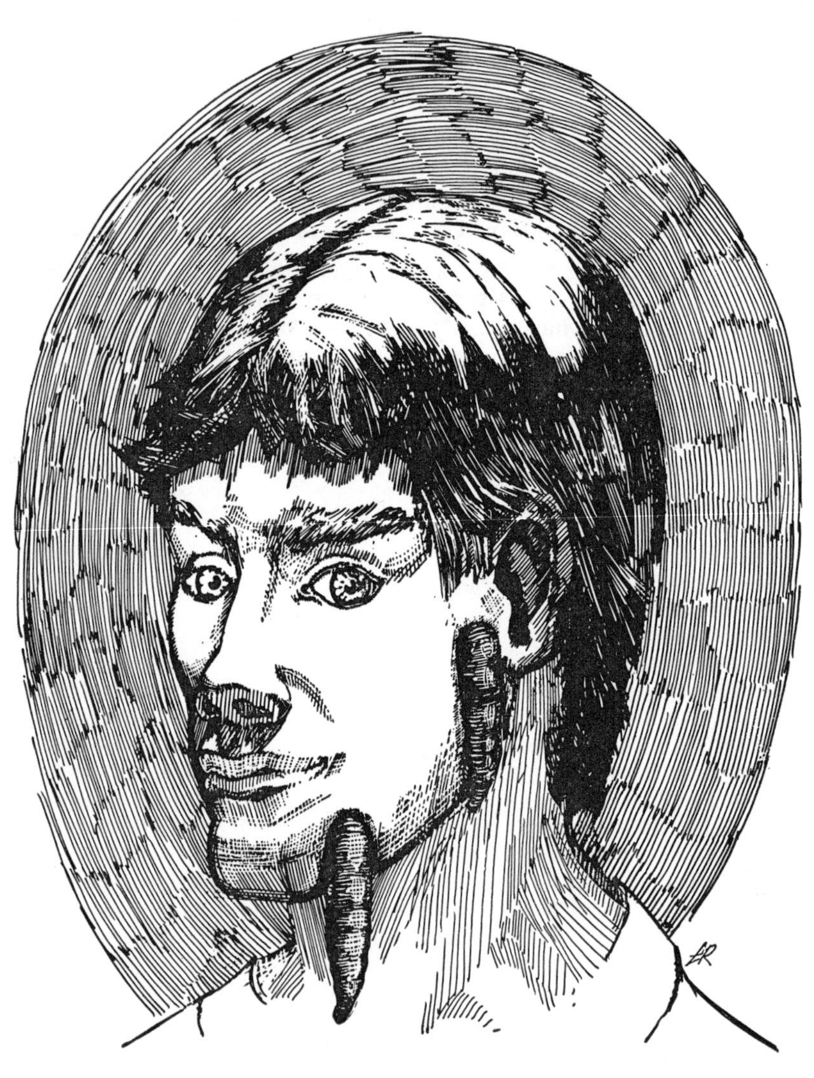

• *Use of Leeches* •

R

RABBITS, CARE AND MANAGEMENT:

The principal thing is always to give more dry than succulent food; weeds and refuse vegetation should be banished, except the roots and leaves of dandelion, sow-thistle, and hog-weed. The most nutritious food is the tops of carrots and parsnips, cabbages, parsley, fine grass, clover, tares, coleworts, and the tops of furze plant, cut up with their dry food. The grains proper for rabbits are oats, peas, wheat, or buckwheat; to these may be added bran, dry clover, pea and bean straw. Rabbits, full grown, which have as much corn as they will eat, never take harm from an abundant supply of vegetable food; but to young rabbits especially very little vegetable food should be given. The greater the impossibility to change the green food, the more necessary to season it. Parsley, fennel, coriander, aniseed, peppermint, bitter chicory, wild thyme, pimpernel, etc., should be mixed twice a week with other green food. Salt as a seasoning mixed with meal once or twice a week.

Rabbits should be fed at daybreak, and from 11 in the morning till 1 in the afternoon, and 1 hour before sunset. The best food for fattening is barley meal, oatmeal, soaked gray peas, and boiled linseed, mixed with meal; but they must be varied. A large quantity of green food is not advisable. Dandelions, thistles, or any plant of the same family are good, but when not to be had give a little water once a day, or a little milk sweetened with sugar. Much exercise is not good for them at this time; but if placed for a few hours a day in fine weather on dry, gravelly ground, and given a little green food, it will promote health.

In selecting for fattening, young males should be sacrificed before the females; they become amorous sooner, and their flesh loses flavor. The rabbit-house should stand upon a dry foundation, and be well ventilated. A spare loft will be a good place. If rabbits are to be kept in a place already built, fill all crevices with pieces of brick and cement; then mix 1 part cement with 2 parts of fine sand and water, till thick like cream; spread on the floor 1½ in. thick. This should be done quickly, for cement dries rapidly, and become as hard as stone, through which vermin cannot penetrate. The sides of the building that have been stopped should be plastered with the same, but thicker than for the floor. Where tiles, stones, or bricks are used for paving see that joints are well filled with cement to avoid filtration of urine under the pavement.

RAG-BAG:

An ornamental rag-bag is thus made: Take an ordinary towel with fringe and a broad red border, cut it in half, sew the edges to pieces of Turkey red the same width and about 20 in. long. The Turkey red should be turned in about 5 in. and a double hem run in it, through which a drawing-string of white tape must be run. On the towel should be sketched in bold letters the word "Rags," which should be worked over with coarse red cotton in vine-stitch. If the lines are worked with 2 lines side by side, it makes the word stand out more boldly from its white background. The fringe of the towel makes a pretty finish to the bottom of the bag.

RANGE, CARE OF THE:

One of the first accomplishments to be mastered by the woman who wishes to become thoroughly conversant with the ins and outs of her kitchen is the making of a range fire. This is one of the tasks that it is popularly supposed may be performed by any body, a faith that is often followed by confusion when the experiment is attempted. The condition of the stove itself is one of the first things to be looked to. Time is wasted in an endeavor to build a hot fire on a substratum of cold ashes and clinkers. The grate must first be cleaned out, and the ash-pan withdrawn, emptied, and replaced. Careless or lazy cooks sometimes neglect to return the pan, permitting instead the hot coals and ashes to fall on the floor of the stove, thus in time seriously injuring it. The stove should be cleaned before the fire is built, the ashes brushed off the top, and the range blacked.

RASHES, HOW TO DISTINGUISH:

Measles appears as a number of dull red spots, in many places running into each other, and is usually first seen about the face and on the forehead, near the roots of the hair, and is often preceded by running of the eyes and nose, and all the signs of a severe cold. Scarlet fever appears first about the neck and chest, but not unfrequently at the bend of the elbow or under the knee, and is usually preceded by a sore throat. It can be distinguished from roseola, a mild disease which is sometimes mistaken for it, by the bright red color of the skin, which appears not unlike a boiled lobster. In chicken-pox the symptom is attended by fever, the spots are small, separate pimples, and come out generally over the whole body.

RASPBERRIES, TO DRY:

Black raspberries and blackberries are dried whole, and care must be taken that they be unbroken; dried red raspberries never sell well.

RATS AND MICE:

(1) When rats refuse to nibble at toasted cheese and the usual baits a few

drops of the highly scented oil of rhodium poured on the bottom of a cage top will always attract them.

(2) Strew pounded potash in their holes. The potash gets into their coats and irritates their skins, and the rats desert the place.

(3) Mix corn-meal or wheat flour with plaster of Paris or carbonate of baryta(1). This forms a hard cake in the rat's stomach and kills. Be careful to keep it out of the reach of children.

(4) Gather any kind of mint and scatter it about the shelves, and they will forsake the premises.

(5) A tincture of Calabar bean is exceedingly efficacious in preserving entomological and other natural history specimens from destruction caused by mice.

(6) Place a quantity of red pepper in cotton and stuff the wad into the holes.

(7) Sprinkle a little calomel on buttered bread and place where the rats can get it, putting a dish of water close by. This does not kill them, but makes them soon disappear.

(8) Once ounce arsenic, 1 ounce lard; mix into a paste with meal, and put about the haunts of the rats. They will eat this greedily. Rat-poisons are objectionable because the rats are apt to die in their holes.

Destruction of Rats: *The following recipe for the destruction of rats has been communicated by Dr. Ure to the council of the English Agricultural Society, and is highly recommended as the best means of getting rid of these most obnoxious and destructive vermin. It has been tried by several intelligent persons, and found perfectly effectual:*

Melt hog's lard in a bottle plunged in water, heated to about 150 degrees Fahr.; introduce into it 1/2 ounce of phosphorous for every pound of lard; then add a pint of proof-spirit of whisky; cork the bottle firmly after its contents have been heated to 150 degrees, taking it at the same time out of the water, and agitate smartly till the phosphorous becomes uniformly diffused, forming a milky-looking liquid. This liquid being cooled, will afford a white compound of phosphorous and lard, from which the spirit spontaneously separates, and may be poured off to be used again, for none of it enters into the combination, but merely serves to comminute the phosphorous, and diffuse it in very fine particles through the lard. This compound, on being warmed very gently, may be poured out into a mixture of wheat flour and sugar, incorporated there-with, and then flavored with oil

(1) A mineral called witherite.

of rhodium, or not, as pleasure. The flavor may be varied with oil of aniseed, etc. This dough, being made into pellets, is to be laid in rat-holes. By its luminousness in the dark it attracts their notice.

RAZOR, CARE OF:

A razor should be strapped before and immediately after using, and will thus be kept in good order for years without any need for the stone. When a razor has lost its edge or become jagged by neglect it may be restored on a hone oiled with kerosene oil; but without the greatest care the edge will be wired and spoiled. A strap of common leather glued to a suitable strip of wood is all that is usually necessary. The practice of pressing on the edge of a razor in strapping generally rounds; the pressure should be directed to the back, which must never be raised from the strap. If you shave from heel to point of the razor, strap it from point to heel; but if you begin with the point, then strap from heel to point. If you only once put away your razor without strapping or otherwise cleansing the edge you must no longer expect to shave well; the soap and damp will soon rust the fine teeth or edge. A piece of plate leather should always be kept with the razors. As you strap your razor, strap the two sides alternately, and keep the back of the razor always on the strap as you turn it from side to side. You thus avoid cutting your strap and turning the edge of your razor.

Razor-strop, to Renovate:

(1) Rub clean tallow over the surface, and then put on it the light top part of the snuff or a dandle and rub it smooth.

(2) Rub well with a piece of soft pewter or lead.

Razor-strop, to Make: Select a piece of satin, maple, or rosewood, 12 in. long, 1 three-quarters in. wide, and three-eights in. thick; allow 3 1/2 in. for length of handle; 1/2 in. from where the handle begins, notch out the thickness of the leather so as to make it flush toward the end; taper the thickness of the leather; this precaution prevents the case from tearing up the leather in putting the strop in; round the wood just enough to keep from cutting by the razor in stropping and turning over the same; now select a proper-sized piece of fine French book-binder's calfskin cover with good wheat or rye paste, then lay the edge in the notch, and secure in place with a small vise; proceed to rub it down firmly and as solidly as possible with a tooth-brush handle, and after the whole is thoroughly dry trim and make the case.

Paste for Sharpening Razors: Take prepared putty, 1 ounce; saturated solution of oxalic acid enough to make a paste; this composition is to be rubbed over the strop, and when dry a little water may be added. The acid having a great attachment for iron, a little friction with this powder gives a fine edge to the razor.

RECEPTIONS:

The practice is to give 1 to 4 receptions during the season. Cards are issued for them, stating the hours, which are usually from 6 P.M. until 11 P.M. It is understood that full dress is not required, and many ladies go attired in dinner or street costume. It is usually supposed in the height of the season that ladies have 2 or 3 invitations for each evening, so that those who attend receptions may leave with propriety after an hour. The hostess receives in the main drawing-room, from whence the guests pass to a refreshment-room, where a table is usually served with salads, oysters, and claret punch; coffee and small cakes are considered necessary.

RED SPIDER:

It is scarcely visible to the naked eye, has 8 legs, its color changes from yellowish to brown and reddish, and on each side of the back is a blackish spot. In the open air it usually attacks kidney-beans. Among trees the young limes mostly suffer, and the mites are found in thousands on the under side of the leaves. These leaves assume a dirty-yellowish or brownish appearance, and in the middle of summer the trees acquire an autumnal hue.

(1) Frequently sprinkling the plants with cold water has been found efficient as a means of destroying these insects.

(2) Repeatedly fumigating the hot-houses with strong tobacco-smoke injures them in some degree.

(3) A tea-spoonful of salt in 1 gallon of water; sprinkle with this; in a few days wash the plant with pure water.

REST, THE GOSPEL OF:

There are plenty of men who work seven days in the week, and during a long life, but if work requires intense and trying application regard rest as of equal importance with labor. Of the smaller habits of leisure, the first to be considered comes after each meal. Men have their lunch brought in to them, and turn to work the moment it is finished. Perhaps they do not even stop working while eating. That is very bad. Man is like the horse; he must have a bait in the middle of the day and a little let-up, if he is to drive through the whole of it. It will pay in the end. Vacations must be taken when needed. It is like burning both ends of the candle to try to do without them.

RETCHING, TO STOP:

Take half a wine-glassful of pure lemon-juice, mix with it just sufficient salt of tartar to destroy the acidity. Give a tea-spoonful of this frequently till the retching ceases.

RHEUMATISM, REMEDIES FOR:

(1) In acute rheumatism oil of peppermint in 10 drop doses on sugar every 4 hours will be found very beneficial.

(2) Take cucumbers when full grown and put them into a pot with a little salt; then put the pot over a slow fire, where it should remain for about an hour; then take the cucumbers and press them, the juice from which must be put into bottles, corked up tight, and placed in the cellar, where they should remain for about a week; then wet a flannel rag with the liquid and apply it to the parts affected.

(3) Procure 1 pint of good alcohol; add 1 pint of water; make it sharp by adding red pepper pods of any kind, broken in small pieces. In 24 hours it will be fit for use. Bathe the affected parts well and frequently, warming it in by the stove, the action of the heat being of great benefit.

(4) *When the joints are stiffened with rheumatism or a settled cold the following applications are said to be capital, and enable the sufferer to move with ease:*

Cut into small bits or grate 1 ounce of castile soap; add a heaping table-spoonful of red Cayenne pepper. Have these in a small pitcher, and then pour on to them 1/2 pint of boiling hot water. Stir until all is dissolved, and add a little cider-brandy or alcohol when bottling. An application of the above brings the blood in a glow to the joints, and on rubbing a little sweet-oil to relax the muscles the patient will be enabled to walk with perfect ease.

(5) For inflammatory rheumatism take 1/2 ounce of pulverized saltpeter put in 1/2 pint of sweet-oil; bathe the parts affected, and a sound cure will speedily be effected.

RHUBARB, TO DRY:

The best method is to strip it of its epidermis. This is a long operation, but both time and expense are spared in the end by the promptness and regularity of the drying. Many cultivators of rhubarb on a large scale have repeated the experiment and have met with the most decisive results.

RICKETS AND SCROFULA(1):

If children have either or both of these diseases a good nutritive diet is a great essential. Then the alkaline bath, a little lime-water, say a teaspoonful 3 times a day, and outdoor exercise are the chief remedies.

RICK-RACK, TO MAKE:

Get pointed linen braid and use either linen thread or coarse cotton. Button-hole a stitch into 8 of the points and draw it carefully into a circle,

(1) Swelling of the neck glands.

and then go around again, putting the needle under every thread; draw it into a wheel, and reverse the work for the other side. When you get the first two done arrange so that it will form insertion, and then attach 2 points together and proceed as before.

RING-BONE, CURES FOR:

(1) Pulverized cantharides(1), oils of spike, origanum, amber, cedar, Barbadoes tar, and British oil, of each 2 ounces; oil of wormwood(2), 1 ounce; spirits of turpentine, 4 ounces; common potash, 1/2 ounce, nitric acid, 6 ounces; sulphuric acid, 4 ounces; lard, 3 lbs. Melt the lard and slowly add the acids; stir well and add the other articles, stirring till cold; clip off the hair and apply by rubbing and heating in. In about 3 days, or when it is done running, wash off with soapsuds, and apply again. In old cases it may take 3 or 4 weeks; but in recent cases 2 or 3 applications have cured.

(2) Pulverized cantharides, oils of origanum and amber, and spirits of turpentine, of each 1 ounce; olive-oil, 1/2 ounce; sulphuric acid, 3 drams; put all except the acid into alcohol; stir the mixture, add the acid slowly, and continue to stir until the mixture ceases to smoke; then bottle for use. Apply to ring-bone or spavin with a sponge tied on the end of a stick as long as it is absorbed into the parts.

RINGS, TO REMOVE TIGHT:

To remove tightly fitting rings from a finger without pain (says the London Lancet) pass the end of a portion of rather fine twine underneath the ring, and evenly encircle the finger from below upward (as whip-makers bind lashes on) with the remainder, as far as the center of the finger, then unwind the string from above downward by taking hold of the end passed under the ring, and it will be found that the ring will gradually pass along the twine toward the tip of the finger.

RING-TOSS GAME, HOW TO MAKE:

Most of the apparatus for ring-toss which is bought in the stores is easily broken. The wooden hoops bound about the room, mar furniture, and soon come apart. This game is an excellent one to have about the house to while away an idle hour or entertain a party of friends. Any boy can make a serviceable set of rings with very little trouble, and at a slight expense, if he will follow the example of sailors and make the rings of rope.

A set of rings should consist of at least 6, better 8, of the same or different sizes, according to the taste of the maker. Rings 7 in. in diameter are very satisfactory. In order to make these cut a length of new three-quarter

(1) A preparation of dried beetles, esp. the Spanish-fly or Blister Beelte-fly used externally as a rubefacient and internally as a stimulant.

(2) A bitter tasting dark green oil from a plant of the Composie family.

in. manilla rope into pieces 2 ft. long. These pieces are bent into rings and the ends fastened firmly together. To make these rings perfectly the ends should be spliced. But few boys are salted enough for a feat of this kind, so they must content themselves with untwisting the rope ends and twisting them together the best they can. The joint, when firmly bound with "marine," (tarred twine), will be firm enough for all practical purposes. The rings are heavy and keep their shape well. Sisters may cover the rings with colored flannel, or wind the rings with ribbons, if they wish to add to the beauty of their brother's work.

The peg should be a simple tapering upright of wood set in a piece of plank 1 1/2 ft. square and 2 in. thick. We need hardly describe a game so well known as ring-toss further than to say that the peg is placed in a corner of the room and the players, standing on a certain line at any agreed distance, attempt to throw the rings so that they shall encircle the peg. Ring-toss parties, with simple prizes for those making the best scores, may be made pleasant entertainments for the winter.

RINGWORM:

This appears in circular patches of little pustules, which form scabs, leaving a red pimply surface, and destroying the bulbs of the hair; it spreads rapidly, and is very infectious. It chiefly affects the neck, forehead, and scalp of weakly children, and may sometimes be traced to uncleanness or contact with the disease.

Treatment:

(1) Shave the part and keep it clean with soap and water, at the same time that an occasional mild saline aperient is administered, and a light nutritious diet, of which rare beef and ripe fruits should form a portion, should be rigorously adhered to. When the scabbing commences, use dressings of tar ointment, or of the ointment of nitrate or red oxide of mercury.

(2) The head should be washed twice a day with soft-soap and warm soft water; when dried, the places to be rubbed with a piece of linen rag dipped in ammonia is from gas tar; the patient should take a little sulphur and molasses, or some other gentle aperient, every morning; brushes and combs should be washed every day and the ammonia kept tightly corked.

(3) *When the disease does not come from direct contagion children are generally in a poor state of blood, and good living, sea-air, and tonic medicines are of great benefit. The following application will frequently be found of much service:*

Wash the part affected with a little lemon-juice; then rub in with the finger a little gunpowder which has been bruised in a mortar.

Do this gently about twice a day. Be very careful not to make the skin sore.

ROACHES:

(1) Cut up green cucumbers at night and place them about where roaches commit depredations. What is cut from the cucumbers in preparing them for the table answers the purpose, and 3 applications will destroy all the roaches in the house. Remove the peelings in the morning and renew them at night.

(2) Red lead, 4 ounces; flour, 1 ounce; powdered sugar, 1 ounce; mix the ingredients well; use by placing some on pieces of paper.

(3) Mix finely powdered borax and fine sugar, half and half, and spread around where the roaches are most troublesome. For a few days it may seem that the remedy is doing no good, but soon they will begin to die, and in a short time will disappear.

(4) Mix up a quantity of fresh burned plaster of Paris (gypsum, such as is used for making molds and ornaments) with wheat flour and a little sugar, and distribute on shallow plates and box boards, and place in the corners of the kitchen and pantry where they frequent. In the darkness they will feast themselves on it and die.

(5) Take flour of sulphur, $^1/_2$ lb.; potash, 4 ounces. Melt in an earthen pan over the fire; pulverize, and make a strong solution in water, and sprinkle the places which they frequent.

ROCKERIES(1), VASES, AND HANG-BASKETS:

These can, if properly made, and furnished with suitable, healthy plants, be made very ornamental additions to the lawn and plazza. Artificial rockeries should partake of a natural appearance as much as possible. Ferns, alpine plants, cypress-vines, vincas, lobelia, dwarf stocks, etc., are good plants for these. Vases and hanging-baskets, whatever their design, should be at least 10 or 12 in. in diameter, and 6 in. or more in depth.

Be sure the drainage is good. Glazed pots and those without outlet for water are not good. The soil should not be over-rich, as it forces the growth too much for beauty and gracefulness. Climbing and drooping vines may, however, be stimulated. A good composition is one third "scouring-sand," the rest dark loam and leaf-mold. The fallings around pine-trees are excellent. For the center plant dracena, or achyranthus, or coleus, or centaurea is good. Next to center, begonias of all sorts, pilea, verbenas, petunia, vicas, sedunes. For edges, *oxalis-lobelia*, and various ivies and grasses. Water regularly.

(1) Rocks and soil arranged as a rock garden.

ROOM, HOW TO DUST:

There are two ways of dusting a room. One is to take a feather brush, and, by briskly whisking off the polished surfaces of wood or marble, disperse into the breathing air the entire quantity of dust particles there accumulated. The other is to carefully wipe with a cotton or silken duster or chamois skin the needful articles, and then shake out the cloth either into the open air or into a fire-place in use, where the draught of air would carry the dust up the chimney. It is very hard work in a house where there is furnace heat or soft coal fires to keep the furniture dusted. An old silk handkerchief makes a good duster.

ROPES, TO SOFTEN:

To make a new rope as limber and soft as an old one, boil it 2 hours in water, and then thoroughly dry in a warm room.

ROSE CULTURE:

Situation: A place apart from other flowers should be assigned to them, if possible sheltered from high winds, but open and not surrounded by trees, as closeness is very apt to generate mildew; where they cannot have a place to themselves, any part of the garden best fulfilling these conditions will answer.

Soil: A most important item in their successful culture. That in which they especially delight is a rich, unctuous loam, that feels greasy when pressed between the fingers. Where this is not to be had the soil must be improved; if light, by the addition of loam, or even clay, well worked in; where heavy, good drainage and the addition of coal ashes in small quantities will help it, but in such places draining is most important.

Planting: Mix some loam and well-rooted manure together, open a good-sized hole, and fill it with fresh soil; plant firmly. Shorten any very long shoots, and, if exposed to winds, secure the plant by short stakes.

Manuring: Roses are strong feeders, and will take almost any amount of manure; pig manure is the best, except in hot soils, when cow manure is preferable; stable manure is generally available and good. Exhibitors generally apply a top-dressing in spring, but it does not improve the appearance of the beds; a good top-dressing may be laid on the beds in autumn, and be dug in the spring.

Watering: When coming into bloom, if the weather be dry, give a good drenching 2 or 3 times a week; continue after blooming to prevent mildew. If greater size be required, liquid manure may be used. Syringe daily for green fly.

Pruning: This may be done any time after the beginning of March, according to the season. Cut out all wood over 2 yrs. old and all weakly shoots. Weak growing kinds should be pruned hard—i.e., down to 3 or 4 eyes; stronger growing kinds may be left longer. Cut to an eye that points outward, so as to keep the inside of the plant open. Teas and noisettes require less cutting back; the tops should be shortened and the weak shoots cut out, and they should not be pruned until May. Use a sharp knife.

ROSE INSECTS, TO DESTROY:

There are a number of insects that trouble the rose, and at one time they were so destructive in this country in some localities that the culture of the rose was almost abandoned. The rose slug is the most common of these and feeds upon the leaves just as the buds begin to develop. They are mostly found on the under side of the leaf, and their appearance is known by the leaves becoming brown, as if scorched or burned.

It is said that an ounce of prevention is worth a pound of cure, and if this is so it would be economy to syringe the plants thoroughly with whale-oil soap-suds, made by using a pound of soap to 8 gallons of water, before the insects appear. Commence this as soon as the leaves develop in the spring, and continue to apply it 2 or 3 times a week till the buds begin to open, after which its use will rarely be found necessary. If roses are neglected till the slugs are numerous, dust the foliage effectually in the morning while the dew is on with white hellebore.

There is another insect known as the rose bug or beetle, which is particularly destructive to greenhouse roses. It is most troublesome while in the larva state, when it works upon the roots, though the mature bug feeds upon the leaves. As yet there has been no remedy found for this pest, except to hunt them and destroy them by hand. It is fortunate for the amateur florist, however, that this insect is confined chiefly to the rose-house or greenhouse, and does not materially affect the outdoor growth of roses.

ROSE SCALES:

These live on the stems and old twigs of rose-trees, which are sometimes entirely covered with them, and look moldy. Brush them off with strong brushes before the rose-trees sprout.

ROSE-WATER, HOW TO MAKE:

Whoever possesses plenty of roses can make this perfume at a slight expense. Gather the roses while free from dew, and put them into a 2-gallon glass jar. Then take a 2-ounce bottle and put in the mouth of the jar so that it will fit closely, and cut some pieces of perfectly clean sponge (that has been boiled to free it from sand and grit) into narrow strips, and soak them in the purest olive oil or Lucca oil. Cotton-seed oil will do if free from any odor. The oil must be perfectly sweet and fresh, or it will spoil the perfume. Place the sponge inside the phial, and turn it upside down in the mouth of the jar, and put it in the hottest sunshine for 4 or 5 days. The heat will distill the rose-leaves, and the aroma will rise and saturate the oil in the sponge.

Throw away the leaves when they are dry, and fill the jar again with fresh rose-leaves. Do this as long as the roses last, and when the bits of sponge are thoroughly saturated squeeze out the oil, or you can leave them in the phial and keep it closely corked. A drop or two of this oil will perfume several ounces of alcohol.

ROSE-WATER, METROPOLITAN:

Take 2 lbs. of rose-leaves, place them on a napkin tied round the edges of a basin filled with hot water, and put in a dish of cold water upon the leaves; keep the bottom water hot, and change the water at the top as soon as it begins to get warm. By this kind of distillation you will extract a great quantity of the essential oil of roses by a process which cannot be expensive, and will prove very beneficial.

ROT, APPLE:

Apples on the trees are affected by a fungus known to botanists as *Spheropsis malorum.* Small pale spots make their appearance on the apple, and in a few days more numerous black pustules or papilla will appear, and thickly scatter over nearly the whole surface of the fruit. When microscopically examined each one of these black papilla is found to contain several oblong pale fungus spores, supported on a short stem or foot-stalk, from which they soon separate. When this fungus rot makes its appearance remove the affected apples at once from contact with the others.

ROT IN SHEEP, TO CURE:

Mix 4 ounces of the best honey, 2 ounces of burnt alum reduced to powder, and 1/2 lb. of Armenian bole(1) with as much train or fish oil as will convert these ingredients into the consistency of a salve. The honey must first be stirred in; afterward the alum and train-oil are to be added.

ROUND SHOULDERS:

To cure round shoulders practice the following exercise several times a day:

Hold the arms at full length in front of the body, the hands touching each other; then throw the arms backward quickly, as trying to make the backs of the hands touch each other behind the back of the body. You should also procure a pair of light dumb-bells, and go through the same exercise.

(1) An astringent earth brought from Armenia.

RUBBER SHOES:

The weight of medical opinion is against the wearing of rubbers except in winter storms, where there is an admixture of slush in the wet under foot. Rubbers make the feet tender by parboiling them and causing them to perspire. Very many persons are almost crippled by them, and make a serious mistake by persisting in wearing them. What is true of rubbers is true of patent leathers. They draw the feet and keep them hot, wet with perspiration, and exposed to chills. Any material which prevents evaporation is bad in direct proportion as it is waterproof. The best protection against wet feet is to grease one's shoes, but as this cannot be done in the city without attracting unpleasant attention the next best preventative is a cork-soled shoe of heavy, very heavy, leather.

RUGS, TO MAKE:

Very pretty, durable bedroom rugs can be made from coarse but tightly woven material, such as is used in coffee-sacks. They may be lined with the same or other heavy, coarse material. Briar-stitch them around the edges with bright colors of coarse woolen yarn, and make a circle in the corner of the same, or some other simple design of fancy work. We use old guano and phosphate sacks. They are made of the strongest and safest material, very thickly woven. To remove the offensive odor, hang the sacks out in one or two hard rains. Soak them afterward in hot suds, and hang them up and expose them to the air and sun a day or two. Then wash them thoroughly and they are ready for use. These rugs are quickly made, easily washed, neat in appearance, and save much wear of carpets.

RUST, TO PRESERVE CAST-IRON FROM:

The Mechanic says cast-iron may be best preserved from rust "by heating it till if touched with flax it causes it to frizzle," and then plunging it into a vat of mixed oil and grease. It is said that "the oleaginous matter actually penetrates the pores and prevents oxidation for a very long time, while it does not prevent painting, if desirable, afterward."

RUST, TO REMOVE FROM POLISHED IRON:

The best method of removing rust from a polished stove or grate is to scrape down to a fine powder some bath-brick, put it into a little oil, and rub the spots well with a piece of flannel dipped in the mixture; after which apply some whiting also well rubbed. This process must be repeated daily until all trace of the rust has disappeared. To prevent the grate or fire-irons from becoming spotted with rust, it is a good plan to rub them over with the fat from the inside of a fowl, and finish them off with whiting. Another method of preserving them from rust is to make a strong paste of fresh lime and water, and with a fine brush smear it as thickly as possible all over the polished surface requiring preservation. By this simple means all the grates and fire-irons in an empty house may be kept for months free from harm without further care or attention.

COCKROACHES, WAYS TO DESTROY:

"These vermin are easily destroyed simply by cutting up green cucumbers at night and placing them about where roaches commit depredations.......Remove the peelings in the morning and renew them at night."

S

SALAD:

To make a good salad is a point of proficiency which it is easy to attain with care. The main point is to incorporate the several articles required for the sauce, and to serve up at table as fresh as possible. The herbs should be "morning gathered," and they will be much refreshed by lying 1 or 2 hours in spring-water. Careful picking and washing and drying in a cloth in the kitchen are also very important, and the due proportion of each herb requires attention. The sauce may be thus prepared:

Boil 2 eggs for 10 to 12 minutes, and then put them in cold water for a few minutes, so that the yelks may become quite cold and hard. Rub them through a coarse sieve with a wooden spoon, and mix them with a table-spoonful of water or cream, and then add 2 table-spoonfuls of fine flask oil or melted butter; mix, and add by degrees a tea-spoonful of salt and the same quantity of mustard; mix till smooth, when incorporate with the other ingredients about 3 table-spoonfuls of vinegar; then pour this sauce down the side of the salad-bowl, but do not stir up the salad till wanted to be eaten. Garnish the top of the salad with the white of eggs, cut in slices; or these may be arranged in such manner as to be ornamental on the table.

SALT AS MEDICINE:

(1) In many a disordered stomach a tea-spoonful of salt is a certain cure.

(2) In the violent internal aching termed colic, add a teaspoonful of salt to a pint of cold water, drink it, and to bed; it is one of the speediest and best remedies known.

(3) The same will revive a person who seems almost dead from receiving a fall, etc.

(4) In an epileptic fit no time should be lost in pouring down salt water, if sufficient sensibility remains to allow of swallowing it; if not, the head must be sponged with cold water until the senses return, when salt will completely restore the patient from his lethargy. In a fit the feet should be placed in warm water with mustard, and the legs briskly rubbed, all bandages removed from the neck, and a cool apartment procured if possible.

(5) In many cases of bleeding at the lungs, when the other remedies fail,

Dr. Rush found that 2 table-spoonfuls of salt completely stayed the blood.

(6) For toothache warm salt water held to the part and renewed 2 or 3 times will relieve in most cases. If the teeth be covered with tartar, wash twice a day with salt.

(7) For swelled neck wash the part with brine and drink twice a day also until cured.

(8) Salt will expel worms if used in food in a moderate degree and aid digestion, but salt meat is injurious if used much.

SALT FOOD:

The excessive use of salt food will produce salt-rheum and the canker, and also affect the hands, causing roughness and cracking. Corn-huskers have need to be careful with their hands; they should do without soap as much as possible, and grease the affected parts at night with unsalted mutton fat well warmed and rubbed in.

SALT FOR POULTRY:

Hens often have a habit of biting and pulling their feathers and greedily eating them until their bodies are bare. This practice, it is believed, is occasioned by a want of salt, as when salted food is given them they make no attempt to continue the habit. Salt pork chopped fine and fed twice a week has been adapted with success, while others put a teaspoonful of salt with 2 quarts of meal or shorts moistened, well mixed, and feed about twice every week. Fowls, like human beings, to be healthy must have a certain allowance of salt.

SALUTATIONS:

Recognition of acquaintances should be quick and salutation gracious. To be complimentary, salutation should be even more than this; it should be flattering, courteous, dignified, and suited to the position of the person addressed. To an old person it should be truly respectful, for there is no such crown as a crown of gray hairs. To a young person it should be reassuring; to a person who is under the pressure of calamity it should be as especially kind, as cordial, as we can make it; but it should always be dignified. We must not give too much. Remember Shakespeare's line: "He bows too low." Do not be servile in your salutation. One may say that the above advice is too redundant; no one could convey a whole paragraph by a bow, but fascinating, kind, gracious-mannered people do all this and more.

The quick recognition is more difficult. How many of us, alas, forget faces. More of us are confused as to when we saw that face last. There is to the dwellers in cities a trying confusion as to degrees of acquaintance, if the memory for people and faces is not extraordinary. Therefore, people who are near-sighted or who have not a memory for faces cannot be quick at recognition. They are always in doubt. Such people have an undeserved unpopularity. People believe them to be cold and haughty, when they are simply confused. But if a person has a truly cordial disposition nothing can prevent their showing it finally. Manner is but the mask of character after all. The true nature will come out.

American etiquette demands that a lady should bow first to a gentleman before he can presume to bow. We differ from this. It comes from England, where an introduction for dancing purposes does not constitute acquaintance. It is for this reason that ladies in England are expected to bow first, while on the Continent it is the gentleman who gives the first sign of recognition, as it should be here, when the recognition is not simultaneous. For example, we will take the case of a mother with many sons. She brings an over-freighted memory to the next meeting, after half a dozen young gentlemen remember that they have dined at her house. She does not remember them at all; they all remember her. Should she bow first to them? No; they should recall themselves to her by a graceful, respectful bow. She will be much obliged to them. All over the Continent it is the man who bows first. In America we can afford to make our own etiquette. It is as much the man's place to bow, with our mode of life, as it is the woman's; far more when the man has received her hospitality.

The one who recognizes first should be the first to show recognition, and in the case of the hostess it is far easier for her guests to remember her than for her to remember all of them. And what harm can it do a woman if a man bows to her? If she wishes to cut him, she can do it as well after he has bowed as before; and if she is polite there are very few respectful bows which she cannot return.

In Europe the salutations of servants and shopkeepers, of couriers and maids, are so much more respectful than here that an American woman is astonished. No doubt there is very much in the polished etiquette of all society abroad which is very grateful to Americans, particularly to women. They like ceremony, politeness, and deference. They like the service so easy and so marked. They like the definiteness of European etiquette. They like fixed social usages. Even a lazy servant affects an American favorably. "He also serves who only stands and waits." There is one thing, however, which an American can well learn—not to be ashamed to take the initiative in hospitality or in politeness. Artificial observances have this merit: they protect the world from "moods," and they start us on our travels at an advantage.

SALVE, YANKEE:

For boils and sores of almost every kind this will be found of great service: Tallow, 1 lb.; linseed oil, 1 lb.; beeswax, 1/2 lb.; Burgundy pitch, 4 ounces; Venice turpentine, 4 ounces; resin 1/4 lb.; oil of lavender, 2 ounces.

Mix all together and simmer over the fire for about 20 minutes. As this makes a large quantity, one half of the above ingredients may be taken.

SCABIES, TREATMENT OF:

With regard to the efficiency of sulphur in the treatment of this disease, Dr. Carl H. Smith, of Kenton, O., writes the Boston Medical and Surgical Journal that he has employed it, mixed with glycerine to the consistence of an ointment, in upward of 500 cases, in civil and army practice, with unfailing success. In 3 or 4 days the disease disappeared, in every instance 1 or 2 applications having been made daily.

SCAB IN SHEEP, OINTMENT FOR:

Scab in sheep is a disease of the skin arising from the presence of a minute insect which buries itself in the skin. The following ointment will cure if applied persistently:

Lard, 2 lbs.; oil of tar, 1/2 lb.; sulphur, 1 lb. Mix the two latter ingredients gradually, then add the former, and rub down altogether. Tobacco-water is also good.

SCALD HEAD:

Children are often troubled with a dirty, yellowish incrustation which forms on the scalp; it usually appears on top of the head and keeps spreading. It is caused by an excessive secretion thrown out on the surface, which thickens into a dry, scaly crust, partially covering the scalp. If any part of this crust be removed the skin underneath exhibits a red, angry appearance. Uncleanliness and keeping the head too warm are generally the cause.

Treatment: In addition to the most particular attention to the preservation of the health and cleanliness, the scales should be removed by thorough washing with soap and water, and, if necessary, by poultices; the hair should also be shaved or cut off as closely as possible; the head should be kept covered with a cloth wet with equal parts of linseed-oil and lime-water.

SCALDS AND BURNS:

The very best thing to be done when any one has received a burn or a scald is to lay on the part that is injured a thick coating of cotton wool or wadding, so as to completely exclude the air. If the above wool happens not to be at hand, scraped potato or turnip will ease the pain.

SCALE IN BOILERS, TO REMOVE:

Petroleum has recently been successfully employed for the removal and prevention of scale in steam-boilers, also for the removal of deposits from water-pipes where the water contains large quantities of lime. It has the effect of penetrating and rotting the scale, causing it to become porous and disengage itself from the surface to which it is attached. It is a very simple remedy, and can be used in small quantities with out any difficulties whatever—say about a quart every week for a 25-horse-power boiler, and in quantities more or less according to the size of the boilers. It may be introduced in the feed-water or through the safety-valve, or in any way most convenient for the purpose; but to be effective it must be pure. The heavy oil used for lubricating purposes in cold situations is the most efficient, as the refined oil of this description is of no use, as it is soon expelled by the heat.

SCARLET FEVER:

Somewhere between the second and tenth day after exposure it begins with languor, pains in the head, back, and limbs, with drowsiness, nausea, and chills; these are followed by heat, thirst, etc. When the redness appears the pulse is quick, and the patient is anxious, restless, and sometimes delirious; the eyes are red, the face swollen, the tongue is covered in the middle with white mucus, and is studded with elevated points of extreme redness; the tonsils are swollen and the throat red. The greatest degree of redness is reached on the evening of the third or fourth day from its beginning, when a gentle moisture appears, the disease begins to decline with itching, and the scarf-skin falls off in branny scales; as the disease advances the tongue becomes suddenly clean, and presents a glossy, fiery-red surface, which is sometimes, with the whole lining of the mouth, raw and tender.

On pressing down the tongue the throat is swollen and of a deep, florid red; on the tonsils may be seen white or gray ulcers; the great amount of mucus in these parts causes also a continual rattling in the throat; the glands under the ear and jaw inflame and occasionally break; the inflammation of the throat almost always runs into ulceration, and abscesses sometimes form in the ear and cause deafness that may be difficult or impossible to cure.

Treatment:

(1) In ordinary cases the treatment should be very simple. The apartment should be kept cool and the bed-covering light; the whole body should be sponged with cool water as often as it is hot and dry, and the patient be permitted to take cooling drinks; when the fever is very high the wet sheet-pack should be thoroughly tried. Give 10 drops of the tincture of belladonna night and morning; the feet and hands should be soaked 2 or 3 times a day in hot water, with a little ground mustard or Cayenne pepper stirred in; if the bowels are costive they should be kept open by gentle laxatives, 1 dram each of rhubarb and magnesia or Rochelle salts, or by injections; the diet should as a rule be liquid, but need not necessarily be low; milk, milk-porridge, chicken or mutton-broth, or beef-tea will be suitable; in many cases tonics, as quinine in 2-grain doses, 5 drops of mineral acids in sweetened water, or 10 drops of muriated tincture of iron, may be required. A useful external application is fat salt bacon, which should be rubbed over the whole surface from neck to heels 2 or 3 times a day; internally nothing is better than equal parts of muriatic acid and honey, applied with a small brush or swab, or diluted with water and used as a gargle. During convalescence great care must be used to prevent catching cold; warm clothing should be worn; quinine in 2-grain doses 3 times daily may be used as a tonic, and lemonade, or cream of tartar water drank freely to excite the free action of the kidneys.

(2) An eminent physician says he cures 99 out of 100 cases of scarlet-fever by giving the patient warm lemonade with gum, arabic dissolved in it. A cloth wrung out in hot water and laid upon the stomach should be removed as rapidly as it becomes cool. In cases where physicians are not easily obtainable simple remedies are not to be despised.

SCHOOL-MASTER, THE GAME OF:

Among stirring games one that is always a success when played with energy is that called the School-master. The one of the party who volunteers to be master of the ceremony places himself in front of his class, who are all seated in a row. If agreeable, he can examine his subjects in all the different branches of education in succession, or may go from one to the other indiscriminately. Supposing he decides to begin with natural history, he will proceed as follows: Pointing to the pupil at the head of the class, he asks the name of a bird beginning with C. Should the pupil not name a bird beginning with this letter by the time the master has counted 10 it is passed on immediately to the next, who, if successful, and calls out, "Cuckoo," or "Crow," etc., in time, goes above the one who has failed. Authors, singers, actors, or any thing else may be chosen if the school-master should think proper as subjects for examination; but, whatever may be selected, the questions must follow each other with great rapidity, or the charm of the game will be wanting.

SCIATICA(1):

Regulate the bowels; apply a hot external application; begin a tonic with anodyne internal remedies. Give one eighth to one sixth grain of morphia internally or by hypodermic injection, or one sixtieth grain of atropia in solution.

A good hot application is made as follows:

Boil a small handful of lobelia in a half pint of water till the strength is out of the herb, then strain it off and add a tea-spoonful of fine salt;

(1) Any painful condition of the hip and thighs.

wring cloths out of the liquid as hot as possible and spread over the part affected.

SCORCHED LINEN, TO WHITEN:

(1) For whitening scorched linen it is often sufficient to wet it with soapsuds and lay it in the hot sun.

(2) Put 1 lb. of white soap into 1 gallon of milk, and boil the scorched article in it.

SCRAP-BOOK FOR PICTURES:

A picture scrap-book, fascinating to both girls and boys, may be made as follows:

Cut tinted pasteboard into leaves of convenient size. On these paste pictures of all sorts that may have accumulated in the house, such as advertising cards, wood-cuts, and the like. Punch holes through these leaves and tie together with bright ribbons. When the pictures are prettily arranged, and interposes with bits of poetry, rhymes, and jingles, the book will hardly fail to prove a source of entertainment.

SCRAPS:

There should be a roomy receptacle for all scraps. Either a trunk or a large drawer may be set aside for pieces, or if both of these are out of the question there should be several piece-bags provided, one for linens, another for wash-goods, another for woolens, another for silks, velvets, and plushes. The remnants of each kind and color should be made into neat rolls, pinned or tied. Smaller bags may hold buttons, hooks and eyes, etc. By the practice of such system as this time and trouble may be saved. The habit of keeping buttons from year to year is worth following, as a set that has been worn one season on a street costume may do duty later on a house-gown or a wrapper.

SCREENS, TO MAKE:

A simple and easily made fire-screen has, instead of the ordinary panel, a rod across the top, from which depends a full curtain of velveteen with a dado of stamped plush studded with small spangles. For every one who has time and taste for embroidery a strip of sateen decorated with needle-work may take the place of the plush. A screen to take in the hand or put in a movable rest is made by covering a long-handled Japanese fan with black satin on which is worked in silver gray silk a representation of a spider's web, which may be drawn from nature without much trouble. The web is worked on a large scale in much the same way that ladies were fond of ornamenting buttons a few years ago—bars radiating from a center, and lines of silk going around with a stitch taken over the bar at each intersection, to prevent the circular effect demanded for the button. The other side of the fan may be covered with plain satin with a flat bow in the center, and the handle may be colored red or black. For screens framed in ebony gilded leather furnishes one of the best of materials.

SCREW IN PLASTER:

It often becomes desirable to insert screws into plaster walls without attaching them to any wood-work; but when we turn them the plaster gives way and our effort is vain; and yet a screw may be inserted in plaster so as to hold light pictures, etc., very firmly. Enlarge the hole to about twice the diameter of the screw, fill it with plaster of Paris, such as is used for fastening the tops of lamps, etc., and bed the screw in the soft plaster. When the plaster has set the screws will hold like iron.

SCREWS, RUSTY, TO REMOVE:

It often happens that screws and nails become so rusted into wood that it is impossible to remove them without damage; whenever this is the case, pour a little kerosene over them, and after soaking a short time the rust will give way. By the same application nuts and bolts that have been fixed by rust for years may be made to turn. The kerosene soon penetrates the interstices.

SCREWS, TO MAKE HOLD:

When screws are driven into soft wood subjected to considerable strain they are very likely to work loose, and many times it is very difficult to make them hold. In every case we have found the use of glue profitable. Prepare the glue thick; immerse a stick about the size of the screw and drive it home as soon as possible. When there is some article of furniture to be repaired, and no glue handy, insert the stick and then fill the rest of the cavity with pulverized resin, then heat the screw sufficient to melt the resin as it is driven in.

Chairs, tables, lounges, etc., are continually getting out of order in every house; and the time to repair the break is when first noticed. If neglected the matter grows still worse, and finally results in the laying by of the article of furniture as worthless. Where screws are driven into the wood for temporary purposes they can be removed much easier by dipping them in oil before inserting. When buying screws, notice what you are getting; for there are poor as well as good kinds. See that the heads are sound and well cut; that there are no flaws in the body or threaded part, and that they have good gimlet points. A screw of one make will drive into oak as easily as others into pine, and endure having twice the force brought against it.

SCURVY:

The symptoms are languor, weakness, and depression of mind; the face and skin are pale and bloated, and the breath is fetid; the gums are swelled, soft, red, and spongy, and bleed; the teeth get loose and often fall out; the skin becomes covered with purple spots, and these sometimes spread and run into each other; ulcerous sores break out on the body which discharge thin, offensive matter; the pulse is weak and soft, and all the secretions have an offensive smell; in bad cases blood is discharged from the bladder, bowels, womb, nose, and mouth, and exertion may be followed by fainting and sudden death.

Treatment: Treatment consists mainly of diet consisting of an abundance of fresh meat and vegetables, with acid fruits, and where the debility is great acid wines and malt liquors; the utmost attention must be paid to cleanliness, and the bowels kept regular.

SEA AND HER CHILDREN, GAME OF:

The players seat themselves in a circle, leaving out one of their number, who represents the sea. Each player having taken the name of some fish, the Sea walks slowly around outside the ring calling her companions one after another by the titles they have adopted. Each one on hearing his or her name pronounced rises and follows the Sea. When all have left their seats, the Sea begins to run about, exclaiming, "The sea is troubled! The sea is troubled!" and suddenly seats herself, an example immediately followed by her companions. The one who fails to secure a chair becomes the Sea, and continues the game as before.

SEA-SICKNESS:

To prevent this observe the following rules:

(1) Do not go on the steamer in a nervous or exhausted condition; have every preparation made at least 24 hours before starting; select a berth as near the center of the vessel as possible; in going to Europe be on the starboard side, and in returning on the port side, which will be the sunny side; go on board sufficiently early to arrange such things as may be wanted for the first day or two, so that they may be easy of access; then undress and go to bed before the vessel gets under way; if subject to nausea, retain the horizontal position the entire passage if necessary; eat regularly and heartily without raising the head for at least 1 or 2 days; on the first night out take some mild laxative medicine, and be careful to keep the bowels open for the remainder of the voyage; after having become so far habituated to the sea as to be able to take meals at the table and go on deck, never think of rising in the morning until something has been eaten; if subsequently during the voyage the sea should become unusually rough, go to bed before getting sick; do not try to keep on deck.

(2) Dissolve 1 ounce of bromide of sodium in 4 ounces water; take 1 tea-spoonful 3 times a day before eating; begin taking this 3 days before embarking.

(3) While sitting avoid resting the feet on the floor. Be seated so that the roll of the ship shall not pitch you forward or backward, but from side to side. Whenever the premonitory symptoms of sea-sickness occur, do not fix attention on any near object; omit reading or writing; go to meals regularly; eat sparingly of plain food.

Relief of Sea-sickness: A distinguished physician writes: "In the greater number of instances I allow the stomach to discharge its contents once or twice, and then if there is no organic disease I give 5 drops of chloroform in a little water, and if necessary repeat the dose in 4 or 6 hours. The almost instant effect of this treatment, if conjoined with a few simple precautions, is to cause an immediate sensation, as it were, of warmth in the stomach, accompanied by almost total relief of the nausea and sickness, likewise curing the distressing headache, and usually causing a quiet sleep, from which the passenger awakes quite well."

SEA-WATER, HOW TO MAKE:

There cannot be a question that by far the simplest plan would consist in the evaporation of the sea-water itself in large quantities, preserving the resulting salt in closely stopped vessels to prevent the absorption of the moisture, and vending it in this form to the consumer; the proportion of this dry saline matter being 56 ounces to 10 gallons of water, less 3 pints. The proportion ordered to be used is 6 ounces to the gallon of water, and stirred well until dissolved.

SEA-WATER, TO MAKE FIT FOR WASHING LINEN:

Soda put into sea-water makes it turbid; the lime and magnesia fall to the bottom. To make sea-water fit for washing linen at sea as much soda must be put in it as not only to effect a complete precipitation of these earths but to render the sea-water sufficiently laxivial or alkaline. Soda should always be taken to sea for this purpose.

SEA-WEEDS, TO COLLECT AND PRESERVE:

Wash the sea-weed in fresh water, then take a plate or dish, (the larger the better), cut your paper to the size required, place it on the plate with fresh water, and spread out the plant with a good-sized camel's-hair pencil in a natural form, (picking out with the pin gives the sea-weed an unnatural appearance, and destroys the characteristic fall of the branches, which should be carefully avoided); then gently raise the position for a few moments, so as to allow the superabundant water to run off; after which place it in the press. The press is made with either 3 pieces of board or pasteboard.

Lay on the first board 2 sheets of blotting-paper; on that lay your specimens; place straight and smooth over them a piece of old muslin, fine cambric, or linen; then some more blotting-paper, and place another board on the top of that, and continue in the same way. The blotting-paper and the muslin should be carefully removed and dried every day, and then replaced; at the same time those specimens that are sufficiently dried may be taken away. Nothing now remains but to write on each the name, date, and locality. You can either gum the specimens in a scrap-book or fix them in as drawings are often fastened, by making 4 slits in the page, and inserting each corner. This is by far the best plan, as it admits of their removal without injury to the page at any future periods, if it be required either to insert better specimens or intermediate species.

Some of the large algae will not adhere to the paper, and consequently requires gumming. The following method of preserving them has been communicated to me by a botanical friend: "After well cleaning and pressing, brush the coarser kinds of algae over with spirits of turpentine, in which 2 or 3 small lumps of gum mastic have been dissolved by shaking in a warm place; two thirds of a small phial is the proper proportion, and this will make the specimens retain a fresh appearance."

SEIDLITZ POWDERS:

Rochelle salts, 2 drams; bicarbonate of soda, 2 scruples; put these into a blue paper, and 35 grains tartaric acid into a white paper. To use put each into different tumblers, fill one half with water, adding a little loaf sugar to the acid, then pour together and drink quick.

SERVANTS' SHOES:

Servants should wear thin shoes in the house, and be told to step lightly, not to slam doors, or drop china, or to rattle forks and spoons. A quiet servant is the most certain of domestic blessings. Neatness, good manners, and faithfulness have often insured a stupid servant of no great efficiency a permanent home with a family. If to these qualities be added a clear head, an active body, and a respectful manner, we have that rare article—a perfect servant.

SEVEN YEARS' ITCH, OR PRURIGO:

Small pimples, almost the natural color of the skin, attended with great itching, at times so intense that those suffering from it scratch and tear themselves until the blood flows; usually worse toward evening.

Treatment: Hot salt water and sulphur baths, or, when it can be had, the line laxatives or cream of tartar and sulphur to keep the bowels open. The itching can be much relieved by bathing with bran water, carbolic acid, soap-suds, etc.

One of the following formula makes a good wash:

(1) Glycerine, 4 ounces; carbolic acid, 1 dram; extract of belladonna, 20 grains; water, $^1/_2$ ounce; mix.

(2) Camphor and chloral hydrate, of each 1 dram; rub together until it becomes liquid; then add cold cream, 2 ounces, and make into an ointment.

SEWER-GAS:

Procure an ounce or two of essence of peppermint in small glass phial. Pour it into the drain or water-closet which communicates most directly with the main drain, if possible into one outside the house. Then pour after it a gallon of hot water. A leakage of sewer-gas will be immediately indicated by an odor of peppermint. The phial should not be brought into the house, but be thrown out of the window or recorked and left; and, if possible, the person who pours the drug into the drain should not come into the house or rooms to be tested for some time, as the odor clings perniciously to the clothes, and may in this way give unnecessary alarm.

SHAMPOO LIQUIDS:

(1) An excellent shampoo is made of salts of tartar, white castile soap, bay rum, and lukewarm water. The salts will remove all dandruff, the soap will soften the hair and clean it thoroughly, and the bay rum will prevent taking cold.

(2) Mix borax, three-quarters lb., with salts of tartar, $^1/_4$ lb., and dissolve 1 ounce of the mixture in 1 pint of water.

(3) Dissolve $^1/_2$ ounce carbonate of ammonia and 1 ounce of borax in 1 quart of water, then add 2 ounces of glycerine, 3 quarts of New England rum, and 1 quart of bay rum; moisten the hair with this liquor; shampoo with the hands until a slight lather is formed, then wash off with clean water.

(4) Soft water, 1 pint; sal soda, 1 ounce; cream tartar, $^1/_4$ ounce. Apply thoroughly to the hair.

SHAVING CREAM:

Take 1 lb. of soft-soap in a jar; add to it 1 quart best alcohol; set the jar in a vessel of boiling water until the soap is dissolved. Perfume with essential oil to suit. This is a good article for shaving, especially for those troubled with pimples on the face. Two or 3 drops rubbed on the face with the end of the finger is enough for shaving. Dip the end of the brush in a little hot water, brush the face briskly, and it will raise a rich lather.

SHEEP, TO PROTECT FROM FLIES:

The months of July and August are the ones when sheep in many localities are subject to a most aggravating annoyance from a fly *(oestrus bovis)* which seems bound to deposit its larvae in the nostrils. It infests wooded districts and shady places where the sheep resort for shelter, and by its ceaseless attempts to enter the nose makes the poor creatures almost frantic. If but one fly is in a flock they all become agitated and alarmed.

They will assemble in groups, holding their heads close together and their noses to the ground. As they hear the buzzing of the little pest going from one to another, they will crowd their muzzles into the loose dirt made by their stamping to protect themselves, and as the pest succeeds in entering the nose of a victim it will start on a run, followed by the whole flock, to find a retreat from its enemy, throwing its head from side to side as if in the greatest agony; while the oestrus, having gained his lodging-place, assiduously deposits its larvae in the inner margin of the nose. Here, aided by warmth and moisture, the eggs quickly hatch into a small maggot, which, carrying out its instincts, begins to crawl up into the nose through a crooked opening in the bone.

The annoyance is fearful and maddening as it works its way up into the head and cavities. The best known preventive is tar, in which is mixed a small amount of crude carbolic acid. If the scent of the acid does not keep the fly away he gets entangled in the tar, which is made soft by the heat of the animal. Any kind of tar or turpentine is useful for this purpose, and greatly promotes the comfort of the sheep and prevents the ravages of the bot in the head.

SHEEP-SKIN MATS:

Wash the skin while fresh in strong soap-suds, first picking from the wool all the dirt that will come out. A little paraffine (a table-spoonful to 3 gallons of water) will aid in removing the impurities. Continue to wash the skin in fresh suds until it is white and clean; then dissolve 1/2 lb. each of salt and alum in 3 pints of boiling water; put it into water enough to cover the skin, which should soak in the solution 12 hours, and then be hung on a line to drain. When nearly dry nail it, wool side in, on a board or to the side of a barn to dry. Rub into the skin an ounce each of pulverized alum and saltpeter, and if the skin is large double the quantity. Rub for an hour or two. Fold the skin-sides together and hang the skin away for 3 days, rubbing it every day or till perfectly dry; then with a blunt knife clear the skin of impurities, rub it with pumice or rotten stone, trim it into shape, and you will have a door-mat that will last a life-time.

If it is to be dyed, have a shallow vessel as large as the skin, in which to prepare the dye, so that the skin can be laid wool-side down smoothly into the vessel, that all parts may be equally immersed in the dye. This should not be more than an inch deep, otherwise the skin might be injured by the hot dye. After coloring, again stretch the skin to dry, and then comb with a wool or cotton card. With these directions all that remains is to prepare the dye. To do this go to a drug-store and purchase the aniline of the color desired, such as aniline yellow, aniline red, aniline crimson, aniline blue, etc. Add to the water enough of the coloring matter to make a proper dye, and follow the instructions above given.

SHEET-IRON STOVES, TO PRESERVE:

Sheet-iron stoves should be rubbed over once a week with a piece of flannel wet with a few drops of oil or melted lard.

SHEET OF PAPER, TO SPLIT:

Get a piece of plate-glass and place it on a sheet of paper, then let the latter be thoroughly soaked. With care and a little dexterity the sheet can be split by the top surface being removed. But the best plan is to paste a piece of cloth or strong paper to each side of the sheet to be split. When dry, violently and without hesitation pull the two pieces asunder, when part of the sheet will be found to have adhered to one and part to the other. Soften the paste in water, and the pieces can be easily removed form the cloth. The process is generally demonstrated as a matter of curiosity, yet it can be utilized in various ways. If we want to paste in a scrap-book a newspaper article printed on both sides of the paper and possess only one copy, it is very convenient to know how to detach the one side from the other. The paper when split, as may be imagined, is more transparent than it was before being subjected to the operation, and the printing-ink is somewhat duller; otherwise the two pieces present the appearance of the original if again brought together.

SHEETS, TO MAKE:

Sheets should be 3 yds. long and 2 breadths wide unless made of full-breadth linen. Linen sheets last longer than cotton ones, and in hot weather are the most comfortable, but in our variable climate cotton sheets are much preferable, especially for delicate or rheumatic people.

SHELF, MANTEL, HOW TO MAKE:

If you have no mantel and need something to take the place of one in your sitting-room or parlor, have a shelf cut about 2 1/4 yds. in length and 1/4 yd. in width out of a pine board; fasten it firmly upon 2 iron brackets with screws, and then screw the brackets to the place upon the wall where the shelf can go and be most useful. If you have the outer corners rounded, the shelf will look better when it is covered. Cover it with a pretty cretonne, tacking the cloth smoothly to the board then make a curtain about 1/4 yd. deep, sew on the edge a cheap jute or fancy cotton fringe of the colors in the cretonne, and tack the upper edge neatly over the top, covering around the edge of the shelf. Over these tacks sew a narrow gimp.

SHIRT-BOSOMS, TO RENDER GLOSSY:

The best recipe for glossed shirt-bosoms is to take 2 ounces of fine gum arabic[1] powder, pour on a pint or more water, and then, having covered it, let it stand all night. In the morning pour it carefully from the dregs into a clean bottle, cork and keep it for use. Add a tea-spoonful of this gum-water to a pint of starch made in the usual way.

SHIRTS, PROPER WAY TO DO UP:

An easy way I have found is to dissolve the starch in a little cold water, then pour on hot—not boiling—water, say 1/2 pint to 2 tea-spoonfuls of starch; wet the bosoms in this, toll them up, let them lie 2 or 3 hours, and iron in the usual way. When cuffs, collars, or shirts are to be ironed so they can be worn some little time without becoming soiled, similar to laundry work, it requires more time and labor.

To polish after ironing, moisten the surface with boiled starch and iron briskly with a smoothing-iron, (I use a nickel-plated one). Cuffs and collars are treated similarly, but on the wrong side first. If they are not yet stiff enough, rub in while ironing more thick starch, cold or hot, and polish them as directed.

When done tip the iron and draw the edge back and forth over the inside of the cuff or collar, which will round it to the shape of the arm or neck. The linen part of turn-down collars, should be finished first, then the other part ironed on the wrong side, as it will turn over the better. Any time when ironing, little specks or soiled spots can be rubbed off with a damp cloth. It will no doubt require some practice to do the above satisfactorily, but I trust that labor and patience will be rewarded with success.

SHOCK:

Prostration, or collapse, which signifies depression of the powers of life, which follows any severe injury. The usual symptoms are that the patient lies cold and half unconscious, with a feeble pulse and imperfect sighing respiration; nausea, and vomiting, hiccough, suppression of urine, and in children convulsions are also very frequent symptoms. The duration of these symptoms is various. Sometimes they pass off quickly; but they remain even for 48 hours before reaction is established.

Treatment: Give stimulants, of which hot brandy and water is the best; and nourishment, such as beef-tea; put blankets, heated bricks, or bottles of hot water under the armpits and between the thighs. Vomiting may be allayed by soda-water with brandy, by sucking ice, by a full dose of opium, by an opiate enema, or by a mustard poultice to the epigastrium. Hiccough may be relieved by small doses of Hoffman's anodyne.

1. A gum from one of several African acacia trees.

SHOE-SOLES, HOW TO PRESERVE:

Melt together tallow and common resin in the proportion of two parts of the former to one of the latter, and apply the preparation hot to the soles of the boots or shoes—as much of it as the latter will absorb. One farmer declares that this little recipe alone has been worth more than $5.

SHORT-SIGHTEDNESS:

This is not always, as is often supposed, a natural defect. It is frequently acquired by the habit in youth of applying the eyes too closely to the object of vision. Thus it is not an infrequent result of the practice, common among children, of bending their heads too near to the books they read. This fatal habit should be carefully guarded against by parents. Even where there seems to be a natural defect it will often yield to a proper regimen of the eyes. Modern oculists reject the old idea that it is good for short-sighted people to make constant efforts to see without artificial aid. Now it is held to be a judicious proceeding to resort as early as possible to the use of glasses, which should be adapted precisely to the wants of the person. These are only to be recognized by a patient trial under the direction of an adept in the art.

SICK-ROOM, THE:

Light in the Sick-chamber: Except in extraordinary cases light is indispensable to the best relief of the sick. It should be softened and subdued, and not glaring. The light should be admitted in large quantities. It is an element of cheerfulness, and on that account should be admitted to as large an extent as the patient can bear without inconvenience. The sun-light has a direct and powerful influence for good upon the physical system, and it is on this account also that its presence should be regarded as a prime necessity. Blinds or curtains may be provided to screen the eyes, if the latter are too weak or sensitive to bear the direct rays; but no substitute can perform its powerful service as a sanitary agent in the sick-chamber.

Cheerful Walls and Cheerful Prospects: The walls should be of a cheerful tint; if possible, some sort of outdoor glimpse should be visible from the bed or chair where the invalid lies, if it is but the top of a tree and a bit of sky. Eyes which have been traveling for long, dull days over the pattern of the paper-hangings till each bud and leaf and quirl[1] is familiar—and hateful—brighten with pleasure as the blind is raised. The mind, wearied of the grinding battle with pain and self, finds unconscious refreshment in the new interest.

Flowers: Many argue that flowers should be carefully kept away from sick people, lest they exhaust the air, or communicate to it some harmful quality. This

1. Quirle, whirl.

may, in a degree, be true of such strong, fragrant blossoms as lilacs or garden lilies, but of the more delicately scented ones no such effect need be apprehended. A well-aired room will never be made close or unwholesome by a nosegay[1] of roses, mignonette, or violets, and the subtle cheer which they bring with them is infinitely reviving to weary eyes and depressed spirits.

Reading Aloud in the Sick-room: "With regard to reading aloud in the sick-room," says Florence Nightingale, "my experience is that when the sick are too ill to read to themselves they can seldom bear to be read to. Children, eye-patients, and uneducated persons are exceptions, or where there is any mechanical difficulty in reading. People who like to be read to have generally not much the matter with them; while in fevers, or where there is much irritability of brain, the effort of listening to reading aloud has often brought on delirium. I speak with great diffidence, because there is an almost universal impression that it is sparing the sick to read aloud to them."

Read Slowly to the Sick: If the patient desires reading, or if reading aloud is not trying to the nerves, it should be done slowly. "People often think that the way to get it over with the least fatigue to him is to get it over in least time. They gabble, they plunge, and gallop through the reading. There never was a greater mistake. Houdin, the conjurer, says that the way to make a story seems short is to tell it slowly. So it is with reading to the sick. I have often heard a patient say to such a mistaken reader, 'Don't read it to me; tell it to me.' Unconsciously he is aware that this will regulate the plunging, the reading with unequal paces, slurring over some part, instead of leaving it out altogether if it is unimportant, and mumbling another."

How to Move a Patient: Sometimes when patients are greatly exhausted, or after severe surgical operations, it may be dangerous to bring them into a sitting position, but they may be safely and easily moved if the body is kept horizontal in the following manner: Place the head of one bedstead against the foot of the other. Having procured two hard-wood poles 6 ft. long and $1^1/_2$ in. in diameter, place one on each side of the patient near the edge of the sheet on which he rests, and roll them firmly into the sheet to within 6 in. of the patients body.

Two persons should stand on each side of the bed, facing the two on the other side, and grasping the poles firmly with both hands, separated about 18 in. apart; they should first pull firmly against each other until the sheet on which the patient lies is converted into a stretcher; then continue to pull, and lifting the body horizontally and moving downward together, they easily deposit the patient in the fresh bed without danger or suffering.

1. Bouquet of flowers.

The sheet on which he has been moved can then be readily slipped out from beneath the body. It is astonishing with what ease a thing can be done when done in the right way.

Cleanliness and Neatness in the Sick-room: The aphorism that "cleanliness is next to godliness" is nowhere more imperative than in the sick-room. Cleanliness absolutely enforced will stamp out any infectious disease, and mitigate all diseases to a marked degree. In enforcing cleanliness in the sick-room we must look to the patients's bed, the patient's body, the nurse and all utensils, vessels, etc.

In the model sick-room there should be two narrow beds of equal height on easy-rolling castors, having hair mattresses, low head-boards, and absolutely free from all abominations, in the way of canopies. The patient may thus have a fresh bed for the night and another for the morning. In the morning the freshly made bed, covered with one sheet, can be trundled up to the bed which has been occupied during the night, and the patient can easily be slid on the same level on to a deliciously fresh bed. The mattress and bedding of the bed vacated can be rolled up, quietly taken into an adjoining room, where, with open windows, they can be shaken, thoroughly ventilated during the day, and made ready for the night.

Directions in Contagious Sickness: *The following general directions are useful to nurses and others in contagious or infectious sickness:*

(1) The sick person should be restricted to one room, or a part of the house separated for the other inmates.

(2) Secure proper ventilation of the sick-room without producing draughts. Smell is an excellent guide as to the state of air; if the air is sweet there is but little dread to be felt.

(3) The virulence of any poison which causes the spread of disease is greatly increased by concentration in close rooms, and decreased by dilution and free circulation of air.

(4) The linen, clothing, bedding, utensils, and every object touched by or in contact with the sick should be isolated, and, such as will permit, should be thrown into boiling water, there to remain at least for half an hour.

(5) The nurse should be restricted to the sick-room or otherwise isolated.

(6) Remember that disease is communicated by both the poisoned air about the sick and by the clothes and other articles used or touched by them.

(7) After the patient leaves the sick-room it should be purified and disinfected. Boil every thing that will admit of it; scald all utensils;

scrub the floors; whitewash ceiling and walls. Empty the room entirely, and leave doors and windows open for at least a day or two.

Important Qualities of a Good Nurse: A good nurse will be full of kindness. She will control by gentleness combined with decision. She will be decisive if no one suspects that she is so at all. It is the triumph of supremacy to become unconsciously supreme. Nowhere is this decision more blessed than in a sick-room. Where it exists in its gentleness the sufferer is never contradicted, never coerced; all the little victories are assumed.

The decisive nurse is never peremptory, never loud. She is distinct, it is true—there is nothing more aggravating to a sick person than a whisper—but she is not loud. Though quiet, she never walks on tip-toe; she never makes gestures; all is open and above board. She knows no diplomacy of finesse, and, of course, her shoes never creak. Her touch is steady and encouraging . She does not potter. She never looks at you sideways. You never catch her watching. She never slams the door, of course, but she never shuts it slowly, as if she were cracking a nut in the hinge. She never talks judicious penetration. She caresses one kind of patient with genuine sympathy; she talks to another as if she were well. She is never in hurry. She is worth her weight in gold.

Twenty-one Brief suggestions to Nurses:

- Be scrupulously neat in person and dress.
- Be cheerful and buoyant to the last degree possible.
- A few drops of hartshorn in the water used for daily bathing will remove the disagreeable odors of warmth and perspiration.
- Never speak of the symptoms of your patient in his presence, unless questioned by the doctor, whose orders you are always to obey implicitly.
- Remember never to be a gossip or tattler, and "always to hold sacred the knowledge which, to a certain extent, you must obtain of the private affairs of your patient and the household in which you nurse."
- Try to give as little trouble to the servants as possible, and make them feel that you have come to help them in the extra work that sickness always brings.
- Never contradict your patient nor argue with him.
- Never whisper in the sick-room.
- If your patient be well enough, and wishes you to talk to him, speak in a low, distinct voice, on cheerful subjects.

- Don't relate painful hospital experiences, nor give details of the maladies of former patients.
- Never startle the patient with accounts of dreadful crimes or accidents that you have read in the newspapers.
- Write down the orders that the physician gives you as to time for giving the medicines, food, etc.
- Give an account of your patient to the physician in as few words as possible.

Hygiene in the Sick-room: Hygiene in the sick-room was discussed in a lecture recently delivered by the Professor of Pathology of the University of Pennsylvania before the nurses of the University Hospital. Dr. Tyson said that no room should be occupied by a sick person which does not have an area of at least 1,700 sq. ft. It should have a southern exposure, and even in summer should receive as much sunlight as possible. Excepting in certain diseases, about which the physicians should give directions, there should be plenty of sunlight admitted to the room all day.

The furniture and hangings of the room should be of such a nature that they could easily be cleaned and washed, and they should be kept in a perfectly clean condition. The constant circulation of air in the room should be a prime requirement, but this should be secured without draft upon the patient. A lighted lamp placed in the fire-place would give a flow of air which would be beneficial in cases where no heat was desired. The general temperature of the room should be from 68 to 70 degrees, and should be constant.

To Change the Air of a Sick-room: Open the windows or doors leading out of doors in the room adjoining sick-room. When the air in this adjoining room is renewed, close the doors and windows and open the door into the sick-room. This changes the air of the room without any draughts or currents endangering the condition of the patient. This may be repeated every hour or oftener, according to need.

SILKS, TO CLEAN WHITE SATIN AND FLOWERED:

(1) Mix sifted stale bread-crumbs with powder blue, and rub it thoroughly all over, then shake it well and dust it with clean soft cloths. Afterward, where there are any gold or silver flowers, take a piece of crimson ingrain velvet, rub the flowers with it, which will restore them to their original luster.

(2) Pass them through a solution of fine hard soap, at a hand heat, drawing them through the hand. Rinse in lukewarm water, dry, and finish by pinning out. Brush the flossy or bright side with a clean clothes-brush the way of the nap. Finish them by dipping a sponge into the size, made by boiling isinglass in water, and rub the wrong side.

Rinse out a second time, and brush, and dry near a fire or in a warm room. Silk may be treated in the same way, but not brushed.

SILVER, CARE OF:

There is wide difference of opinion as to the best material for cleaning silver. The whiting and plate-powder, it is alleged, remove the dirt or tarnish and a minute portion of the metal at the same time, a serious consideration in plated-ware, but of less importance in solid silver, where the infinitesimal amount lost is hardly discernible even after long service. In fact, nearly all the preparations advertised for this purpose are made on the same basis, ground chalk disguised in various ways. The silver-soap sold a few years ago was good for a while, but has deteriorated of late. Electro-silicon is the most valuable preparation for cleaning silver, and is easily used. With all, the chamois-skin rubbing must finish the work.

Cleaning: The first essential in cleaning silver is plenty of hot water. The pieces should be washed clean in almost boiling suds to begin with. Nor must the water be allowed to grow cold. If there is a butler's pantry it will be an easy matter to let off the cooled suds and fill up with fresh hot water. If an ordinary dishpan is used, the tea-kettle must be kept constantly on the stove in readiness to replenish the pan. Best of all is the double dishpan, holding boiling water in both divisions, the one clear, the other suds. As each piece is drawn from the suds and rubbed with whiting, electro-silicon, or silver-soap, it may be dropped into the clearer water on the other side. When the dishpan is of the ordinary style the silver should be scoured piece by piece and placed unwiped on a waiter. All done, the dishpan should be filled anew with hot water, the contents of the tray emptied into this, and each piece rinsed off, wiped dry, and laid aside to await a final polishing with the chamois-skin.

Tarnishing: It is liable to tarnish from many causes, some of which can be avoided. Flannel is apt to obtain sulphur, and should not be used to mop up silver articles. Clean, soft tissue-paper first, then a bag of canton flannel, form a good covering. Want of sufficient ventilation in a house shows itself very quickly by the tarnish on the silver, caused by foul air and coal-gas. Iron and steel oxidize in damp air, according to the rule that the presence of water favors chemical change. A little oil coating will exclude the air, and hence no oxidation can take place.

Of 9 silver polishes which have been examined, 5 contained alcohol and ammonia for the liquid portion, 4 alcohol and sassafras extract. The solid portion in all cases was chalk, with in one case a little of the jeweler's rouge. The caution to be observed in the use of these preparations is in regard to the fineness of the material. A few coarse grains will scratch the coating of the silver. Precipitated chalk or well washed diatomaceous earth seem to be of the most uniform fineness.

SILVERING ON MIRRORS, TO REPAIR:

Pour upon a sheet of tin-foil 3 drams of quicksilver to the square foot of foil. Rub smartly with a piece of buckskin until the foil becomes brilliant. Lay the glass upon a flat table face downward, place the foil upon the damaged portion of the glass, lay a sheet of paper on the foil and place upon it a block of wood or a piece of marble with a perfectly flat surface; put upon it sufficient weight to press it down tight; let it remain in this position a few hours. The foil will adhere to the glass.

"SIMON SAYS," GAME OF:

In this game an imaginary Simon is the presiding genius, and the orders of no one but Simon are to be obeyed. The leader of the company generally begins by saying, "Simon says, 'Thumbs up,'" when every one must immediately obey the command of Simon or incur the penalty of paying a forfeit. Simon may then say, "Wink your left eye," "Blow your nose," "Kiss your neighbor," or any thing equally absurd. Whatever Simon says must be done. No command, however, not prefaced by the words "Simon says" is to be regarded. With the idea of winning forfeits, the leader will endeavor to induce the company to do certain things not authorized by Simon; indeed, the fun of the game consists in every one doing the wrong thing instead of the right one, and in having a good collection of forfeits.

SKIN, CARE OF THE:

The skin is not only a covering and a protection for the body, but also the medium of perspiration. This perspiration consists of 99 parts of water, and 1 part of solid matter. It is called insensible because the vapor is not recognized by the senses, except where its flow is excessive and interrupted, forming drops on the surface which are called in common language sweat. The daily exhalations through the skin aggregate about an average weight of 2 lbs. The skin also possesses a remarkable absorbing power, and to such a degree that substances may be imbibed through its pores as a medicine, or as a partial relief from thirst and hunger. As an exhalant and absorbent the skin in its functions has been compared to the lungs. Some writers on physiology describe it as "the third lung of the body." By carefully conducted experiments it has been found that the skin acts in the same way as the lungs in absorbing oxygen from the air, and giving off carbonic acid to an appreciable amount.

The Pores of the Skin: These are fine tubes about 1-300 in. in diameter and 1/4 in. in length, which run through the cutis, and then curl up in little balls. They are very numerous. In the palm of the hand there are about 2,800 in a single square inch. On the back of the neck and trunk, where they are in the fewest, there are yet 400 to the square inch. The entire number on the body of an adult is estimated about 2,500,000. The mouths of these pores may be seen with a pocket lens along the fine ridges which cover the palm of the hand. Through these pores the body throws off its excess of water and various impurities from the blood, and imbibes oxygen and other substances with which the skin comes into contact.

Keeping the Skin Clean: In view of the nature and functions of the skin, the great importance of keeping it clean and healthy is apparent. It should be one of the chief themes in the list of our duties in caring for the health of the body to keep its pores open. To this end the bath, clean bed-linen, and clean, fresh clothing become not only as luxury but a necessity. The skin, so commonly neglected, claims, and should receive the careful attention of parents and instructors.

The Condition of the Skin: The skin is the envelope of the whole human structure, has a wonderful influence upon the external aspect. It is, as it were, the atmosphere which surrounds that microcosm or little world of human being, Man. Upon its purity depends greatly the look of every part and feature which can only be seen through it. If the skin is not kept in a wholesome condition by a proper diet and regimen, there can be no beauty. A dingy integument will spoil the grace of proportion and delicacy of line of the most regularly cut face and perfectly molded form.

Washing the Face: Washing the face in acid buttermilk is a country cosmetic still in favor for sunburn, freckles, and scaly skin. The juice pressed from cucumbers is altogether preferable, and though of old repute is a fashionable London preparation. The juice of milkweed also is a proprietary lotion for the face, sold by modish cosmetic artists abroad. These vegetable lotions, being gummy, protecting, and detersive, refine the skin, and, unlike spirituous washes, do not bring out the hair on the cheeks. A seraglio[1] secret to take away wrinkles is to heat an iron shovel red hot, throw on it a spoonful of myrrh in powder, and smoke the face over it, covering person and shovel with a sheet to keep in the fumes. Repeat this 3 times, heat the shovel again, and pour on it 2 spoonfuls of white wine, steaming the face with it 3 times. This rite is to be repeated night and morning until the effect is gained.

Plantain water is very softening for the face, but vaseline rubbed on the skin of neck and face every night faithfully will keep wrinkles at distance for long years beyond their usual appearance. It should be generously applied, left for the skin to absorb a few minutes, and the excess wiped gently off with a soft cloth. As vaseline is 25 cents a pound, which lasts a year, this is the cheapest as well as the safest general cosmetic. This should always be applied before going into the hot sun for long walks or rides, as well as domestic work in heated rooms.

The skin must always be washed clean with warm water and fine

[1] To close away or confine.

soap, and well dried before using any application, and man or woman should always go to bed with face and neck thoroughly and freshly washed. Sleeping with the imperceptive dust of the day in the skin, clogging and griming it, is a great cause of wrinkles.

SKIP-JACK, GAME OF:

The Skip-Jack is best made of the forked bone, commonly called the "merry-thought" of a fowl. The merry-thoughts should be preserved whole, and a piece of catgut or 2 strings twisted together be tied round its 2 arms, a thin piece of stick ought to be just long enough to extend beyond the arch of the bone. If the strings have been sufficiently twisted it will be found that the stick placed between them will now act as a spring. The Skip-Jack is thus complete, and it will be made to skip by carrying out the following instructions. Push the stick up so that its free end may rest under the merry-thought, just where the stick touches the bone; apply a small bit of cobblers' wax, so that the end of the stick may adhere to the bone; then place the toy on the ground, and in as few seconds the spring of the stick will have overcome the adhesion of the wax, it will get free, and the Jack will skip to a considerable height.

SLEEP:

A great part of the pleasure of life consists in alternate rest and motion. Those who neglect the latter can never relish the former. Sleep is as necessary as the air we breathe or the food we eat. It quiets the restless child and recruits the tired laborer, contributing to nature's processes in the growth of the immature and restoration to all, as well in mind as body. The more uninterrupted it is, the more salutary its effects. The requisite quantity varies with the individual, dependent upon age, temperament, and habit. The rapid development of the infant demands a large part of the 24 hours, gradually diminishing through childhood and adolescence, till adult age is reached, when an average of 7 or 8 hours is sufficient. Less activity in old age, a smaller quantity by several hours suffices, unless, as it is sometimes the case in extreme old age, the requirement of the infant is observed.

To promote sleep and enhance its enjoyment a bed is needed. The modern bed is, and should be, a firm mattress, filled with curled hair, wool, or moss, singly or variously combined, excelsior,[1] or the familiar shuck, supported by wooden slats, stout cloth, woven wire, or springs. The use of opium, alcohol, and chloral to produce sleep is most pernicious; dangerous results follow the use of all. There are persons who certainly seem to require much more than the average quantity of sleep, as there are certainly those to whom much less is necessary. Children disposed to lie abed should generally be indulged, and not compelled to get up.

1. Thin wood shavings used for packing.

Beds: The best kind of bed to sleep in is one that is moderately hard and that has a reasonably hard pillow. One physician said that he personally preferred a hair pillow, because it does not allow the head to sink in it and become too warm. As for the size of the pillow, it is a rule that full-blooded persons prefer a high pillow, because they are more comfortable with their heads high. There are, and always have been, superstitions about the necessity for sleeping with the feet toward the equator, with the head toward the north for North Americans and Europeans, and the head toward the south for South Americans, Africans, and Australians. It scarcely seems worth while to discuss the modicum of reason that may lurk in such a proposition.

SLEEP AND HEALTH:

Sleep is a necessity: Without it we would suffer speedy dissolution. Every act that we perform, every movement we make, every thought that passes through our minds, every emotion that stirs our souls, breaks down a certain amount of nervous tissue, and leaves us weaker than before. These broken cells can be repaired during sleep only. The system, exhausted by physical and mental labor during the day, must be built up and strengthened for the next day's work during the dark still hours of night, while the senses are locked in slumber and the mind and muscles are all relaxed, for at no other time is this process of building up carried on.

How We Go to Sleep: The muscles which move the arms and legs usually become relaxed before those which maintain the body in an erect position. In relation to the social senses, that of sight is the first lost, the eyelids forming a barrier between the retina and the external world; but, independently of eyelids, if they had been removed by the surgeon, or could not be closed by disease, this is still the first sense whose function is abolished. Some animals, as the hare, do not shut their eyes when asleep; and in cases of somnambulism the eyes remain open, although the sense of sight is temporarily abolished and their acuteness is much lessened. Taste is the next to disappear, and then smell; hearing follows, and touch is the most persistent of the senses. So, conversely, a person is most easily awakened by the sense of touch; next in order by sounds, and then by smell.

Position During Sleep: The recumbent position has much to do with sleep. Undoubtedly sleep may occur in the sitting posture, and even while standing; but these cases are exceptional. It is certain also that sleep in bed is generally sounder with a low pillow than with a high one. If, therefore, there be a state of wakefulness at night, the head should be kept low; if, on the contrary, there is undue sleepiness, the head should be kept high. The degree of sleep and its amount may be regulated by simply taking care that the head is in the right position. If prolonged recumbency is a necessary part of the treatment, the tendency to sleep too much during the day and too little at night may be thus corrected.

Why High Pillows are Injurious: It is often a question among people who are unacquainted with anatomy and physiology whether lying with head exalted or on a level with the body is the more unwholesome. Most, consulting their own case on this point, argue in favor of that which they prefer. Now, although many delight in bolstering up their heads at night and sleep soundly without injury, yet it is a dangerous habit. The vessels in which the blood passes from the heart to the head are always lessened in their cavities when the head is resting in bed higher than the body; therefore, in all diseases attended with fever the head should be pretty nearly on a level with the body, and people ought to accustom themselves to sleep thus and avoid danger.

Sleeping on the Back or Side, Which? It is not best to sleep mainly on the back, but it is well to alternate, and sleep occasionally on either side, not always on the right nor always son the left, but on both. The right side is better of the two sides to lie upon for any length of time, as it leaves the action of the heart free, and precludes the probability of undue pressure on any of the large blood-vessels; but generally the body may be allowed to select its own position.

Amount of sleep Necessary: It is impossible to lay down rules regulating the amount of sleep necessary for each individual; some persons need much more than others. The amount necessary depends much upon the age, health, temperament, and climate.

Best Hours for Sleeping: Sleep obtained 2 hours before midnight, when the negative forces are in operation, is the rest which most recuperates the system giving brightness to the eye and a glow to the cheek. The difference in the appearance of a person who habitually retires at 10 o'clock and that of one who sits up until 12 is quite remarkable. The tone of the system, so evident in the complexion, the clearness and sparkle of the eye, and the softness of the lines of the features, is, in a person of health, kept at "concert pitch" by taking regular rest 2 hours before 12 o'clock, and thereby obtaining the "beauty sleep" of the night. There is a heaviness of the eye, a sallowness of the skin, and an absence of that glow in the face which renders it fresh in expression and round in appearance, that readily distinguishes the person who keeps late hours.

Are Feather Beds Unhealthy? Feathers make a very unhealthy bed, because they retain the heat and keep the temperature of the body too high, thus debilitating the skin and rendering the system liable to contract colds; they also retain the moisture and waste matter thrown out by the lymphatic, which is absorbed, producing disease. A dry straw bed, or, what is better, a hair mattress, should be used.

Sleep Procured by Medicine: Is rarely as beneficial as that secured naturally. The disturbance to the nervous system is often sufficient to counterbalance all the good results. The habit of seeking sleep in this way without the advice of a physician is to be deprecated. The dose must be constantly increased to produce the effect, and thus great injury may be caused. Often, too, where laudanum or morphine is used, the person unconsciously comes into a terrible and fatal bondage. Especially should infants never be dosed with cordials, as is the common family practice. The damage done to helpless childhood by the ignorant and reckless use of soothing-syrups is frightful to contemplate.

Sleeping Hints: Sleep is the best known form of rest, and yet it is only partial, for scarcely any part of the body is completely at rest. The heart beats, the blood courses, the lungs and skin are active. In sleep the volume of blood in the brain is diminished. Remedies which diminish the amount of blood in the brain (as bromide of potassium) are promotive of sleep. Sleep is a good thermometer of health. Whatever improves the sleep of an invalid betters his condition. Sleep with the mouth shut. Will to do it and persevere and you will succeed. Wash the body before sleeping, especially after a day of dust or sweating. Exhalations through the skin are more abundant while asleep than when awake; therefore the bed should be well aired before it is made up. In youth more sleep is needed than in old age, when nature makes few permanent repairs, and is content with temporary expedients. In general, one should sleep until he naturally wakes. "I have nothing to say about feather beds," says a recent writer. "None of our family like them, but I would willingly provide one for an elderly person to whom habit has made it seem a necessity."

Soft or Hard Beds? On this question there are wide differences of opinion, some persons advocating soft and others hard beds. The difference between them is that the weight of a body on a soft bed presses on a larger surface than upon a hard bed, and consequently more comfort is enjoyed. Hard beds should never be given to little children, and parents who suppose that such beds contribute to health by hardening and developing the constitution are surely in error. Eminent physicians—both here and in England—concur in this opinion, and state that hard beds have often proved injurious to the shape of infants. Birds and animals cover their offspring with the softest materials they can obtain, and also make soft beds for them; and the softness of a bed is not evidence of its being unwholesome. But if it is not kept sweet and clean by daily airings and frequent beatings—whether it is hard or soft—it is surely injurious to health.

Warm or Cold Sleeping-rooms? There is an old notion, and a foolish one, that it is better to sleep in a cold room than in a moderately warm one. Given good ventilation, and a fire in a sleeping room in cold weather is healthy. There is no gain in the chilliness of dressing and undressing in a temperature near the freezing-point, but the shock to the system is positively injurious. Cold bed-chambers always imperil health and invite fatal diseases. Robust persons may safely sleep in a temperature of 40 or under, but the old, the infantile, and the frail should never sleep in a room where the atmosphere is much under 50 degrees Fahr.

Are Plants in Sleeping-rooms Injurious? Dr. J. C. Draper, in a paper in the *Galaxy*, furnishes a very clear and able discussion in reference to this question. We condense and quote: "Though the air is dependent for the renewal of its oxygen on the action of the green leaves of plants, it must not be forgotten that it is only in the presence and under the stimulus of light that these organisms decompose carbonic acid. All plants, irrespective of their kind or nature, absorb oxygen and exhale carbonic acid in the dark. The quantity of noxious gas thus eliminated is, however, exceedingly small when compared with the oxygen thrown out during the day. When they are flowering, plants exhale carbonic acid in considerable quantity, and, at the same time, evolve heat. In this condition, therefore, they resemble animals as regards their relation to the air; and the number of plants placed in a room would, under these circumstances, tend to vitiate the air. While the phanerogamia or flowering plants depend on the air almost entirely for their supply of carbon, and are busy during the day in restoring to it the oxygen that has been removed by animals, many of the inferior cryptogamia, as the fungi and parasitic plants, obtain their nourishment from material that has already been organized. They do not absorb carbonic acid, but, on the contrary, they act like animals, absorbing oxygen and exhaling carbonic acid at all times. It is therefore evident that their presence in a room cannot be productive of good results."

The Best Way to Sleep: The best thing to do with one's head is to keep it cool; with one's feet is to keep them warm. The bedroom window should be open in summer and winter. It is a great thing to keep air constantly changing in a bedroom. This practice will cure a great many headaches which have resisted all other remedies; it will prevent a great many more than might otherwise assail humanity. Beds should be made up with the head toward the window, so that the strong light of day shall not wake or disturb or strain the eyes of the sleeper.

How to Get Sleep: How to get sleep is to many persons a matter of high importance. Nervous persons who are troubled with wakefulness and excitability usually have a strong tendency of blood on the brain with cold extremities. The pressure of the blood on the brain keeps it in a stimulated or wakeful state, and the pulsations in the head are often painful. Let such rise and chafe the body and extremities with a brush or towel, or rub smartly with the hands to promote circulation and withdraw the excessive amount of blood from the brain, and they will fall asleep in a few moments.

A cold bath, or a sponge bath and rubbing, or a good run, or a rapid walk in the open air, or going up or down stairs a few times just before retiring, will aid in equalizing circulation and promoting sleep.

These rules are simple and easy of application in castle or cabin, and may minister to the comfort of thousands who would freely spend money for an anodyne to promote "Nature's sweet restorer, balmy sleep."

Sleep-walking, or Somnambulism: Children are most subject to sleep-walking. When adults are affected with it the cause may generally be traced to mental exhaustion, over-excitement, or emotional feeling.

The most preferable method of awakening a somnambulist is by dashing cold water on the face. It is well to occasionally administer an aperient, and also to rectify any errors of diet, if necessary, and to remove, by the exercise of judicious and kindly advice and change of scene, undue excitement or morbid feeling.

The other precautions such as securing the feet during sleep, guarding the exits of the bed-chamber, etc., are obvious.

SLUGS ON PLANTS, TO DESTROY:

(1) Any choice plants may be preserved from the ravages of slugs by placing a few pieces of garlic near them. No slugs will approach the smell of garlic. Fruit-trees may be protected from slugs by tying a piece of hair-line or bind a bit of hair-cloth round their stems; if the trees are against the wall, the hair-line should be fastened all along the bottom of the wall close to the brick-work, and no slugs can pass it.

(2) Greenhouse slugs often become a nuisance in the greenhouse. A certain remedy is to sprinkle salt freely along the edges of the bench or table, the crossing of which is sure death to the slug. Slugs are very voracious, and their ravages often do considerable damage, not only to the kitchen-garden, but to the flower-beds also.

SMELLING-BOTTLES, TO FILL:

Take equal parts of sal-ammoniac crushed to a coarse powder and pearlash(1) mixed together, and perfume it with 2 or 3 drops of some essential oil, like neroli or lavender. Strength is increased by holding the bottle in the warm hand. Concentrated acetic acid can be used instead of salts of ammonia, and then the bottle should be first filled with a few crystals of sul-

(1) Crude carbonate of potash obtained from the ashes of plants.

phurate of potash, and some small bits of sponge moistened with the acid, and the perfume can be dropped upon them.

SMELLING-SALTS:

Sub-carbonate of ammonia, 8 parts; put it in coarse powder in a bottle, and pour on it oil of lavender, 1 part; mix.

SMILAX, HOW TO GROW:

Smilax is an exceedingly graceful vine with glossy, green-ribbed leaves, and is not more extensively used than any other plant for decorating parlors, the hair, and for trimming dresses. With a little care it can be grown successfully as a house-plant. The vine does not require the full sun, but will grow well in a partially shaded situation. It can be trained on a small thread across the window or around the pictures.

Grown from both seeds and bulbs. Pot the bulbs as soon as received, watering but little until you see signs of growth. They grow very rapidly, and should always have strings to twine on. Give plenty of fresh air, but be careful and not let a direct draught of cold air blow upon the vines, as they are very tender when young. Give them a warm place and they will amply repay all care. When growth is complete the foliage will turn yellow. Then gradually withhold water and allow the bulbs to dry. They then can be put in some cool dry place. After they have been in this dormant state 6 or 8 weeks they will begin to show signs of life, and then are ready for another season's growth.

SNAKE AND INSECT BITES, ANTIDOTES FOR:

(1) The general treatment should be the same as that pursued in cases of hydrophobia. Various internal remedies may be recommended, of which the best is carbonate of ammonia in doses of 10 to 20 grains every hour. Friction to the surface of the body with pieces of flannel dipped in hot alcohol is also beneficial.

(2) Sweet-oil is of a very good remedy. The patient must take a spoonful of it internally and bathe the wound for a cure. To cure a horse it requires 8 times as much as for a man.

(3) The application of carbolic acid immediately on the receipt of the injury prevents both local and general poisoning. The pure acid, however, if applied in too great quantity, is liable to produce sloughing(1) and even dangerous symptoms; hence it is best used in the proportion of two parts of acid and one of alcohol. Given internally, or applied to the wound at a late period, it produces no effect. It is believed to act, not by neutralizing the poison, but by

(1) The shedding off of dead tissue or skin.

causing contraction of the small vessels, and thus preventing its absorption.

Bites of Venomous Insects: Among the symptoms following the bites of scorpions, tarantulas, centipedes, spiders, bees, hornets, etc., are headache, vertigo, dimness of sight, and feverishness. Sometimes the wound is not much inflamed, while in other cases it becomes red, painful, and swollen, ending in suppuration.

Treatment of Insect Bites:

(1) Cleanse the wound and sponge it thoroughly with a strong solution of ammonia, and afterward cover it with linen or other suitable cloth, wet with solution of ammonia.

(2) Poison from bees, hornets, spider-bites, etc., is instantly arrested by the application of equal parts of common salt and bicarbonate of soda, well rubbed in on the place bitten or stung.

SNEEZING, COUGHING, ETC., HOW TO CHECK:

Dr. Brown-Sequard, in one of his Boston lectures, says: "There are many facts which show that the morbid phenomena of respiration can be also stopped by the influence of arrest. Coughing, for instance, can be stopped by pressing on the nerves on the lip in the neighborhood of the nose. A pressure there may prevent a cough when it is beginning. Sneezing may be stopped by the same mechanism. Pressing in the neighborhood of the ear, right in front of the ear, may stop coughing. It is so also of hiccough, but much less so than may stop coughing. Pressing very hard on the top of the mouth, inside, is also a means of stopping coughing."

SOAP-BUBBLES, GAME OF:

Few things amuse children more than blowing bubbles. Dissolve 1/4 ounce of castile soap or oil soap cut up in small pieces in three-fourths pint of water, and boil it for 2 or 3 minutes, then add 5 ounces of glycerine. When cold this fluid will produce the best and most lasting bubbles that can be made.

SOAPS AND WASHING FLUIDS:

Hard Soap: Five pails soft-soap, 2 lbs. salt, and 1 lb. resin. Simmer together, and when thoroughly fused turn out in shallow pans so as to be easily cut.

Soft Soap: Boil 25 lbs. of fried grease in 2 pails of strong lye. Next day add another pailful of hot lye; also on the following day, if there is grease on the top of the soap. Afterward add a pailful of hot water each day until the barrel is filled.

Common Hard Soap: Put in an iron kettle 5 lbs. soda, and 3 gallons soft water; let it soak over night; in the morning pour off the water, then add 3$^1/_2$ lbs. of grease, boil till thick, turn into a pan until cool, and then cut in bars.

Labor-saving Soap: Take 2 lbs. sal-soda, 2 lbs. yellow bar-soap, and 10 quarts of water; cut the soap into thin slices and boil together 2 hours; strain, and it will be fit for use. Put the clothes to soak the night before you wash, and to every pail of water in which you boil them add 1 lb. of soap. They will need no rubbing, merely rinse them out, and they will be perfectly white and clean.

Honey Soap: Cut thin 2 lbs. of yellow soap into a double sauce-pan, occasionally stirring it till it is melted, which will be in a few minutes, if the water is kept boiling around it; then add $^1/_4$ lb. of palm-oil, $^1/_4$ lb of honey, 10 cents' worth of true oil of cinnamon; let all boil together another 6 or 8 minutes; pour out and stand it by till next day; it is then fit for immediate use.

Washing Fluid: Five lbs. of sal-soda, 1 lb. of borax, $^1/_2$ lb. of fresh unslaked lime, 4 ounces of liquid ammonia. Pour 1 gallon of boiling water upon the soda and borax; when it has dissolved and has cooled, add the ammonia. Slake the lime in 1 gallon of hot water, and let it stand until entirely settled, when the clear fluid must be carefully poured off. Turn it upon the solution of soda and borax, and add to the mixture 8 gallons of cold water. Put the clothes to soak the night before washing-day, with 6 table-spoonfuls of this fluid to a tubful of clothes.

SOCKS AND STOCKINGS:

The best socks to wear are those that are made of merino(1). That prevents evaporation if the foot perspires, and so keeps the feet from getting cold. In warm weather there is no objection to cotton socks; but the thin silk hose that are to be found in all the furnished stores are neither warm nor healthful. In winter every one should wear some sort of woolen socks, it is so essential that the feet should be kept warm.

There is a theory, held by some folks, that thin socks are warmer than thick ones, because thick ones make the feet perspire, and therefore render them liable to chilliness.

According to a very distinguished traveler, who happened to be crossing Siberia in one of those government sleighs which one can get if he can first get an imperial order, and which travel night as well as day, he found his feet getting always very cold, though he traveled sleeping under immense piles of furs. The natives told him to put dry hay in his boots to absorb the perspiration, and after that he slept in comfort. According to this reasoning silk socks might be preferable to woolen, but many doctors hold

(1) Wool of the Spanish merino sheep.

that very thin silk serves no particular purpose beyond covering the feet. It fits so closely, and is possessed of so little warmth, that the cold induced by close fitting and thin covering is not overcome.

All theories, therefore, can only be met by wearing in winter what best suits the nature of the individual after he has experimented with the light of the information given above.

SODA-WATER POWDERS:

A pleasant cooling, summer drink. The blue paper contains carbonate of soda, 30 grains; the white paper tartaric acid, 25 grains.

Directions: Dissolve the contents of the blue paper in half a tumbler of water, stir in the other powder, and drink during effervescence. Soda powders furnish a saline beverage, which is very slightly laxative, and well calculated to allay the thirst in hot weather. One pound of carbonate of soda, and 13½ ounces of tartaric acid supply the materials for 256 powders of each sort.

SOFT-BOILED EGGS:

Although one of the simplest articles of food, there is nevertheless art in preparing a soft-boiled egg, so great an art that every householder is advised to provide herself with an egg-boiler. This is a little apparatus made of block-tin, furnished with a receptacle for hot water and a two-storied waiter for holding at least one dozen eggs. On top of the handle, around which the lid fits closely, rests a three-minute glass, enabling one to judge precisely of the time that his egg has been boiling, provided always that the water is assuredly boiling when poured over the eggs. The taste of the person for whom the eggs are cooked must be ascertained and particularly attended to, if satisfaction is to be expected from the process. For most persons 1½ minutes is allowed for having them just right; but others, again, like only 1 minute and yet others 2. When soft-boiled eggs are served there should be placed conveniently a pat of fresh butter, the pepper-crust, salt-cellar, and a plate of cold loaf-bread.

SOILED CLOTHES:

Soiled clothes should never be kept in a bedroom closet. They render it unsavory, with an odor that clings when the offending cause has been removed. The hamper for these should stand in the bathroom, or in a corner where there is a free circulation of air. They should never be put where they are liable to fall a prey to mice or cockroaches. These will scent food that has been spilled upon garments, or even the starch in them, and make a feast of it, devouring the fabric at the same time.

SORE THROAT, CUES FOR:

(1) Powdered potash held on the tongue and allowed to dissolve is very good for sore throat when there are "white spots."

(2) For clergymen's sore throat use fluid extract Callinsonia and simple syrup, equal parts. Take a tea-spoonful 3 or 4 times a day.

(3) Take the whites of 2 eggs and beat them in with 2 spoonfuls of white sugar; grate in a little nutmeg, and then add a pint of luke warm water. Stir well and drink often. Repeat the prescription if necessary. A practical physician thinks it will cure the most obstinate case of hoarseness in a short time.

(4) One of the best of cures is a cold-water compress. Before going to bed wet a cotton rag in cold water and wring it partially dry. Put it closely around the throat, and wrap around it a large piece of flannel to keep the moisture in. In the morning bathe the throat in cold water and rub briskly with a coarse towel to prevent catching cold.

(5) Every body has a cure for this trouble, but simple remedies appear to be most effectual. Salt and water is used by many as a gargle, but a little alum and honey dissolved in sage tea is better. Others use a few drops of camphor on loaf-sugar, which very often affords immediate relief. An application of cloths wrung out of hot water and applied to the neck, changed as often as it begins to cool, has the most potency in removing inflammation.

SOUP:

It is always well to begin the dinner, as every Frenchman does, with soup. This quiets the excessive craving of the stomach, but does not completely satisfy the hunger; and by thus subduing its voracity prevents it from inordinate indulgence in food that is less easy of digestion. So also is there a good reason why the sweet thing should be eaten at the close of the dinner. All saccharine food has the effect of quickly satiating, and if taken at the commencement of a meal would satisfy the appetite so completely as to indispose it for the other more substantial articles of diet.

SPAVIN (1) AND RING-BONE CURE:

Venice turpentine and Spanish flies, of each 2 ounces; euphorbium and aqua ammonia, of each 1 ounce; lard, 1 1/2 lbs. Pulverize all and put into the lard; simmer slowly over coals, not scorching or burning, and pour off free of sediment. For ring-bones cut off the hair, and rub the ointment well into the lumps once in 48 hours. For spavin once in 24 hours for 3 mornings. Wash well previous to each application with suds, rubbing over

(1) A disease of horses where a deposit or infusion of lymph develops in the hock joint.

the place with a smooth stick to squeeze out a thick yellow matter. This has removed very large ring-bones.

SPONGES, TO CLEANSE:

Sponges can be cleansed by washing them in ammonia and water (use the proportion of a tea-spoonful to 2 quarts) and afterward in a solution of muriatic acid—1 part acid to 25 parts water. Sponges are not kept clean without care. They should be thoroughly rinsed, then aired and dried, after every using, and unless they can be kept thus scrupulously neat they should be banished. For our own use a small piece of Turkish toweling or a neatly hemmed piece of old table-cloth, which can go through the regular laundry process, seems neater. Buttermilk is excellent for cleaning sponges. Steep the sponge in the milk for some hours, then squeeze it out and wash it in cold water. Lemon-juice is also good.

SPRAINS, REMEDY FOR:

(1) Put the white of an egg into a saucer, keep stirring it with a piece of alum about the size of a walnut until it becomes a thick jelly; apply a portion of it on a piece of lint or tow large enough to cover the sprain, changing it for a fresh one as often as it feels warm or dry; the limb is to be kept in an horizontal position by placing it on a chair.

(2) Sprains are always promptly relieved by allowing the coldest water to fall upon the part steadily, until no discomfort is experienced. Repeat as often as necessary. Keep the sprained joint elevated if about the hands, and horizontal if about the feet, so as to pomote the flow of blood from the parts by gravity, and live for a few days on fruits and coarse bread mainly.

(3) In case of sprain or bruise, after it has been well bathed with extremely hot water, the extract of witch-hazel heated, poured on flannel, and bound on the part will relieve the pain as quickly as if it really contained magical properties.

(4) The white of an egg into which a piece of alum about the size of a walnut has been stewed until it forms a jelly is capital remedy for sprains. It should be laid over the sprain upon a piece of lint, and be changed as it becomes dry.

(5) Rub sprains, bruises, and lameness with a paste made of salt and the white of an egg.

Sprained Ankle or Wrist: Wash the ankle very frequently with cold salt and water, which is far better than warm vinegar or decoctions of herbs. Keep the foot as cool as possible to prevent inflammation, and sit with it elevated on a high cushion. Live on low diet, and take every day some cooling medicine, such as Epsom salts. It cures in a few days.

SPRING MEDICINES:

It is a popular error that certain seasons of the year call for the taking of certain forms of medicine, even when there seems to be no change from health. Thus "a good spring medicine" is now called for by many otherwise sensible people as regularly as our ancestors asked their physicians for their annual or quarterly blood-letting. The "spring medicine" is a "something to purify the blood," and this means an active cathartic, as a rule. The purity of the blood is probably not affected by any such drugs. It becomes "impure" by reason of some special poison, like that of ague, typhoid fever, measles, small-pox, or the like, entering the life current and increasing therein, or by reason of the lungs, kidneys, or skin not properly acting, as a rule.

SPRINGS, HOW TO FORM:

The finest spring can be made by boring, which is performed by forcing an iron rod into the earth by its own weight, turning it round, and forcing it up and down by a spring-pole contrivance. The water will sometimes spout up several feet above the surface. Iron pipes are put down in the hole after the water is found. Depressed situations having a southern exposure, with rising ground toward the north, are the best situations in which to find water.

SQUASHES, TO KEEP:

Squashes are injured by the lightest frosts, and should be kept in a warm, dry store-room rather than in a cellar; if hung up by the stem in a cool place they will keep for many months.

SQUINTING:

Squinting frequently arises from the unequal strength of the eyes, the weaker eye being turned away from the object to avoid the fatigue of exertion. Cases of squinting of long standing have often been cured by covering the stronger eye, and thereby compelling the weaker one to exertion.

STAINS, REMOVING:

Grease-spots: Cold rain-water and soap will remove machine-grease from washable fabrics.

Stains from Acids: Can be removed by spirits of hartshorn, diluted. Repeat if necessary.

Wine-stains: May be taken out of articles by holding the spots in milk while it is boiling. Sal-volatile, or hartshorn, will restore colors taken out by acid. It may be dropped upon any garment without doing harm.

Iron-rust: Dip the rusty spots in a solution of tartaric or citric acid; or wet the spots with lemon-juice and salt, and expose it to the sun.

Mildewed Linen: This may be restored by soaping the spots while wet, covering them with fine chalk scraped to powder, and well rubbed in.

To Remove Mildew: Remove mildew by dipping in sour buttermilk and laying in the sun.

Coffee-stains: Pour on them a small stream of boiling water before putting the article in the wash.

Grass-stains: Wash the stained pieces in clean, cold, soft water, without soap, before the garment is otherwise wet.

Tea-stains: Clear boiling water will remove tea-stains and many fruit-stains. Pour the water through the stain, and thus prevent its spreading over the fabric.

Medicine-stains: These may be removed from silver spoons by rubbing them with a rag dipped in sulphuric acid, and washing it off with soap-suds.

Fruit-stains: Freezing will take out all old fruit-stains, and scalding with boiling water will remove those that have never been through the wash.

For Fruit and Wine Stains: Mix 2 tea-spoonfuls of water and 1 of spirit of salt, and let the stained part lie in this for 2 minutes, then rinse in cold water, or wet the stain with hartshorn.

Ink-stains: Ink-stains may sometimes be taken out by smearing with hot tallow, left on when the stained articles go to the wash.

How to Take Marking-ink out of Linen: A saturated solution of cyanuret of potassium applied with a camel's-hair brush. After the marking-ink disappears the linen should be well washed in cold water.

Ink in Cotton, Silk, and Woolen Goods: Saturate the spots with spirits of turpentine, and let it remain several hours; then rub it between the hands. It will crumple away without injuring either the color or texture of the article.

Ink-stains on Mahogany: Put a few drops of spirits of niter in a tea-spoonful of water, touch the spot with a feather dipped in the mixture, and when the ink disappears rub it over at once with a rag dipped in cold water, or there will be a white mark not easily effaced.

Ink-stains on Silver: The tops and other portions of silver ink-stands frequently become deeply discolored with ink, which is difficult to remove by ordinary means. It may, however, be completely eradicated by making a little chloride of lime into a paste with water, and rubbing it upon the stains. Chloride of lime has been misnamed "the general bleacher," but it is a foul enemy to all metallic surfaces.

Ink and Iron Mold: This may be taken out by wetting the spots in milk, then covering them with common salt. It should be done before the garment has been washed. Another way to take out ink is to dip it in melted tallow. For fine, delicate articles, this is the best way.

To Remove Paint-stains on Windows: It frequently happens that painters splash the plate or other glass windows when they are painting the sills. When this is the case melt some soda in a very hot water and wash them with it, using a soft flannel. It will entirely remove the paint.

Stains on the Hands: A few drops of oil of vitriol (sulphuric acid) in water will take the stains of fruit, dark dyes, stove-blacking, etc., from the hands without injuring them. Care must, however, be taken not to drop it upon the clothes. It will remove the color from woolen, and eat holes in cotton fabrics. To remove ink or fruit stains from the fingers, take cream of tartar, 1/2 ounce; powdered salt of sorrel(1), 1/2 ounce; mix. This is what is sold for salts of lemon.

To Extract Grease-spots from Books: Gently warm the greased or spotted part of the book or paper, and then press upon it pieces of blotting-paper, one after another, so as to absorb as much of the grease as possible. Have ready some fine, clear, essential oil of turpentine heated almost to a boiling state, warm the greased leaf a little, and then with a soft, clean brush apply the heated turpentine both sides of the potted part. By repeating this application the grease will be extracted. Lastly, with another brush, dipped in rectified spirits of wine, go over the place carefully, until the paper becomes smooth and clean.

Removing Tar-spots: The old remedy for removing tar is butter; tar is soluble in fat, and especially in butter; when this is left on the tar-spot for some time, both butter and tar are easily washed out by a sponge, with soap and water. It is the same with resinous wagon-grease. A creamy mixture of powdered extract of liquorice, with oil of aniseed, will easily dissolve tar, resin, pitch,

(1) Rumex Acetosa, a plant containing a large quantity of bioxalate of potash.

Venice turpentine, etc. It is afterward washed out with soap and warm water.

To Remove Grease from Coat-collars: Wash with a sponge moistened with hartshorn and water.

To Extract Grease from Papered Walls: Dip a piece of flannel in spirits of wine and rub the greasy spots gently once or twice.

To Clean Wall-paper: Tie a soft cloth over a broom, and sweep down the walls carefully.

STAIR-CARPETS, HOW TO LAY:

To save your stair carpets from wearing out at the edge, they should always have a strip of paper put under them at and over the edge of every stair, which is the part where they first wear out, in order to lessen the friction of the carpet against the boards beneath. The strips should be within an inch or two as long as the carpet is wide, and about 4 or 5 in. in breadth, so as to lie a distance from each stair.

STAMMERING, CURES FOR:

(1) Where there is no malformation of the organs of articulation stammering may be remedied by reading aloud with the teeth closed. This should be practiced for 2 hours a day for 3 or 4 months. The advocate of this simple remedy says, "I can speak with certainty of its utility."

(2) A simple, easy, and effectual cure of stammering is simply, at every syllable pronounced, to tap at the same time with the finger; by so doing, the most inveterate stammerer will be surprised to find that he can pronounce quite fluently, and by long and constant practice he will pronounce perfectly well.

(3) *The effectual cure mainly depends upon the determination of the sufferer to carry out the following rule:*

Keep the teeth close together, and before attempting to speak inspire deeply; then give time for quiet utterance, and after every slight practice the hesitation will be relieved. No spasmodic action of the lower jaw must be permitted to separate the teeth when speaking.

STARCHING, FOLDING, AND IRONING:

To Prepare Starch: Take 2 table-spoonfuls of starch dissolved in as much water; add a gill of cold water; then add 1 pint of boiling water, and boil it half an hour, adding a small piece of spermaceti, sugar, or salt; strain, etc. Thin it with water.

Flour Starch: Mix flour gradually with cold water so that it may be free from lumps. Stir in cold water till it will pour easily; then stir it into a pot of boiling water, and let it boil 5 or 6 minutes, stirring it frequently. A little spermaceti will make it smoother. This starch will answer very well for cotton and linen. Poland starch is made in the same manner.

Starching Clothes: Muslins look well when starched and clapped dry while the starch is hot, then folded in a damp cloth till they become quite damp before ironing them. If muslins are sprinkled they are apt to be spotted. Some clap muslins, then dry them, and afterward sprinkle them.

Folding Clothes: Fold the fine articles and roll them in a towel; then fold the rest, turning them all right side outward. Lay the colored articles separate from the rest. They should not remain damp long, as the colors might be injured. Sheets and table linen should be shaken and folded.

Gloss for Linen: "Starch Luster" is a substance used for washing purposes, which, when added to starch, causes the linen to which it is applied to assume not only a high polish, but a dazzling whiteness. A portion, of the size of a copper cent, added to $^1/_2$ lb. of starch, and boiled with it for 2 or 3 minutes, will produce the best results. This substance is nothing more than stearine, paraffine, or wax, colored by a slight admixture of ultramarine blue, which may be added at will.

To Make Flat-irons Smooth: Rub them with clean lard and wipe dry; or rubbing them with a little beeswax while hot will have the desired effect. Rub them with fine salt and it will make them perfectly smooth.

To Preserve Irons from Rust: Melt fresh mutton suet, smear over the irons with it while hot, then dust it well with unslaked lime, powdered, and tied up in muslin. When not used wrap the irons in baize, and keep them in a dry place. Use no oil on them at any time except salad-oil.

To Remove Starch or Rust from Flat-irons: Have a piece of yellow beeswax tied in a coarse cloth. When the iron is almost hot enough to use, but not quite, rub it quickly with the beeswax, and then with a clean, coarse cloth. This will remove it entirely.

Ironing: In ironing a shirt first do the back, then the sleeves, then the collar and bosom, and then the front. Calicoes should be ironed on the right side, as they thus keep clean for a longer time. In ironing a frock first do the waist, then the sleeves, then the skirt. Keep the skirt rolled while ironing the other parts, and set a chair to hold the sleeves while ironing the skirt, unless a skirt-board be used. Silk should be ironed on the wrong side, when quite damp, with a iron which is not very hot, as light colors are apt to change and fade. In ironing velvet turn up the face of the iron, and after dampening the wrong side of the velvet draw it over the face of the iron, holding it straight. Always iron lace and needle-work on the wrong side.

To Clear-starch Lace, etc.: Starch for laces should be thicker and used hotter than for linens. After your laces have been well washed and dried, dip them into the thick, hot starch in such a way as to have every part properly starched. Then wring all the starch out, and spread them out smooth on a piece of linen; roll them up together and let them remain for about a half an hour, when they will be dry enough to iron. Some think that laces should never be clapped between the hand, as it injures them. Cambrics do not require so thick starch as net or lace. Some people prefer cold or raw starch for book-muslin, as some of this kind of muslin has a thick, clammy appearance if starched in boiled starch. Fine laces are sometimes wound round a glass bottle to dry, which prevents them from shrinking.

Ironing Laces: Ordinary laces and worked muslin can be ironed by the usual process with a smoothing or sad iron; finer laces cannot be. When the lace has been starched and dried, ready for ironing, spread it out as smooth as possible on an ironing-cloth, and press over it, back and forth, as quickly as you can, a smooth, round glass bottle containing hot water, giving the bottle such pressure as may be required to smooth the lace. Sometimes you may pass the laces over the bottle, taking care to keep them smooth. Either way is much better than to iron.

Gum Arabic Starch: Get 2 ounces of fine white gum arabic and pound it to powder. Next put it into a pitcher and pour on it a pint or more of boiling water, (according to the degree of strength you desire), and then, covering it, let it set all night. In the morning pour it carefully from the dregs into a clean bottle, cork it, and keep it for use. A table-spoonful of gum-water stirred into a pint of starch that has been made in the usual manner will give to lawn (either white or printed) a look of newness to which nothing else can restore it after washing. It is also good (much diluted) for thin white muslin and bobbinet.

STINGS OF INSECTS, ETC:

The sting of a bee is generally more virulent than that of a wasp, and with some people attended with more violent effects. The sting of a bee is barbed at the end, and consequently, always left in the wound; that of a wasp is pointed only, so that they can sting more than once, which a bee cannot do. When stung by a bee, let the sting, in the first place, be instantly pulled out; for the longer it remains in the wound the deeper it will pierce, owing to its peculiar form, and emit more of the poison. The sting is hollow, and the poison flows through it, which is the sole cause of the pain and inflammation. The pulling out of the sting should be done carefully, and with a steady hand, for if any part of it breaks, in all remedies then, in a great measure, will be ineffectual.

When the sting is extracted suck the wounded part if possible, and very little inflammation, if any, will ensue. If hartshorn drops are immediately afterward rubbed on the part, the cure will be more complete. All notions of the efficacy of sweet-oil, bruised parsley, burnet, tobacco, etc., appear on various trials to be totally groundless. On some people the stings of bees and wasps have no effect; it is therefore of little consequence what remedy they apply to the wound. However, the effect of stings greatly depends on the condition of body a person is in; at one time a sting will take little or no effect, though no remedy is used, which at another time will be very virulent on the same person. We have had occasion to test this remedy several times, and can safely vouch for its efficacy. The exposure to which persons are subjected during the hot summer months will no doubt render this advice very useful; its very simplicity making it more acceptable. Press the barrel of a watch-key over the part so as to expose the sting, which must be removed. Lay a rag moistened with hartshorn and oil over the part. Give 6 or 8 drops of hartshorn in 2 ounces of infusion of camomile, and cover up in bed.

STOCKINGS, TO MEND:

Stockings should always be mended with cotton of the same color. A single thread must be used. The doubled cotton may close the gap more quickly, but it produces a lump that is apt to make the wearer of the stocking thoroughly uncomfortable. There are some unfortunates who claim that their skins are too sensitive to permit of their wearing mended hose. If the repairing is skillfully done there is no reason why there should be any suffering from this cause. The thread should be run through the fabric some distance on each side of the hole as well as back and forth across it. Worn places should also be darned before a real break appears.

The old custom of running the heels of stockings before they were put on at all is almost obsolete, but its revival might not come amiss in large families where there are plenty of small feet to tread out the heels of stockings, while the rest of the foot and the leg are still good. The heel-protectors that are sold at most large shoe-stores save wear to the stocking. So does the habit of changing the hose often enough to prevent their becoming stiff with dirt, or perspiration. Mothers of little children occasionally sew a piece on the inside of the stocking knee to prevent the skin showing as the outer covering becomes frayed.

STOMACH, INFORMATION ABOUT THE:

(1) The position of the stomach is more nearly vertical than horizontal.

(2) An empty stomach, if in good tone, is always tubular.

(3) A tubular stomach should be the rule on rising.

(4) Non-irritating liquids pass directly through the tubular stomach.

(5) They do likewise if the stomach contains food, and in such cases pass along the lesser curvature.

(6) The morning mucus contained in the stomach hinders or retards digestion.

(7) Water drank before meals dilutes and washes out this mucus, stimulates the gastro-enteric tract to peristalsis, and causes hyperamia of its lining membrane, thus greatly aiding the process of digestion as well as elimination.

(8) Cold water should be given to those who have the power to react, while warm or hot water must be administered to all others.

(9) Salt added to the water is very beneficial in preventing the formation of unabsorbable parapeptone.

(10) It is perfectly proper to drink water before, during, and after meals.

STONES, TO REMOVE FROM FIELDS:

(1) Heat the stone to a high degree by means of a fierce fire applied to one part of it only, which will cause it to expand; when the stone has been thus made intensely hot, pour water upon it to make it crack, the effect being increased with powerful blows given with very heavy hammers.

(2) Pierce the stone in the direction of its veins, and introduce into the hole a cleft cylinder of iron; then drive a wedge of the same metal in between the two halves of the cylinder.

(3) A quantity of water may, during the winter season, be introduced into a hole made in the stone to a sufficient depth, the aperture to be then closed with a stopper closely driven into it. The water contained in this hole, expanding as it freezes, exerts a force sufficient to break in pieces the strongest stone.

STOVES IN SUMMER:

It is a great mistake to remove in warm weather from all the rooms of our houses all heating apparatus. As a matter of fact, in the latitude of New York, and in many places south of that latitude on the sea-coast, there are many days in the summer when artificial heat is a necessity to the comfort of a great many people. Invalids, elderly people, young children, really suffer from cold in the summer time. The dews of evening and early morning dampen not the feet only, but the entire apparel of persons exposed to them, and render the warmth of a fire not only pleasant to the sensibilities, but requisite to the preservation of health. There should be in one room, accessible to all members of the family, a grate, fire-place, or stove, where, on the shortest notice, a fire can be kindled and damp feet dried, and purple fingers and faces made rosy again.

Coal-oil stoves are many of them made with heaters, and these are useful in this climate on account of their portability and the quickness with which they will when lighted warm a room. "An ounce of prevention is worth a pound of cure." Many an attack of chills, of fever, or rheumatism, would be saved if those exposed and liable to such attacks could at the right time have access to abundance of artificial heat. Then, too, we have a great many damp days in summer, especially along the sea-coast, when mildew and mustiness in our furniture and dry-goods would be saved by heating our houses thoroughly and expelling the accumulated moisture. Open grates and fire-places are the pleasantest methods of heating in the summer time; but where these are not in reach, stove-heat is not to be despised or neglected.

STUMPS, TO BLOW OUT;

The cheapest and most effective way to get rid of stumps in a field is to blast them out with cartridges of giant powder. This is put up in cartridges about 10 in. long by 1½ in. in diameter, and these can be cut into pieces of the size required with a knife. A piece 2 in. long is sufficient to throw out a good-sized stump. A hole is punched under the stump with a crowbar; the explosive, with the proper fuse and fulminating cap attached, is put into the hole; water is poured in as tamping, and the fuse is fired. The explosion throws the stump out in several pieces, leaving the hole to be filled up afterward.

STUMPS, TO BURN:

In the autumn or early winter bore a hole 1 or 2 in. in diameter, according to the girth of the stump, and about 18 in. deep; put into it 1 or 2 ounces of saltpeter; fill the hole with water and plug it close; in the ensuing spring take out the plug and pour in about a gill of kerosene oil and ignite it. The stump will smoulder away, without blazing, to the very extremity of the roots, leaving nothing but ashes.

STY IN THE EYE:

(1) Sties are little abscesses which form between the roots of the eyelashes, and are rarely larger than a small pea. The best way to manage them is to bathe them frequently with warm water or warm poppy-water if very painful. When they have burst use an ointment composed of 1 part of citron ointment and 4 of spermaceti, well rubbed together, and smear along the edge of the eyelid. Give a grain or two of calomel with 5 or 8 grains of rhubarb, according to the age of the child, twice a week. The old-fashioned and apparently ab-

surd practice of rubbing the sty with a ring is as good and speedy a cure as any process of medicinal application, though the number of times it is rubbed or the quality of the ring and direction of the strokes have nothing to do with its success. The pressure and the friction excite the vessels of the part, and cause an absorption of the effused matter under the eyelash. The edge of the nail will answer as well as a ring.

(2) Take a fig, cut it once or twice in two, put it in a cup, pour boiling water on it, and let it stand until cool, not cold, then bathe the eye with the water quite frequently.

(3) Put a tea-spoonful of tea in a small bag, pour on it just enough boiling water to moisten it, then put it on the eye pretty warm. Keep it on all night, and in the morning the sty will most likely be gone; if not, a second application is sure to remove it.

SUFFOCATION, TO AVOID:

To avoid suffocation in a house on fire steep a handkerchief or towel in water and tie it round the head covering the mouth and nostrils. In that condition a person will be in a position to breathe freely and walk in the densest smoke to be met with in a burning building.

SUNBURN AND FRECKLES:

To get off the freckles, to cause the sunburn to disappear, you have got to put on your face and neck, and on your arms, darkened by battling with the waves, a mixture of 2 parts of Jamaica rum to 1 of lemon-juice; dabble it well on the surface, let it dry, and wash it off in the morning in your hot bath. Besides whitening the skin, which the lemon does, the rum gives it a vigor and makes a rosy flush come to the surface. You will gain no good from this by doing it or 1 or 2 nights; keep it up for 2 weeks at the least, and remember that when your skin has that depressed, worn-out look that comes from sitting up too late at night nothing will invigorate it like a few drops of Jamaica rum put into the water with which you wash your face.

Wash for Sunburn: Take 2 drams of borax, 1 dram of Roman alum, 1 dram of camphor, $^1/_2$ ounce of sugar candy and 1 lb. of ox-gall. Mix and stir well for a fortnight, till it appears clear and transparent. Strain through blotting-paper, and bottle up for use.

SUN CURE, THE:

Hidden among the mountains of Carinthia lies a little wooden-roofed village of Veldes, or Bledu, in the irresponsible language of its Slavonic inhabitants. It stands on the shores of a small lake of deep blue water. By the lake hotels and villas congregate. These are one and all brilliant and festive dwellings. To this romantic little shrine sun-worshippers come during the summer to offer sacrifices, while a larger number of pleasure-seekers flock in from Trieste, from all parts of Germany, Poland, and the north of Italy. What I lost in the society of the amiable and the wealthy I never knew, for they lived down on the lake side in the "air-hut colony," while I remained in the village high above the lake. The "air-huts" are little wooden dwellings for the sun-cure patients, consisting of 1 large room which has 3 walls instead of 4. The flat roof of the bath-house has been inclosed by a tall fence, so that only the sky is visible from the inclosure. Here, with heads carefully shaded from the hot rays, each in a wooden compartment, the patients frizzle for about 1 or $1^1/2$ hours. This process is soothing, strange as it may appear. The sun-god rewards his devotees.

Now and then a voice calls above the divisions for a glass of water, now and then a sigh over the heat escapes a worshiper; otherwise the place is quiet and sleepy and reposeful. Reading or mental exertion of any kind is forbidden, and indeed severely punished by headache or exhaustion. Uninspired must be the drowsy observations that mingle now and then with the humming of the flies, and no one attempts to break this rigid law. Even the execrations wring from the sufferers by the persistent attacks of these insects ought to be of the mildest character possible, considering the provocation. Much had to be endured from the active colony that had established themselves at the sun bath. During the last 10 or 20 minutes the faithful are wrapped up in blankets like mummies; a tepid bath and a rubbing follows, and then the long-suffering one is released, but only to repeat the process in the afternoon. Through the opposite actions of the cool air in the morning and of the sun and midday great things to the advantage of the patient are said to occur. Dr. Rikli traces a large number of illnesses, nervous and other, to the want of vigorous skin action and the consequent strain on the other parts of the body to do the work which the lazy skin is neglecting to do.

SUNDAY DINNER, THE:

The custom of preparing Sunday's food on Saturday, and making a cold dinner an inseparable accompaniment to the day of sacred rest, has happily become a thing of the past. Even the most strait-laced now consider cooking plain meals one of those works of necessity and mercy against which there is no law. A few conservatives who cannot quite relinquish ancient usages compromise by serving the Sunday roast cold, but flanking it with a variety of hot vegetables. While there is an ounce of absurdity in condemning one's family to eat food that has been cooling for 24 hours, there is yet a degree of unkindness insisting upon a more elaborate repast on what is supposed to be tbe easiest day of the week than is demanded on any other.

A little extra labor on Saturday will reduce Sunday's work to a minimum, and yet provide as tempting fare as any one, except a very critical gastronomist, need exact. Soup should be made on Saturday. The stock can be prepared then, and nothing left for the next day but the thickening and seasoning. Even this may be done on Saturday, along with the straining and clearing, and the soup be none the worse for it—rather better, indeed. The meat may be skewered ready for the pan; or if fowls are to be served they may be drawn and trussed, the bread crumbed for the stuffing, and the seasoning mixed with this. The stuffing itself must not be inserted until just before the fowls go into the oven, as it becomes soggy if left in too long before cooking. If salads are desired, the mayonnaise can be mixed on Saturday, and will be benefited by a night on the ice.

SUNLIGHT AND HEALTH:

Sunlight is one of the most powerful forces in nature, kindling the whole vegetable world into being, and making animal life possible by its extraordinary chemical agency.

SUNLIGHT AND HUMAN LIFE:

Sir James Wylie says that "the cases of disease on the dark side of an extensive barrack at St. Petersburg have been uniformly for many years in the proportion of 3 to 1 to those on the side exposed to strong light." Dr. Forbes uses the following language: "It may be enunciated as an indisputable fact that all who live and pursue their calling in situations where the minimum of light is permitted to penetrate suffer seriously in bodily and mental health. The total exclusion of the sunbeam induces the severer forms of chlorosis, green sickness, and other anemic conditions depending upon an impoverished and disordered state of the blood. Under these circumstances the face assumes a death-like paleness, the membranes of the eyes become bloodless, and the skin shrunken and turned into a white, greasy, waxy color; also emaciation, muscular debility and degeneration, dropsical effusion, softening of the bones, general nervous excitability, morbid irritability of the heart, loss of appetite, tendency to syncope and hemorrhages, consumption, physical deformity, stunted growth, mental impairment, and premature old age. The offspring of those so unhappily trained are often deformed, weak, and puny, and are disposed to scrofulous affections."

SUNLIGHT AND SLEEP:

Sleepless people—and they are many in America—should court the sun. The very worst soporific(1) is laudanum, and the very best; sunshine. Therefore, it is very plain that poor sleepers should pass many hours in the day in sunshine, and as few as possible in the shade.

SUN-SCALD:

When apple-trees are commencing to open their leaf buds, the ter-

(1) Sleep inducer.

minal ones frequently already opened, there is susceptibility to sun-scald. The edges of the terminal leaves will turn to a dark color and the bark from green to black, on the south or south-west side first, and from hour to hour curves around the tree. The best relief is to at once severely crop off below the parts affected.

SUN-STROKE, MOST DANGEROUS TIME FOR:

About the third or fourth day from the commencement of a heated term sun-strokes usually appear. The sufferers in most cases are exposed to the heat for some days preceding the attack. In the summer of 1866 the majority of sun-stroke cases—generally laboring men—were brought to Bellevue Hospital in the morning or early in the day.

Premonitory Symptoms of Sun-stroke: The symptoms of sun-stroke are usually headache, vertigo, dimness of vision, nausea, often developing into coma, or even delirium or convulsions, ending in many cases in insanity, softening of the brain, or death.

Hints for the Prevention of Sun-stroke: *For the prevention of sun-stroke the following are hints, especially when there is a tendency to a hot brain:*

Wear a light-colored, well ventilated hat. Avoid meats and other heating foods. Eat plenty of fruit. Wet the hair on the temples and top of the head often, but not behind. If the hot brain pressure is felt coming on, dash cold water on the face and temples, or in the absence of that, clasp and squeeze both temples with the fingers to crowd the blood back, and rub the back of the neck powerfully to draw the blood from the brain. Where special danger is apprehended, wear a cool, wet bandage around the forehead and head.

Treatment of Sun-stroke after Recovery: After consciousness has returned, mustard plasters or blisters are to be applied to the back of the neck. As soon as convenient the patient should be sent to a cool district in the country, and kept free from excitement. The brain must rest from all work. Exercise in the open air and nourishing diet are essential; regular habits must be rigidly enforced. A continuance of this treatment for several months prevents, or at least lessens, the danger from nervous affections which follow sun-stroke.

SUN-STROKE, PREVENTION AND TREATMENT OF:

Sun-stroke is caused by excessive heat, and especially if the weather is "muggy." It is more apt to occur on the second, third or fourth day of a heated term than on the first. Loss of sleep, worry, excitement, close sleeping-rooms, debility, abuse of stimulants predispose to it. It is more apt to attack those working in the sun, and especially between the hours of 11 o'clock in the forenoon and 4 o'clock in the afternoon. Have as cool sleeping-rooms as possible. Avoid loss of sleep and all unnecessary fatigue. If working indoors and where there is artificial heat—laundries, etc.—see that the room is well ventilated. If working in the sun wear a light hat, (not black, as it absorbs the heat), straw, etc., and put inside of it on the head a wet cloth or a large green leaf; frequently lift the hat from the head and see that the cloth is wet. Do not check perspiration, but drink what water you need to keep it up, as perspiration prevents the body from being over-heated. Have, whenever possible, an additional shade, as a thin umbrella when walking, a canvas or broad cover when working in the sun. When much fatigued do not go to work, especially after 11 o'clock in the morning on very hot days, if the work is in the sun.

If a feeling of fatigue, dizziness, headache, or exhaustion occurs, cease work immediately, lie down in a shady and cool place; apply cool cloths to and pour cold water over the head and on the neck. If any one is overcome by the heat send immediately for the nearest good physician. While waiting for the physician give the person cool drinks of water, or cold black tea or cold coffee, if able to swallow. If the skin is hot and dry sponge with or pour cold water over the body and limbs, and apply to the head, pounded ice wrapped in a towel or other cloth. If there is no ice at hand, keep a cold cloth on the head, and pour cold water on it as on the body. If the person is pale, very faint, and pulse feeble, let him inhale ammonia for a few seconds, or give him a tea-spoonful of aromatic spirits of ammonia in 2 table-spoonfuls of water with a little sugar.

SWEATS, TREATMENT OF:

A mixture of 3 parts of salicylic acid and 87 parts silicate of magnesia is said to be not only a remedy for sweating of the feet, but, when rubbed over the whole body, on the authority of Dr. Kohnhom, a cure for night sweating by consumptives(1).

SWEEPING:

The preparation of the apartment for sweeping and its restoration to order afterward take more time than is consumed in the actual broom-work. The bric-a-brac must be carefully dusted and put in a safe place, the movable furniture brushed and wiped off and carried from the room, and the larger pieces kept for the service alone. The draperies must be unhooked from the rings, shaken out of the window, and brushed off with a whisk-broom. Small rugs must also be brushed and shaken. Doing all this at first is much better than postponing it until the sweeping is done. There will be quite enough to look after then without having another task to attend to when the weary reaction comes that usually follows vigorous exertion.

Some exceptionally neat housewives insist upon their parlors receiv-

(1) Caused by consumption (tuberculosis).

ing a complete cleaning once each week. Unless the drawing-room is also the family sitting-room, and it as such consistently occupied, this is hardly necessary. The room should be carefully dusted every morning, the floor gone over with a carpet-sweeper twice a week, and the regular sweeping, in which furniture, draperies, and bric-a-brac are removed, done once a fortnight. To attempt this important task the sweeper should array herself in appropriate garb. A rather short dress of some wash material, loosely fitted about the waist and sleeves so as to give the arms free play, a neat cap that will cover the hair entirely, easy shoes, and a pair of old gloves deprived of their finger-tips, form a comfortable and sensible uniform. Thus equipped, the dust is not to be feared, and the exercise, as exhilarating under proper circumstances as any form of calisthenics, will be really enjoyed.

For various reasons Friday is the best day for doing the bulk of the week's sweepings. The house must be made clean as late in the week as possible before Sunday. Saturday has its own appropriate duties, which leave no room for general sweeping. Performing the work earlier in the week allows space for becoming dirty again before the Sabbath puts a temporary ban upon labor. Even taking into account the desirability of getting the house into the state of apple-pie order dear to the heart of the true housekeeper, there is yet no necessity for doing it in such a manner that the other inmates of the home feel that they would prefer dirt to cleanliness at such a price.

SWEET-POTATOES, TO KEEP:

There is no better way than to pack them in dry sand in boxes, and keep the temperature of the place where they are stored at from 45 degrees to 60 degrees Fahr. Where one has but a few, dig when thoroughly ripe; handle them as carefully as if they were eggs; dry them well, and then pack in half-barrels or small boxes, and place them in the kitchen near the stove or some other warm place. The sand will absorb heat during the day and give it off slowly at night. In this way danger from freezing is obviated.

SWEETS:

Sweets are one of the curses of human civilization. They are the source of an untold amount of indigestion. They ferment very readily. They develop acidity, which diminishes the alkalinity of the blood, the blood being properly always alkaline, and to the effects of their use rheumatic subjects are particularly sensitive. Sweets do not include desserts merely, but they are found in the most unexpected places to the uninitiated. They are in—and they are the most pernicious principle—wines of all sorts, beers, and fruits. All fruits are sweet. The fact that an apple is sour does not remove it from this category. The same is true of all wines, claret even included. They are best regarded as the subjects of indulgence only, but on principle must be heartily condemned. If you have a sweet tooth pull it out.

SWELLED BREAST:

The swelling of the breasts to an enormous size is very common during the earlier months of pregnancy in plethoric(1) women. Boys and girls about the age of puberty are subject to slight swelling and tenderness, which soon disappears of itself if not interfered with. The breasts of new-born infants also are sometimes found to be swollen and hard.

Treatment: When the breasts are found to be hard and swollen they should be gently bathed with warm hog's lard, and a piece of folded linen saturated with it laid over them. If this means does not cause the swelling to subside, apply a warm poultice, changing it every 3 hours till the abscess breaks and discharges its matter, when it will speedily heal.

SUNBURN AND FRECKLES:

"To get off the freckles, to cause the sunburn to disappear, you have got to put on your face and neck, and on your arms, darkened by battling with the waves, a mixture of 2 parts of Jamaica rum to 1 of lemon-juice; dabble it well on the surface, let it dry, and wash it off in the morning in your hot bath. Besides whitening the skin, which the lemon does, the rum gives it a vigor and makes a rosy flush come to the surface."

(1) Having a superabundant body.

S—452

T

TABLE-COVERS:

(1) Handsome table-covers are made of alternate squares of half-squares of basket flannel and of velveteen; one made of 2 shades of brown is very pretty, and one of brown and lemon-color is particularly effective. The spread should be lined; it is not necessary that the entire lining should be of expensive material; unbleached factory cloth will answer, provided that the facing is deep. No border is requisite, but if one prefers to have it, this should be of velveteen, and the facing of a contrasting color. If the blocks are neatly put together, no needle-work is necessary to adorn the spread, but, of course, this point must be determined according to the taste and means of the maker.

(2) A simple but very handsome scarf for a small table is made by taking 3 strips of broad ribbon; have the center strip of a contrasting color; for instance, if the 2 outer pieces are of the somber or shaded ribbons, let the center be of cardinal; turn the ends back to make them pointed, and put a tassel on each point; baste the ribbon to a lining of silesia(1), old silk, or even to canton flannel, and where the edges join work fancy stitches. A great variety of scarfs could be made in this form, and be ornamented by putting sprays of flowers in embroidery or painted on each point, or a vine or a scroll could be worked with good effect on the center stripe.

(3) Small round tables can be covered with a pretty gray cloth; draw it over the edge and fasten it on the under side with carpet-tacks; finish the edge with macrame lace; do not fasten it on with tacks; take a needle and strong thread and blind-stitch it on. The lace should be lined with satin, of any color that will harmonize with the other furniture. Line a piece of the lace and fasten it around your shelf in place of the lambrequin, and you will like it much better. Take a piece of board the length of your shelf, cover it with the satin, paint a vine upon it; begin at the lower left-hand corner and let it extend almost to the upper right-hand corner; place this on your shelf against the wall, and you have a nice background for vases and small statuary.

(4) The first, for a table longer than wide, is of olive-green felt, trimmed

(1) A kind of thin coarse linen cloth.

with a band of cardinal plush about a finger wide, and put on with yellow embroidery silk in any of the fancy stitches. A worsted fringe composed of the different shades of olive-green, tipped with a dash of red, serves as a finish to the bottom. The lining is of olive-green canton flannel, although I had intended it to match the plush band but, not being able to get any thing near the color, had to fall back upon the olive-green. The second is a scarf of olive-brown plush-lined with cardinal silk. On one end is embroidered pink and white flowers, with their leaves in the different shades of green, and on the other side red and yellow flowers with their leaves. The cardinal lining extends beyond the plush on the long sides in 3 small folds, so as to form a finish. The short sides below the embroidery are finished with red silk balls about 1 in. apart. The third cover is for an octagon-topped stand. It is of English red plush, nailed tightly over the top. While from the sides hang scalloped lambrequins, 1 scallop to a side, each of which is embroidered in patterns of pink primroses, pond-lilies, forget-me-nots, fine white flowers, leaves, etc. A fancy fringe, the predominant color of which is red, finishes the bottom of each lambrequin. Instead of plush for the last 2 tables, felt or canton flannel may be used with very pretty effect.

TABLE ETIQUETTE:

There is nothing so disagreeable as careless and untidy table manners, and to acquire graceful and pleasing habits while eating sometimes takes years of practice, but it can be done; we see every-where ladies and gentlemen, and sometimes children, who show their good breeding by their conduct at the table. To begin to make yourselves like these, the first thing to do is to sit down and think how you really behave at the table. Are your hands and nails and face clean, and hair brushed back smoothly? Do you seat yourself quietly, and remember to put on your napkin? Do you sometimes put your knife in your mouth instead of a fork or a spoon? Do you pour your tea in your saucer instead of drinking from the cup? How do you pass your plate if you are to be helped a second time?

The best way is to hold your knife or fork in your hand, and then it will not fall on the cloth. Then about passing articles of food: Do you reach over another person's plate, or stand up to reach something not near at hand, and knock over a glass or cruet in the attempt? Do you eat fast and loud, and put large pieces in your mouth, or speak with food unchewed, or pick your teeth? O, I hope none of these, for any one of them would make you appear impolite and uncultivated. And then you remember not to whisper, yawn, or stretch, or touch the hair, or blow the nose. If it is necessary to use your handkerchief, do it so quietly that no one will notice it; but this should be done before you come to the table. And if there are bones, cherry-pits, and things that cannot be swallowed, do not spit them on the plate, but put them on your spoon and then on your plate.

Will you think of these hints the next time you sit down to your dinner and avoid them? And remember that courtesy at the table is as indispensable as away from it, and if you practice it at home you will not have to put it on when you are away, it will be so natural and easy for you.

TAKE CARE, GAME OF:

A flower-pot is filled with sand or earth; a little stick with a flag is placed in it. Every child playing has to remove a little sand from the pot, with a stick without upsetting the flag, crying at the same time, "Take care!" The one who upsets the flag pays a forfeit. It becomes an anxious matter when the sand has been removed several times.

TAN AND SUN-BURN:

Ladies who spend the summer in the country and at the sea-side may be glad to know of some simple remedies for tan and sun-burn. When the face is burnt by exposure it is best to bathe it with a little cold cream; this simple and pleasant wash will remove the discoloration and swelling as if by magic, and leave the skin cool and smooth.

To prevent tan and sun-burn, take the juice of a fresh lemon and rub it in thoroughly before going into the open air, allowing it to dry on the face; at night dust a little oatmeal upon the skin, and next morning, after washing it off, apply a little cold cream or buttermilk. Such a simple and harmless treatment will be found much more effectual than the use of cosmetics, which close up the pores and dry and roughen the finest complexion in a frightful way and in a short space of time.

During the height of summer the hands, face, and neck should, after being well washed in soft water at least once in 24 hours, have always well rubbed into them a very little cold cream or other pleasant emollient. This should be done by using a minute quantity and thoroughly rubbing it in, in which case not the slightest unpleasantness or after greasy effect will be apparent.

If after severe exposure the skin has been scorched by the sun, there is no case in which the old adage of a stitch in time saving nine has more force.

On retiring to rest the hot and reddened skin should be freely bathed with tepid water, and then anointed with a compound of borax, 10 grains; lime-water, 2 ounces; finest French oil of jasmine and oil of sweet almonds, each 1 ounce. If this be not at hand, fresh cream may be substituted, or even new milk. The tender surface must be only gently dabbed, not rubbed with any degree of force, in applying any of these. No soap whatever must be used for 2 or 3 days in washing the scorched skin—only tepid water; and if any detergent be necessary, a little almond meal or oatmeal. After each time of washing a little of the recipe, or of milk or cream, as attainable, must again be gently dabbed on the skin.

If, in spite of these precautions, any peeling of the skin and tan or brownness should ensue, apply this mixture every morning after washing: Chloride of ammonia, 2 drams; spirit of wine, 1 ounce; attar of roses, 10 drops; French rose-water, 1 pint; Venetian talc in finest powder, 1 ounce. Dissolve the chloride in the rose-water, and the attar in the spirit; mix the 2 solutions and add the talc.

With those whose skins have an inflammatory tendency, it is of the greatest importance during the summer to avoid a stimulating and heating diet, and to adopt a regimen largely composed of cooling foods, such as a liberal allowance of fruits—stewed, baked, or raw; salads, green vegetables, fish, poultry, and white meats.

TAPE-WORM, CURE FOR:

(1) Take at one dose ether, two-thirds ounce; 2 hours after this take caster-oil, 1 ounce. The worm is discharged entire or almost so, and always with the head intact.

(2) Take equal parts of tincture of assafetida(1) and tincture absinthil(2), in tea-spoonful doses, night and morning. No fasting is necessary.

TAR FROM THE HANDS, TO REMOVE:

We recommend rubbing the hands with the outside of fresh orange or lemon peel and wiping dry immediately. It is astonishing what a small piece will clean. The volatile oil in the skins dissolve the tar, so that it can be wiped off.

TEA:

Tea is adulterated with leaves of the sycamore, horse-chestnut, and plum; with lie teas, which is made up of tea-dust, sand, and gum to give it consistency; also with leaves of the beech, bastard plane, elm, poplar, willow, fancy oak, hawthorn, and sloe. It is colored with black-lead, rose, pink, Dutch pink, vegetable red and yellow dyes, arsenite of copper, chromate and bichromate of potash. Green teas are more adulterated than black. They are colored with Prussian blue, turmeric, Chinese yellow, etc., flavored with sulphate of iron, catechu gum, la veno beno, and Chinese botanical powder.

Tea-leaves that have been once used are collected, "doctored," and again sold as fresh tea. Obtain some genuine leaves of tea, moisten them, and lay them out with gum upon paper. Press them between the leaves of books, until dry. When you suspect a sample of tea, damp and unroll the

(1) A bad smelling gum resin obtained from plants of the parsley family.
(2) Absinth; a strong spirituous liquor flavored with wormwood and other plants containing absinthin.

leaves, and gum and dry them as genuine ones; you will then be able by comparison to detect the admixture.

Preparation: A silver or metal tea-pot is better than an earthen-ware one for drawing out the flavor and strength of the tea. The amount of tea used must depend upon the quantity required. The old-fashioned allowance is a very sensible one, i.e., 1 large tea-spoonful for each of the company, and 1 for the tea-pot.

Before making the tea pour 1/2 pint of boiling water into the tea-pot, and let it stand 2 or 3 minutes. Pour it out and immediately put in the tea. Close the lid and let it remain for a minute to heat, then pour upon it 1/2 pint of boiling water. Let it stand for 3 minutes, add sufficient boiling water to fill the tea-pot, and the tea will be ready for use. Be careful not to drain all the liquor from the pot so long as it is necessary to continue to add boiling water, or the tea will be very weak, and if it is desirable to add a little fresh tea let it be brewed separately in a tea-cup before it is added to that which is already made, as its strength will not be drawn out if it is put on the old leaves.

Perhaps it is unnecessary to say that unless the water is really boiling when it is put upon the tea there will be no good tea. Boiling after the tea is made injures the flavor, either by deadening or making it rank. Another way is to make a strong infusion by pouring boiling water upon tea and let it stand 20 minutes, putting into each cup no more than is necessary to fill about one third full; then each cup is filled with hot water from an urn or kettle; thus the tea is always hot and equally strong to the end. In preparing tea a good economist will be careful to have the best water, i.e., the softest and least impregnated with foreign mixture, for if tea be infused in hard and in soft water the latter will always yield the greatest quantity of the tanning matter, and will strike the deepest black, with sulphate of iron in solution.

TEETH, CARE OF THE:

Dissolve 2 ounces of borax in 3 pints of water; before quite cold add thereto 1 tea-spoonful of spirits of camphor; bottle the mixture for use. One wine-glass of the solution, added to 1/2 pint of tepid water, is sufficient for each application. This solution, applied daily, preserves and beautifies the teeth, extirpates tartarous adhesion, produces pearl-like whiteness, arrests decay, and induces a healthy action in the gums.

Camphorated Dentifrice: Prepared chalk, 1 lb.; camphor, 1 or 2 drams. The camphor must be finely powdered by moistening it with a little spirits of wine, and then intimately mixed with the chalk.

Myrrh Dentifrice: Powdered cuttle-fish, 1 lb.; powdered myrrh, 2 ounces.

A Wholesome Condition: A wholesome condition of the teeth is not only essential to good looks, but to daily comfort and permanent health. Chewing of the food, so necessary to a good digestion, cannot be properly performed with weak and diseased masticators, which are, in fact, the frequent cause of dyspepsia and other affections of the stomach. Local disease of the most tormenting kind, such as *tic-douloureux* and the various painful face, head, and ear aches, and disorders of the eye, as well as fatal cancer and tedious ulcers of the tongue and lips, are often due to no other cause than a decayed and ragged tooth.

Want of Cleanliness: This is, perhaps, the most direct of the preventable causes of the most common dental disease, viz., decay; for this is always the result of chemical action, progressing from without inward. Food allowed to remain in the crevices and interstices of the teeth soon decomposes, aided as it is by the heat and the moisture of the mouth; and acid being generated attacks the tooth structure, gradually but surely decomposing it, and this decay so formed is capable of again reproducing itself by its attack upon the sound bone beneath it. Time only is needed for the complete destruction of the structure, rapidity of which is retarded or not by the circumstances of constitution, vital force, etc.

Deposit of Tartar Injurious: An earthly substance, commonly known as tartar, is in greater or less quantities deposited on all teeth, which, if allowed to accumulate and harden, works great mischief by pressing the gums from their normal position, causing inflammation in them, and instead of being firm are spongy, bleeding from the slightest pressure. The roots of the teeth being thus partially exposed, they gradually become loose and sore, and often teeth which are so perfect in formation as to resist the action of decaying agents, perfectly sound themselves, lose so much of their vital connection with their sockets as to drop out. So insidiously do both of these diseased conditions progress, especially the latter, that many are just startled from the complacent reflection on the fact of never having had toothache to lament over irrecoverable loss.

How to Care for Permanent Teeth: The value of the permanent teeth depends largely upon healthfulness of the first or temporary set. The milk-teeth should be cared for and preserved till nature is ready to supply their places with the permanent organs, so that the arch of the mouth may be preserved, and that the roots may be absorbed and the material therein may not be lost to the system in the development of the new tooth. Irregularity of the second set would be almost unknown if by frequent visits to a competent dentist the first teeth were retained until nature should have no further use for them and then removed.

Care for Teeth Early: The child should be taught at 5 to dampen the brush in water every morning, rub it over a cake of castile soap, and then brush the teeth well, inside and out, front and rear, until with the aid only of the saliva the mouth is full of soap-suds; then rinse with tepid water, twirling the brush sideways over the back part of the tongue so as to cleanse it fully of the soap and leave a good taste; after each meal the mouth should be well rinsed with tepid water, as also the last thing on retiring. The mouth maintains a temperature of 98 degrees, hence if any food lodges about or between the teeth it begins to rot very soon, giving out an acid which immediately begins to eat into the tooth preparatory to an early decay; if solid particles are observed to lodge between the teeth the child should be taught to use a very thin quill to dislodge it, but not without, for the more a quill is used the greater space between the teeth, which is a misfortune, as it necessitates the use of a tooth-pick for all after life, consuming a great deal of valuable time.

How Often Should the Teeth Be Washed? Grown people should clean their teeth at least 5 times in the course of 24 hours—on rising in the morning and going to bed at night, and after each meal. A brush as hard as can be borne without pain should be used, and the best of all appliances is pure soap and water, always lukewarm.

Use of Aromatic Water: It is the custom in some parts of England and France to rinse the mouth with warm aromatic water after eating. It is well to remember that this precaution not only tends to keep the teeth clean, but to clear the voice of those about to sing or converse.

Cracking Nuts with the Teeth: No one, young or old, should turn their jaws into nut-crackers, and it is dangerous even for women to bite off, as they often do, the ends of thread in sewing.

Teething: Young children, while cutting their first set of teeth, often suffer constitutional disturbance. At first they are restless and peevish, but not unfrequently these symptoms are followed by convulsive fits, and sometimes under this condition the child is either cut off suddenly or the foundation of serious mischief to the brain is laid. The remedy, or rather safeguard, against these circumstances consists merely in lancing the gum covering the tooth which is making its way through.

Toothache Cures:

(1) Relief from toothache or neuralgic affections arising from teeth in any stage of decay may often be obtained by saturating a small bit of clean cotton or wool with a strong solution of ammonia, and applying it immediately to the affected tooth. The pleasant contrast instantaneously produced sometimes causes a fit of laughter, although a moment before extreme suffering and anguish prevailed.

(2) One dram of collodium flexile(1) added to 2 drams of carbolic acid is a most excellent application. A small portion should be inserted into the cavity of the tooth by means of a bit of lint.

(3) Powdered alum and salt mixed in equal quantities, and placed on a small piece of damp cotton, and put into the cavity, sometimes gives permanent relief.

Artificial Teeth: When teeth become so troublesome as to habitually disturb the nervous system they should be removed. Many diseases are caused, and most others greatly aggravated, by toothache. "Stop the ache, or remove the tooth," should be universally obeyed. Thousands of persons suffer for years in great discomfort to themselves and to all around them, until their constitutions are permanently impaired, when the removal of a single tooth would bring permanent relief.

TELESCOPIC GIANT, GAME OF:

A good way to make a giant is to fasten a hat to the top of a broom or a long stick, and then a little below the hat to fix a small hoop to form the shoulders. A very long mantle of some description must then be firmly fastened on as gracefully as possible, under which a gentleman, the taller the better, must take his post, holding in his hand the stick. As may be imagined, the result is exceedingly ridiculous, owing to the giant being able to make himself tall or short as may suit his inclination. At one moment he may shoot himself out to a great height, then become quite small, clattering and gesticulating all the time to make the affair more comical.

THISTLES, CANADA, TO KILL:

The best way is to let them grow until they blossom, then cut them off near the top of the ground; the stalk will then be hollow, and the water will get in the hollow and rot them, so they will never sprout again. If they are cut off with a hoe or plow, the ground will close over them and there will come two sprouts for one.

THROAT, SORE:

Sore-throat is one of the commonest affections, and is met with in every grade, from a simple dryness and slight heat, or sensation of rawness and hoarseness, to a total loss of voice from ulceration of the vocal cords and constant soreness, with expectoration of a puriform secretion, sometimes with difficulty got rid of. From the frequency of the affection among clergymen and public speakers it received the name of "clergyman's sore throat."

(1) A solution used to protect skin and other sensitive surfaces, made from gun-cotton dissolved in ether.

Treatment: Use gargles of alum and sage tea, flaxseed, and slippery-elm infusions, mild liquid diet, and a mild cathartic, as calomel, aloes, rhubarb, of each 5 grains; mix and take in syrup or capsule at bedtime; if it does not operate by morning, take $^1/_2$ ounce of Epsom salts or castor-oil. Pour a few drops of spirits of camphor on a lump of sugar, and allow it to dissolve in the mouth every hour.

Wet compresses to the throat are the best remedies known; double a towel 2 or 3 times, so as to make a pad that will fit snugly under the chin and over the throat, and let it extend around from ear to ear; bind a thickly folded towel over the wet pad, having the towel wide enough to overlap the edges of the pad; it may be put on cold or warm; when cold it soon becomes warm from the heat of the skin, and is really a warm vapor-bath; when the pad is taken off the throat should be washed in cold water to close the pores, and then well dried with a towel.

TIES, TO WASH:

To wash gentlemen's neckties let them soak a little; then wash with soap and hot water; rinse in cold water, slightly blued; dry; dip once more in cold water; starch and wring them thoroughly, then iron.

TIGHT LACING AND HEALTH:

Physical Effects of Tight-pressed Garments: The free and easy expansion of the chest is obviously indispensable to the full play and dilatation of the lungs; whatever impedes it, either in dress or in position, is prejudicial to health, and, on the other hand, whatever favors the free expansion of the chest equally promotes the healthy fulfillment of the respiratory functions. Stays, corsets, and tight waistbands operate most injuriously by compressing the thoracic cavity, and impeding the due dilation of the lungs, and in many instances they give rise to consumption.

Effect on Respiration: Referring to this subject, a writer states that men can exhale at one effort from 6 to 10 pints of air, whereas in women the average is only from 2 to 4 pints. In 10 females, free from disease, whom he examined, about the age of 18, the quantity of air thrown out averaged $3^1/_2$ pints, while in young men of the same age he found it to amount to 6 pints. Some allowance is to be made for natural difference in the two sexes, but enough remains to show a great diminution of capacity in the female, which can be ascribed to no other cause than the use of stays.

Absurdity of Tight Lacing: There would be no tight lacing if girls could be made to understand this simple fact—that men dread the thought of marrying a woman who is subject to fits of irritable temper, to bad headaches, and other ailments we need not mention, all of which every body knows are the direct and inevitable product of the compression of the waist. When a

Swiss once saw a fine-looking Englishman he exclaimed, "What a pity he has not the goiter." So, we are so accustomed to mutilated waists that when we see a naturally formed woman we are apt to say, "What a pity she has not a small waist."

If we look at the beautiful specimens of ancient statuary we find no small, contracted chests, no did Powers take for his model one of our fashion-plates. If they are correct he certainly showed a plentiful lack of taste. Furthermore, it destroys all gracefulness of carriage. When any muscles of the body are cramped the movements cannot be easy; there is a certain wiggle—a "divine wiggle." How is the human race to have health with this mode of dressing. Only fashion makes us think it is beautiful, or tolerate it for a moment. We would not otherwise endure the misery it imposes, but so accustomed are some to suffering that they are hardly conscious of it, they don't know when they are dressing tight, don't know when the breathing is oppressed.

TIMBER, TO CUT:

To clear land of a small growth of trees without the aid of a stump-puller, and at the same time have the land in immediate condition for tillage and cropping, the timber should be cut out by the roots; i.e., until the weight of the tree breaks what are left and causes it to fall. The tree can be left for a heavy wind to prostrate it. Just after the frost leaves the ground in the spring is a good time, as the soil is easily removed from about the roots, which should be cut off below the surface of the ground, so that they will not materially interfere with cultivation. Trees and brush may be cut at any time that they will not be liable to throw up a growth of shoots. When only the roots are left in the soil, but little trouble need be anticipated from this source. After 2 or 3 plowings they will decay.

TOBACCO, THE MISUSE OF:

For tobacco the broadest advice must be as in the case of alcohol—Don't. Still the man who smokes or chews must know whether it is hurting him or not, and how much. Those who find themselves exceedingly nervous after smoking, and who find their heart's action violently accelerated and rendered uneven by tobacco, do not need to be told that it is a habit they should stop or moderate. The old fellows whose lives have been spent for no better result than the publication of a death notice asserting that they lived a century and smoked to the day of their death were never seriously affected by tobacco, but their cases and that of the average man are widely different. Smoking is hurtful, and chewing is more so.

There are men who take a sentimental view of a cigar, and fancy themselves enjoying part of the poetry of life by smoking. Let such confine their rhapsodies to evening, and finish their dinner with a cigar. That will hurt them only a fourth as much as 4 cigars, and only a third as much as 3. As for chewing tobacco, the less said about it the better, beyond the fact that is the most harmful form of the tobacco habit as well as the nastiest vice man has ever popularized. Not even an insane man associates chewing with sentiment, no poet has sung the vice, no man has fallen so low as to boast of being its victim.

There are men who fancy that they are such adepts at chewing as to be able to do it without betraying the fact; some even fancy that they have talked to ladies but they are all twice wrong, first in chewing and second in thinking to hide it. Some doctors recommend substitutes for tobacco to aid chewers to break the habit. They prescribe slippery-elm, camomile flowers, and coca leaves, but the best and amplest substitute is a strong will and earnest inclination.

TOILET MATS:

Very pretty and useful toilet mats may be made of white enameled cloth, cut in sizes or shapes to suit the fancy. Punch small holes one-eighth in. from the edge and the same distance apart. Into these crochet a border of colored split zephyr, using white knitting cotton of suitable size for the outer scallop, which should be edged with worsted.

TOILET SOAP:

As eminent physician has declared that "if the skin be moderately active, 3 or 4 days suffice to form a layer which may be compared to a thin coating of varnish or sizing." As this accumulation increases and decomposition follows it is not necessary to describe the result. What agency but soap can remove it? Many good authorities declare that water alone is sufficient, except at rare intervals. There are oil glands as well as excretory ducts, and for no idle purpose has nature produced these tiny human oil-wells.

Inunction, or the external use of oil, has a recognized place among the prescriptions of some famous modern physicians, who in this way seek to restore that necessary property of which the body has been deprived by the excessive use of soap or by disease. They claim that it enables the patient to resist cold, that its nutritive qualities convey heat to those organs which require it, that it gives a sense of exhilarating freshness, and that it is not only soothing in cases of nervous depression, but it is capable of strengthening weak lungs. For this purpose almond-oil, cocoa-nut, olive-oil, or vaseline are daily applied by the aid of vigorous rubbing. To all such treatment, and in most cases where inunction is not required, the daily application of soaps is injurious. Plenty of soft water, a coarse wash-rag, hand friction and a Turkish towel, with soap applied at rare intervals, and the skin should retain the delicate smoothness of an infant.

Those milk-baths indulged in by the ancient Roman emperors and empresses owed their emollient properties to the oil contained in the milk. Every old nurse knows, too, that weakly children are sometimes injured by too frequent ablutions. Dry rubbing is often the safest opiate for a nervous little one, answering many of the purposes of soap.

TOMATOES, TO DRY:

To every gallon of peeled tomatoes put 1 tea-cupful of salt, and 1 table-spoonful of pounded black pepper. Boil all well until it becomes a marmalade. Then sift 1 pint of flour and let it cook a few moments longer, in order that the mixture be thickened. Now take off the tomatoes, and spread them over dishes slightly greased. Dry them in the sun 3 or 4 days, then roll them into balls; sprinkle with flour, and expose to the sun a week or two longer. Put away in paper bags. One ball the size of a small apple is enough for a tureen of soup in winter.

TOMATOES, TO KEEP:

Pick the green tomatoes before the vines freeze; place in a cool, dry place, where air can be admitted and the frost can be kept out.

TONGUE, THE:

The tongue, though not wont to make a frequent appearance before the public, demands no less care for the proper performance of the duties of its private station. Upon its surface there is apt to gather a fur which is not easily removed by the ordinary rinsing of the mouth. There is an instrument of silver, called a tongue-scraper, which was never absent from the toilet-cases of our grandmothers, but is now almost obsolete, that is well adapted to this purpose, and should be used every morning to remove the covering of thickened mucus which accumulates in the course of the night. This fur, if left, gives a sensation of pastiness and fullness to the mouth, and not only destroys the delicacy of the taste and the disposition for food, but thickens the voice.

TONIC, A SPRING:

It is quite the usual thing in springtime to have a "spring fever," to be "bilious," to "take something to cleanse the blood." The advertising columns of almost every journal advise what is best to be taken. Let us give a bit of advice "free gratis, for nothing."

Take a glass of water, pure as you can get it, and as you sew, or read, or write, or work sip a tea-spoonful at intervals, making a glass of water last half an hour. Do this before breakfast and also before going to bed, sipping thus in 24 hours 3 glasses of water.

This will be as good as a trip to Carlsbad. The waters of the springs, there, which taste so horrid that the only way to get them down is to sip them, are good for the patients only because they are sipped, and not because they are nauseous. Pure limpid waters, so the learned say, would answer the purpose exactly as well. The doctors at Carlsbad—and there is a great drove of them—insist particularly that the waters shall be sipped.

But they do not insist that the patients shall stay at home and sip water. Of course, the change of scene and air and mode of life has much to do with change in health, but leaving all that out of the question, one might as well sip pure water at home as the waters of Carlsbad, and with what a trip to Carlsbad would cost visit the Yellowstone wonders.

TOOTHACHE REMEDIES:

(1) As toothache is nowadays an inevitable accompaniment of teeth, it is well to know what to do for it. Oil of cloves on a bit of cotton wool is good to insert in the cavity, and after a little, when it seems to lose its virtue in that particular place, it is well to mix it with an equal quantity of oil of cinnamon, oil of peppermint, or creasote. It is best to swallow as little as possible of these fiery liquids; therefore the cotton should be pressed quite dry before applying to the aching nerve. It sometimes occurs that the pain in that special tooth will stop, but a sound one, or the ear or temple, will ache harder than the decayed tooth. This plainly shows neuralgia, and medicine is needed which will quiet the nerves before relief can be expected, although temporary ease may be obtained by applying to the face a mustard-plaster or a succession of cloths wrung from hot water, or, better still, a solution of hops and vinegar, or, as some people advise, a warm and moist buckwheat cake, well sprinkled with Cayenne pepper.

(2) The mother whose child suffers from toothache must find a corner in the medicine-chest for a vial of powdered alum saturated with sweet spirits of niter. This mixture put in the cavity, if there is one, or rubbed on the gum, if there is not, will give immediate ease.

(3) The worst toothache, or neuralgia coming from the teeth, may be speedily cured by application to the defective tooth of a bit of cotton saturated with ammonia.

(4) A little horse-radish scraped and laid on the *ærisi* of the side affected will in many cases give speedy relief. Another way is to place a little scraped horse-radish in the mouth or the tooth and just around the gum. It relieves rheumatic pains in the gum and face also. The mouth may afterward be rinsed with a little camphorated water, lukewarm.

(5) Six parts of sal volatile(1) and 3 of laudanum, mixed; apply to the tooth with lint.

(6) Powdered gum camphor, 1 ounce; chloral hydrate, 1 ounce. Rub them together in a wedgewood mortar until they liquefy. Apply to the cavity on a small piece of cotton.

(1) A mixture of ammonium carbonate and ammonium bicarbonate.

TOOTH-POWDERS:

(1) One dram of pulverized charcoal, 1 dram of pulverized orris root, 1 dram of pulverized castile soap, 6 grains of pulverized camphor, and a sufficient quantity of alcohol. Powder the soap, then mix in the camphor reduced to a stiff paste with alcohol, then add orris root and charcoal. If it is liked, bergamot or oil of sassafras can be added as a flavor.

(2) Take 1/2 ounce of powdered chalk, 1/2 ounce of cream of tartar, 1 dram of powdered myrrh, 1 dram of orris root, and 2 drams of powdered bark; mix well together to make it of a pale red color, add a little powder of myrrh, and put into bottles for use.

(3) Burn some rock alum, beat it in a mortar, and sift it fine; then take some rose-pink, mix well together to make it of a pale red color, add a little powder of myrrh, and put into bottles for use.

(4) Six ounces prepared chalk, 1/2 ounce cassia powder, 1 ounce orris; mix well; put in small pots and label.

TORPID LIVER MYTH, THE:

A notion that is widely prevalent is that relative to inaction of the liver. The term "torpid liver" is in every one's mouth, and is held to account for every bad lack of muscular exercise, excitement over bad ventures on the market, or other form of dissipation. The liver is quite an important organ, and has much to do with the secondary processes of digestion—those which go on after the stomach and pancreas have done their work—but it is innocent of most of the sins laid at its door. The bile is manufactured in large amounts daily, but we know positively of but few uses to which it is put in the body, and of still fewer drugs that could, at will, stimulate this huge gland to secrete more bile; it is very uncertain that any benefit would result from "arousing it from its torpor."

TRACING-PAPER:

Mix together by a gentle hand 1 ounce of Canada balsam and 1/4 pint of spirits of turpentine; with a soft brush spread it thinly over one side of good tissue-paper. It dries quickly, is very transparent, and is not greasy, therefore does not stain the object upon which it may be placed.

TREE OF LEAD:

Dissolve 1 ounce of sugar of lead(1) in a quart of clean water, and put it into a glass decanter or globe. Then suspend in the solution, near the top, a small piece of zinc of an irregular shape. Let it stand undisturbed for a day and it will begin to shoot out into leaves and apparently to vegetate. If left undisturbed for a few days it will become extremely beautiful, but it

(1) Neutral plumbic acetate.

must be moved with great caution. It may appear to those unacquainted with chemistry that the piece of zinc actually puts out leaves, but this is a mistake, for if the zinc be examined it will be found nearly unaltered. This phenomenon is owing to the zinc having a greater attraction for oxygen than the lead has; consequently, it takes it from the oxide of lead, which re-appears in its metallic state.

TRICHINA:

Trichina is the term applied to a minute, slender, and transparent worm, scarcely one twentieth of an inch in length, which has recently been discovered to exist naturally in the muscles of swine, and is frequently transferred to the human stomach when pork is used as food. Enough of these filthy parasites have been detected in 1/2 lb. of pork to engender 30,000,000 more, the females being very prolific, each giving birth to from 60 to 100 young, and dying soon after.

The young thread-like worm at first ranges freely through the stomach and intestines, remaining for a short time within the lining membrane of the intestines, causing irritation, diarrhea, and sometimes death, if present in sufficient numbers. As they become stronger they begin to penetrate the walls of the intestines in order to effect a lodgement in the voluntary muscles, causing intense muscular pain and severe enduring cramps, and sometimes tetanic symptoms. After 4 weeks' migration they encyst themselves permanently on the muscular fiber and begin to secrete a delicate sac, which gradually becomes calcareous. In this torpid state they remain during the person's life-time.

TRICKS OF MANNERS:

Avoid them by all means. Many good and kind people, with many excellences of character, render themselves disagreeable—nay, odious—to others, merely from lack of—shall it be said?—lack of delicacy, or want of observation. They pick their teeth, or, worse still, suck them, smack their lips at table, or make other disagreeable noises when drinking or taking soup. If they help themselves to any dish on the table they bring it up beside their own plate, edges touching, and perhaps plunge the spoon into the heterogeneous mass in the plate, or clean it off with their own knives, a proceeding most exasperating to persons of fastidious natures.

Others clean their ears, pare their nails, hawk and clear their throat, forgetting that in the privacy of their own rooms they should attend to all such matters of personal cleanliness. Still others, particularly young men, loll in their chairs, or beat a tattoo on window panes, table, or any thing convenient. Another disagreeable habit, uncommonly annoying to the sensitive nerves, is that of rocking backward and forward, crickety-creak, crickety-creak, and keeping time with the monotonous sound by regularly raising the palm of the hand on the chair arm. If all guilty of these tiresome peculiarities of manner were only to consider the effect which they have upon others, the avoidance, the dislike which they incur on account of them, they surely would make a sturdy effort to correct them.

TURNIPS, TO KEEP:

Of all the roots turnips are the most affected by heat. They will sometimes grow in a cellar of not over 40 degrees temperature. There is a natural heat about the roots, and when they are piled together this accumulates and the roots sprout. A little frost does not hurt turnips. Place them in small lots in stalls where the frost can get at them, and cover with straw to prevent thawing.

TWO HATS, GAME OF THE:

A similar game to this of the Two Hats is that known by the name of the Game of Contrary. One of the company comes forward holding in his hand two hats, one of which he places on his own head, the other he gives to one of his friends. The person to whom the hat is given must, from the moment he receives it, make every action of his to be exactly opposite to that of the owner of the other hat.

For instance, should the later sit down, his victim must immediately stand up; should he place the hat on his head, his friend must stand bareheaded; should he take it off, the other must put his hat on. This principle of contrary must be carried out to the very utmost, not only as far as the hats are concerned, but in every other way imaginable. When once the game is entered upon, opportunities will readily present themselves of carrying out the original idea, i.e., that dictated by the rule of contrary.

TYPHOID FEVER:

The symptoms are languor, alternate flushes of heat and chills, pain in the head, difficulty of breathing, frequent weak and sometimes intermitting pulse, the tongue dry and covered with brown fur, the forehead covered with sweat, while the hands are dry and glow with heat, the patient talking wildly. Consult a physician the instant such symptoms manifest themselves.

Typhoid Fever from Impure Water: M. Dujardin Beaumetz, in a recent communication to the Paris Academy, gives the case of a family who took a house for the season at a fashionable resort. They were warned not to drink the well-water, as it was supposed to be impure. They drank mineral-water until the last day, when, in the hurry of packing, they neglected to send for mineral-water and concluded to try the well-water. They drank of it, and 6 died; 4, who had previously had typhoid fever, were made sick, but recovered. A microscopic examination of the well-water revealed the presence of the bacillus supposed to be the cause of typhoid fever.

U-V

ULCERS, TO PREVENT AND CURE:

(1) Dried and pulverized clay applied to an ulcer will cure it in a short time, and leave no scar.

(2) Petroleum has been used with good results as an external application to ulcers and wounds. It may be used undiluted or diluted with equal parts of oil or glycerine.

(3) Ulcers caused by cyanide of potassium, so much used by photographers, may be guarded against by rubbing the hands, when soiled with it, with a mixture of photo-sulphate of iron reduced to a very fine powder, and linseed oil.

UNDERCLOTHING:

Woolen materials make the best underclothing. Silk is good, but not so good as wool, especially for sufferers from rheumatism. Silk is too close and hard a fabric, and doesn't hold as much air as wool. The secret of beneficial clothing to keep the person warm is that it must be something whose meshes will hood air, which is the best non-conductor of heat. The men of the last generation were very partial to red flannel, and this is still recommended by persons who have only a vague and mysterious idea of why they recommend and use it. The fact is that in our grandfathers' days red flannel was a little more harsh and rough than flannel of any other color, and it titillated and rubbed the skin in such a way as to keep it warm. But under the manufacturing processes of to-day all flannels are alike in that respect.

Any underclothing that is made with a goodly proportion of wool will do. Very thin wool keeps the body cooler in the summer, and, if there is much perspiration, prevents the taking of cold by graduating the evaporation. Silk does not absorb like wool, so that perspiration is liable to be condensed and make the undershirt positively wet, and hence before long, inevitably cold and chilling. We have known duck-hunters, clothed heavily in flannels, to fall overboard in the morning and shoot for the rest of the day without discomfort. They could not have done that in silk.

To some skins wool is positively irritating. If you turn a microscope on a woolen garment and a silk garment, the reason will be easily seen—one is so much rougher than the other. In order to enable yourself to wear it, if it is very desirable, wear first a light under-shirt of linen and a heavy woolen one over it. Then you will have warmth and comfort to the skin.

But it is important to have all underclothing loose. To be warm it should not be tight against the body. If it is so, the cold air strikes it and the body simultaneously, whereas, if the garment is loose, a cushion of air, an air space, offers an extra shield against sudden changes of temperature. Two undershirts of one thickness are warmer than one of double that weight.

Flannel should always play an important part in every adult man's clothing as a protection for the stomach. The eminent desirability of always having a thickness of flannel round the bowels should be impressed upon every man. A mere band will do; a cholera band it is often called. It is only necessary to tack a piece of flannel with safety-pins to one's undershirt, or the wearer may have the bands regularly made to button in place. Flannel worn in this way is a preventive of colds and of the possible chilling of the large blood-holding organs in that part of the body. If these are chilled the least that follows is arrested digestion, while much more serious consequences sometimes ensue.

VACATION, DANGERS OF THE SUMMER:

There is a need to be very careful about the use to which a summer vacation is put. The idea may never have been publicly advanced before, but it is none the less likely that as much harm as good is done to New Yorkers by the misuse of the summer trip to the country. Men who plan to go to bed in a sleeping-car as deskmen and wake up nimrods are far too plenty. So are clerks and salesmen, pent up in shops for 11 months, who expect to benefit themselves by becoming mountain-climbers on the spur of the opportunity.

The whole field of summer recreation which tempts dyed-in-the-wool city men to transform themselves at a day's notice to horsemen, fishermen, hunters, 20-mile pedestrians, oarsmen, and athletes is a field strewn with mistaken and hurtful intentions. There may be nothing of value to the young in this reflection; it is next to impossible to kill a boy, a drunkard, or a cat.

Young fellows under 25 have reservoirs of health and animal spirits, upon which they draw checks to meet even extraordinary taxes upon their system. They are buoyed up by the very novelty of life, the intoxication of first acquaintances with the beauties of nature, the strangeness of country customs, and the sense of sudden freedom. There are few young fellows to whom it would be worth while to give advice. It is a dispensation of untoward fate that they can only get wisdom with years.

But the man of 35 and upward, whose constitutional elasticity is lessening as his cares increase, is the one who needs to govern his summer recreation with judgement. He still retains youthful spirits and thinks himself a young buck. He is the one who may hurt himself very seriously by overdoing the summer's pleasure. No longer does a view of the country fill and sustain him as of old; no longer can he empty his mind of that business which has now grown important, or of those home responsibilities that now concern a family instead of himself and his landlady as before. If he tries to hunt and walk, or climb, or ride and row as he used to do, and persists in it, he may seriously injure himself, or he may only deprive himself of any real good of his vacation.

The change of climate alone—of which few man make much account—is often striking in itself, and the addition of any other strain will be too much. The thing for a bushy city man of sedentary habits to do on his vacation is to rest. Let him go to the most beautiful spot he knows of, and the purest air and within reach of wholesome, well-cooked food, and there sit him down and vegetate for a while. Let him exercise in moderation as he did in town, but no more. It has been well said that in mature age a man is fitted for contemplation and reflection. There comes a time "when the top of a mountain looks best as viewed from a valley."

VEGETABLES, TO CHOOSE:

In buying vegetables, particular attention must be given to their appearance; even this is often deceiving, as the dealer will brighten up the stale vegetables by the use of water; if the out end of asparagus is brown and dry and the heads bent on one side, the asparagus is stale; to be sure that the mushrooms are genuine, sprinkle a little salt on the spongy part or gills of the sample to be tried; if they turn yellow they are poisonous; if black there are wholesome; allow the salt to act before you decide on the question; false mushrooms have a warty cap, or else fragments of membrane adhering to the upper surface; they are also heavy, and emerge from a fulva or bag. They grow in tufts or clusters in woods, on the stumps of trees, etc., whereas the true mushrooms grow in pastures. False mushrooms have an astringent, styptic, and disagreeable taste; when cut they turn blue; they are moist on the surface, and generally rose or orange in color; the flesh is white, and the stem is white, solid, and cylindrical.

When peas are young the shells are green; when newly gathered they are crisp; when old they look yellow, and when plump the peas are fine and large.

To test a potato, take a sound one, paying no attention to its outward appearance, and divide it into two pieces; then examine the exposed surfaces; if there is much water it will be soggy when boiled; in regard to color, a yellowish white indicates a good potato; if it is a deep yellow it will not cook well. Rub the two pieces together and a white froth will appear around the edges and upon the two surfaces; this signifies the presence of starch, and the more starch the better the potato; test the strength of the starchy element by releasing the hold upon one piece after rubbing it against the other; if it clings to the other it is a good sign.

When watermelons are to be bought, look for small specks, scales, or blisters on the outer cuticle or rind; these are multiplied an enlarged as the fruit matures. A ripe melon will show them thick over the surface; a partial development only indicates half ripened fruit; a full crop of blisters reveals its perfect ripeness.

VENTILATION:

As houses are generally made it is better to draw down the upper sash of window, for the reason that the warmest air, particularly during the winter, collects near the ceiling, and injurious matters are carried up into it from the floor. Drawing down the sash will afford a double means of ventilation—permitting the warm and noxious air at the top to escape, and the outer air to enter at the bottom of the sash through the lower one. When the weather is cold it is not necessary that the upper sash be lowered much; an inch or two would be sufficient for a room of the average size; i.e., 14 or 15 ft. square. A room which is used for the general assembling of the family—what is called the living room—should not be less than that in dimension.

VERMIN, TO FREE THE HOUSE FROM:

We will begin with the most offensive, the bed-bug. Scores of methods have been tried to rid the house of these, and in some cases there would seem no remedy, when beds, bedding, walls, and even furniture are infested; yet patience and perseverance have effected what seemed an impossibility.

When closets and floors are the lurking-places, use strong sassafras tea, dashing it into every corner and crack, under the bare boards, into the floor seams, and every crevice. Let it lie in one place while doing another, and do not be too careful in wiping off the surface. After doing this fill up all the cracks or holes with soap or putty.

Should this not prove effectual, as it generally does, after one or two applications, try carbolic acid and water, 1 table-spoonful of acid to 4 quarts of water, or a little stronger if used only for holes and cracks. This was used in South America every 2 weeks to keep the very troublesome insects there.

For bedsteads do not rely on salt and water; coal-oil mixed with the oil used in lubricating machinery is also excellent, as it retains the offensive properties of the coal-oil, which evaporates too freely when used by itself. Still, though this mixture has proved effectual in one instance, carbolic acid and corrosive sublimate have stood the test of years.

Carbolic soap would be a good service in stopping up cracks and crevices. A good coat of varnish put over the bedstead, and into the seams and corners, is an excellent temporary remedy. Where the insects, through neglect, have accumulated in great numbers, coal-oil destroys them at once in their haunts, and prevents the danger of scattering them about as when the brush or cloth is used. The oil will prevent their returning for 2 or 3 weeks, if used freely.

Red precipitate and lard, if put into the holes made for screws or other fastenings, will keep out the insects for a year of two, but will not prevent their infesting other parts of the bed and bedding.

Corrosive sublimate and carbolic acid are best put on with a sharp-pointed feather, such as a goose-feather, so that all cracks can be reached by the liquid. Any good druggist can furnish the solution. When hair mattresses are thoroughly permeated by fumes of carbolic acid they will remain free from the inroads of bugs for years. This fumigation is frequently done by the manufacturers, and proves a great recommendation to their work.

Copperas mixed with whitewash upon the cellar walls will keep vermin away. Bugs are constantly brought into houses by travelers, in books from libraries, old papers, etc., not to mention other riders in street-cars, so that extreme vigilance is required to prevent their inroads. When railway cars are taken to pieces for repairs these insects are found by scores, secreted about the seats. Their increase is so rapid that if they did not destroy each other they would soon render a house uninhabitable, were no means taken to destroy them. In cities they have been seen forming a procession from one house to another. They will also precipitate themselves voluntarily from the ceiling to the bed. These insects, which by daylight seem sluggish and stupid, at night are as active as ants.

VINEGAR FOR THE SICK-ROOM:

There is a French legend that during the plague at Marseilles a band of robbers plundered the dying and the dead without injury to themselves. They were imprisoned, tried, and condemned to die, but were pardoned on the condition of disclosing the secret whereby they could ransack the houses infected with the terrible scourge. They gave the following recipe, which makes a delicious and refreshing wash for the sickroom:

Take of rosemary, wormwood, lavender, rue(1), sage and mint, a large handful of each; place in a stone jar and pour over the whole 1 gallon of strong cider vinegar; cover closely, and keep near the fire for 4 days; then strain and add 1 ounce of powdered camphor. Bottle and keep tightly corked. The vinegar is very aromatic, cooling, and refreshing in the sick-room, and is of great value to nurses.

VIOLET POWDER:

Wheat starch, 6 parts by weight; orris-root powder, 2. Having reduced the starch to an impalpable powder, mix thoroughly with the orris-root, and then perfume with attar of lemon, attar of bergamot, and attar of cloves, using twice as much of the lemon as either of the other attars.

(1) Rue-oil; from the rue plant, used as a stimulant, an antispasmodic and an emmenagogue.

U—474

VACATION, DANGERS OF THE SUMMER:

"The whole field of summer recreation which tempts dyed-in-the-wool city men to transform themselves at a day's notice to horsemen, fishermen, hunters, 20-mile pedestrians, oarsmen, and athletes is a field strewn with mistaken and hurtful intentions. There may be nothing of value to the young in this reflection; it is next to impossible to kill a boy, a drunkard, or a cat."

W-Z

WAISTCOATS:

It is hygienically absurd that man's dress should be so voluminous in front and so thin behind. The least protection is that which is given to the spine and the center of the back, underneath which lie the roots of the lungs. Every man who is interested in properly caring for himself should see to it that the backs of his waistcoats be made of cloth or flannel. A good thickness of either material will at least give the back as much covering as the front gets, though no harm would be done if it had more.

WALL-PAPER, HOW TO HANG:

There are many house-keepers who have one or more rooms they would like to re-paper, but are kept from doing as much of this kind of work as they would like to on account of the expense of getting a professional paper-hanger to put the paper on. Any one who takes the pains to notice can soon learn to put on paper as well as the best paper-hangers. In the first place, you can often find among the cheap papers one or more lots that look just as well and are as good quality as the more expensive ones. When you have got your paper home, trim off the edge on the right side, as it is better for an inexperienced hand to commence at the left side of the door or window, and go toward the left.

When you are ready to begin, make your paste with boiling water, and let it boil about as long as common starch, and it should be no thicker than starch after it is cold. Let it cool, and strain it through a common salt-sack to take out the lumps. Then take a piece of washing-soda large as a walnut with the hull off, dissolve it in water, and put it in the paste, and you need not use any glue or any thing else whatever.

Let an assistant hold the paper up the wall, so that it will match with the piece already on, and cut it off half an inch shorter than needed, as it will stretch that much. Lay the paper wrong side up on a large table, let your help hold one end while you put on the paste quickly and evenly with a whitewash brush. Be sure to get every part covered. Take hold of the upper end, while your assistant takes the lower end, fasten it at the top, then sweep it down with a soft broom or brush, prick all windy places with a pin, and pat gently with a soft cloth. If it should become fast at the bottom too soon for the rest, pull it out carefully from the wall and replace it again. Paper put on with washing-soda in the paste will not crack and come loose on greasy walls, as it often does without it. Try this plan, and your rooms will look nice and new with but little expense.

WALL-PAPER, METHOD OF CLEANING:

Cut into 8 half quarters a quartern loaf 2 days old; it must neither be newer nor staler. With one of these pieces, after having blown off all the dust from the paper to be cleaned, by the means of a good pair of bellows, begin at the top of the room, holding the crust in the hand and wiping lightly downward with the crumb, about half a yard at each stroke, till the upper part of the hangings is completely cleaned all round. Then go round again, with the like sweeping stroke downward, always commencing each successive course a little higher than the upper stroke had extended, till the bottom be finished. This operation, if carefully performed, will frequently make very old paper look almost equal to new. Great care must be taken not by any means to rub the paper hard, nor to attempt cleaning it the cross or horizontal way. The dirty part of the bread, too, must be each time cut away, and the pieces renewed as soon as it may become necessary.

WALLS, TO REPAIR CRACKS IN:

Equal parts of plaster of Paris and white sand, such as it used in most families for scouring purposes, mixed with water to a paste, applied immediately and smoothed with a knife or flat piece of wood, will make the broken place as good as new. The mixture hardens very quickly, so it is best to prepare but a small quantity at a time.

WARTS, TO REMOVE:

Warts are not only very troublesome, but disfigure the hands. They may be cured so as to leave no scar.

(1) Take a small piece of raw beef, steep it all night in vinegar, cut as much from it as will cover the wart, and tie it on; or if the excrescence is on the forehead, fasten it on with strips of plaster. It may be removed during the day and put on every night. In one fortnight the wart will die and peel off. The same prescription will cure corns.

(2) Apply the juice from the milk-weed *(Asclepias cornuti)* to the wart once and it will assume a chalky state, disappear, and not return.

(3) Pass a pin through the wart, apply one end of the pin to the flame of a lamp; hold it here until the wart fries under the action of the heat. A wart so treated will leave.

(4) If the wart is hard, a good method is to cut it off with a knife or scissors, and apply a little caustic(1) to the roots.

(1) Any substance which, on being applied to the flesh, destroys animal tissue.

(5) If the wart has a narrow neck, tie a silk thread or horse-hair around it, and it will soon drop off. A little caustic applied to the roots will prevent it from growing back.

(6) Dr. Lawrence says the easiest way to get rid of warts is to pare off the thickened skin which covers the prominent wart; cut it off by successive layers; shave it till you come to the surface of the skin, and till you draw blood in 2 or 3 places. When you have thus denuded the surface of the skin, rub the part thoroughly with lunar caustic. One effective operation of this kind will generally destroy the wart; if not successful, however, cut off the black spot which has been occasioned by the caustic, and apply it again; or you may apply acetic acid, and thus you will get rid of it.

THE WASH:

When the clothes come from the wash they should be sorted by some one who is sufficiently skilled and observant so that no defect escape her eye. Each garment should be opened and inspected, and then re-folded in the original creases. The firmness of the threads holding buttons should be tested with a little tug, button-holes scanned, bindings, seams, and trimmings scrutinized closely.

Each piece that needs even a stitch should be laid aside. The adage that a stitch in time saves nine verifies itself weekly in the experience of the housekeeper. A large basket may hold all the mending except the stockings. These should have their own bag. Being smaller than the other pieces, they are more apt to become mislaid. As they are examined they should be paired. Those that need mending may be drawn into one another and consigned to the darning bag, while such as are in good order may be turned, rolled tightly, and put away.

WASHING FLUIDS:

(1) Good hard soap, 1/2 bar; saltpeter, 1 ounce; borax, 1 ounce; soft water, 4 quarts; dissolve over a slow fire; when partly cool, add 5 ounces spirits of ammonia.

(2) Take 1 lb. of sal soda and 1/2 lb. of unslaked lime; put them into 1 gallon of water and boil 20 minutes; let it stand till cool, then drain off and put into a strong jar or jug; soak your dirty clothes over night, or until they are wet through; then wring them out and rub on plenty of soap, and in one boiler of clothes, well covered with water, add 1 tea-cupful of washing fluid; boil briskly for half an hour, and then wash them thoroughly through 1 suds; rinse, and your clothes will look better than with the old way of washing twice before boiling.

(3) *For Woolen Goods:* Ammonia, 4 ounces, white Castile soap, 4 ounces;

alcohol, 2 ounces; glycerine, 2 ounces; ether, 2 ounces; dissolve the soap in 1 quart soft water over the fire, and add 4 quarts water; when nearly cold add the other ingredients; bottle and keep well corked. Use a cupful of the fluid in each pail of warm water; put the clothes in and stir them around; then rinse in warm water and iron.

(4) Sal soda and borax, 1/4 lb. each; gum camphor, 1 ounce; alcohol, 1/2 pint; dissolve the soda and borax in 1 gallon of boiling rain-water; pour in 2 gallons of cold rain-water, add the camphor, first dissolved in the alcohol; stir well and bottle for use; 4 table-spoonfuls of the preparation are to be mixed with 1 pint of soft-soap, and the clothes soaked over night before putting them into the suds.

WASHING MADE EASY:

To save your linen and your labor pour on 1/2 lb. of soda 2 quarts of boiling water in an earthenware pan; take 1/2 lb. of soap, shred fine, put it into a saucepan with 2 quarts of cold water, stand it on a fire till it boils, and when perfectly dissolved and boiling add it to the former. Mix it well, and then let it stand till cold, when it has the appearance of a strong jelly. Let your linen be soaked in water, the seams and any other dirty part rubbed in the usual way, and remain till the following morning. Get your wash-boiler(1) ready and add to the water about a pint basin full. When lukewarm put in your linen and allow it to boil 20 minutes. Rinse it in the usual way, and that is all which is necessary to get it clean and keep it in good color. The above recipe is invaluable to housekeepers. Give it a trial.

WASTE-PAPER FOR HOUSEHOLD USES:

Few housekeepers have time to blacken their stoves every day or even every week. Many wash them in either clean water or dish-water. This keeps them clean, but they look very brown. After a stove has been blackened it can be kept looking very well for a long time by rubbing it with paper every morning. If I occasionally find a drop of gravy or fruit-juice that the paper will not take off, I rub with a wet cloth, but do not put on water enough to take off the blacking.

I find that rubbing with paper is a much nicer way of keeping the outside of my tea-kettle, coffee-pot, and tea-pot bright and clean than the old way of washing them in suds. The inside of coffee-pots and tea-pots should be rinsed in clear water, and never in dish-water. Rubbing with a dry paper is also the best way of polishing knives and tinware after scouring. This saves wetting the knife-handles. If a little flour be held on the paper in rubbing tinware and spoons, they shine like new silver. For polishing windows, mirrors, lamp-chimneys, etc., I always use paper in preference to any cry cloth.

(1) A large pot, heated by a fire for cleaning clothes.

Preserves and pickles keep much better if brown paper instead of cloth is tied over the jar. Canned fruit is not so apt to mold if a piece of writing-paper, cut to fit the can, is laid directly on the top of the fruit. Paper is much better to put under a carpet than straw. It is warmer, thinner, and makes less noise when one walks over it. A fair carpet can be made for a room not in constant use by pasting several thicknesses of newspapers on the floor, over them a coat of wall-paper, and give it a coat of varnish. In cold weather I have often placed paper between my bed-quilts, knowing that two thicknesses of paper are as warm as a quilt. If it is necessary to step on a chair always lay a paper on it; this saves rubbing the varnish. Children easily learn the habit of doing so.

WASTE-PIPES, HOW TO CLEANSE:

A simple, inexpensive method of cleaning the waste-pipe of washstands, bathtub, or kitchen, the stoppage of which often entails great expense, is said to be as follows: Just before retiring at night pour into the pipe enough liquid potash lye of 36 degrees strength to fill the "trap," as it is called, or bent portion of the pipe just below the outlet. About a pint will suffice for a washstand, or a quart for a bathtub or kitchen sink. Be sure that no water runs into it till next morning. During the night the lye will convert all the offal in the pipe into soft-soap, and the first current of water in the morning will remove it entirely, and leave the pipe as clean as new. The so-called potash lye is not recommended for this purpose. The lye should be kept in heavy glass bottles or demijohns(1) covered with wicker-work and plainly labeled, always under lock when not in actual use.

WATCH, CARE OF A:

A watch, even of very good quality, can only give satisfaction if it is treated according to its subtle construction. Its possessor must prevent it from falling or being knocked about. A jump from a street car has more than once caused a good timepiece in the jumper's pocket to change its rate. A watch must be kept clean and in a clean place. Dust and small particles of the pocket lining gather continuously in the pockets, and even the best-fitting case cannot prevent particles of dirt from finding their way to the wheels and pivots of the movement. Watch-pockets should be turned inside out and cleaned at regular intervals.

A watch ought to be wound regularly at about the same hour every day. The best time to do it is in the morning, for two reasons: First, because the hours of rising and dressing are more regular with most people than their hours of disrobing and retiring; secondly, because the full power of the main-spring is more likely to reduce to a minimum the irregularities caused by the movements of the owner during the day.

When not carried in the pocket a watch should always hang by its

(1) A large bottle of glass or earthenware.

ring in the same position that it is worn. As a rule watches will run with a different rate when laid down. Only high-grade watches are adjusted to positions, and will show only a few seconds difference in 24 hours, while common watches will be out of time several minutes in one night. Ladies often complain that their watches do not run regularly. This may be on account of smaller size and more difficult regulating, but the main reason for the faulty rate is to be found in the fact that ladies do not always carry their watches, and consequently often forget to wind them.

Never leave a hunting-case watch open during considerable length of time. A careful observer will find in the morning a layer of dust on the crystal of a watch that has been open during the night. That dust will find its way into the movement. The dust on the outside of the case will be unconsciously rubbed off by the wearer, and when the watch is closed the dust inside of the case must remain there. Main-springs cannot be prevented from breaking. Like china, they are made to go to pieces. But breakage will occur less frequently if the watch is wound carefully.

Do not take it from your warm pocket and hang it against the cold wall. Protect it from direct contact with the cold object by an ornamental piece of cloth, plush or velvet being preferred. The regular running or rate of a watch depends entirely upon its construction and lower or higher grade of perfection and finish. It is useless to worry one's self about the irregularities of a watch of ordinary quality. Watch movements of low or even middle prices cannot be expected to have a steady and regular rate. They may run fairly well for every-day use, but nobody should require them to be absolutely correct. No absolutely correct timepiece has yet been made.

The rate of a watch will change from the moment it is carried. Although it has been correct on the rack, the watch when delivered to its purchaser changes its rate. It will run fast or slow, the watchmaker being unable to foretell which. A watch ought to be cleaned every two, or at the utmost every three, years, if it is not to be spoiled. The oil will change. It will become thickened by the dust that cannot be kept out of the best-closing case. The dust will work like emery, and grind the surfaces of the pivots of the train. The best of movements will be spoiled if this requirement is neglected. Even after being cleaned and put in order they will not recover their former exactness.

Many times it has been observed that a watch ran well for years, and that it was unreliable after having been cleaned. The reason is to be found in the fact that the pivots and their thick oil fit the jewel holes, and the cleaned pivots and their clean oil do not fit the same jewels. Any body who has the misfortune to drop his watch in the water will find it to his advantage to put it immediately in pure alcohol, (not whisky or gin), and to leave it there until the watchmaker can take it apart and put it in order. Of course delay is not advisable in such cases.

WATER—ITS RELATION TO HEALTH:

How Water Becomes Polluted: The pure water, after falling from the clouds, filters through the soil and carries from the rocks and soil certain soluble parts, the nature and amount of which depend upon the nature of the rock and soil. It is always contaminated by passing through a drainage area of polluted ground. In this respect the increasing density of population and the encroachment of civilization upon the primeval state of the earth's surface have largely altered the conditions for a supply of pure water. Not only in crowded centers of population and industry, but also in some agricultural districts, the soil is more or less contaminated with sewage and all kinds of effete or decaying matters.

Well-water Often Dangerous: Few wells, as ordinarily constructed, are free from surface pollution. Their walls are open from bottom to top for the inflow of the water from the contaminated soil and surface-water around. A densely crowded population soon impregnates the surface soil with filth, which drains into the water-course below, especially if such water is near the surface; the walls of the wells are so constructed as not to prevent the inflow. "Artesian wells," and "deep-driven wells" from which the surface water is excluded furnish the best water (except pure rain-water) which can be obtained without the expense of lengthy and tightly closed conduits, in which the water is brought from a distance and from unpolluted reservoirs.

Caution in Locating Wells: Every well should be widely separated from barn-yards, cess-pools, pens, sinks, and similar places, and should not be simply stoned up with loose stones or bricks, so that any surface liquid that filters through the soil has free access; but its walls should be made water-tight with cement, so that nothing can reach it except that which has been filtered throughout dense beds of unpolluted ground below. If this precaution is neglected, the best and deepest well may be continually contaminated by infiltration from the surrounding surface. If at any time no good drinking-water can be had, or its purity appears doubtful, the only way to remove its dangerous qualities is to filter the water through thick layers of fine sand, or, better, through ground charcoal or animal charcoal.

Care in Constructing Cisterns: Cisterns should be constructed of suitable material, carefully built and covered, and so placed that no foul air can pass through or over the water they contain. The overflow-pipes from cisterns should be free from connection with any other pipes. Roofs and gutters supplying cisterns must be frequently inspected, and some simple contrivance should be adopted to insure their careful cleansing before the water is allowed to run into the cistern. Cistern water ought to be frequently examined, and be kept free from color, odor, or other indications of impurity.

How to Examine Suspected Water: A simple method of examination is by dissolving a lump of loaf-sugar in a quantity of the suspected water in a clean bottle, which should have a close-fitting glass stopper. Set the bottle in the window of a room where the sunlight will fall on it. If the water remains bright and limpid after a week's exposure, it may be pronounced fit for use; if it becomes turbid, it contains enough impurity to be unhealthy. Such water should not be used for drinking purposes until it has been boiled and filtered, after which it should be aerated by any simple process, such as pouring several times from one vessel into another in the open air.

WATER, TO CLARIFY:

The use of alum to purify water dates back a long time. It is difficult to give any general rule as to the amount of alum to be used, as amounts of impurity in water vary. The larger the amount of alum, added, the more quickly will the separation of the impurities take place. It will be better to err on the side of too large an amount, for even then the amount of alum added will be insufficient to impart any detrimental properties to the water. The average quantity required is 2 grains of alum to a gallon of water. The alum should be dissolved in a little hot water and thoroughly stirred into the water to be purified. Let it stand 48 hours and rack off.

WATER-PIPES, TO PREVENT FREEZING:

(1) The tying up of the ball-tap with straw or flannel during severe weather will in general prevent the freezing of water-pipes. The surest method is to have the main pipe higher than the cistern or other receptacle, and, being thus of a regular incline, the pipe will immediately be exhausted when the supply ceases. When water remains in the pipes, if each tap be left dripping, the circulation of the water will prevent it from freezing.

(2) When the frost begins to set in, cover the water-pipes with hay or straw bands, twisted tight round them.

(3) In pumping up the water, let all the water out of the pipe when done; but if this is forgotten, and it should be frozen, take a small gimlet and bore a hole in the pipe a little distance from the place where it is let off, which will prevent its bursting. Put a peg into the hole when the water is let off.

WAX FLOWERS:

There is no art more easily acquired nor more encouraging in its immediate results than that of modeling flowers and fruit in wax. We do not mean that it is easy to attain the highest perfection in this art, but that, compared with other pursuits of a similar nature, the difficulties to be surmounted are comparatively few, and the first rewards of perseverance come very speedily and are surprisingly agreeable. The art, however, is attended by this drawback, that the materials required are somewhat expensive. But then the flowers produced are of value, and this is a set-off against the cost. The materials required for commencing wax-flower making will cost from $5 to $10, and no progress can be made without this outlay at the start.

The materials may be obtained at most fancy repositories in large towns; and persons wishing to commence the art would do well to call at those places and inquire the particulars and see the specimens of materials; because in this, as in every other pursuit, there are novelties and improvements being introduced which no book can give an idea of. Those who reside in places where they cannot obtain the requisite materials may procure information by writing to any of the many dealers in those articles in New York.

There are some small works published which profess to teach the art, but they are, in fact, written by professors, and the chief aim of them is to sell the materials which they are written to advertise. Those who wish to pursue the subject further than our instructions will take them may be able to refer to either or all of the works mentioned. Printed instructions are, however, of comparatively little value, except at the starting to supply the simplest elements of the art.

The petals, leaves, etc., of flowers are made of sheets of colored wax, which may be purchased in packets of assorted colors. The stems are made of wire of suitable thicknesses, covered with silk, and overlaid with wax, and the leaves are frequently made by thin sheets of wax pressed upon leaves of embossed calico. Leaves of various descriptions are to be obtained of the persons who sell the materials for wax-flower making. Ladies will often find among their discarded artificial flowers leaves and buds that will serve as the base of their wax models.

The best guide to the construction of a flower—far better than printed diagrams or patterns—is to take a flower, a tulip, a rose, or a camellia. If possible, procure 2 flowers nearly alike, and, carefully picking one of them to pieces, lay the petals down in the order in which they are taken from the flower, and then cut paper patterns from them, and number them from the center of the flower, that you may know their relative positions.

The perfect flower will guide you in getting the wax petals together and will enable you to give not only to each petal, but to the contour of the flower, the characteristics which are natural to it. In most cases they are merely pressed together and held in their places by the adhesiveness of the wax. From the paper patterns the wax petals or other portions of the flowers may be cut. They should be cut singly by a scissors rather loose at the points, and the scissors should be frequently dipped into water to prevent the wax from adhering to the blades. The scraps of wax that fall from the cuttings will be found useful for making seed-vessels and other parts of the flowers.

Very few and very simple instruments are required, and these may be purchased at the place where the wax sheets, etc., are obtained. With regard to the leaves of flowers, where the manufactured foundations of them cannot be obtained, patterns of them should be cut in paper, and the veinous appearance may be imparted to the wax by pressing the leaf upon it. In the construction of sprigs it is most important to be guided by sprigs of the natural plant, as various kinds of plants have many different characteristics in the grouping of their flowers, leaves, and branches. It would be possible to extend these instructions to an indefinite length, but nothing would be gained thereby.

The best instruction of all is to take a flower and copy it, observing care in the selection of good sheets of wax, and seeing that their colors are precisely those of the flowers you desire to imitate. For the tints, stripes, and spots of variegated flowers you will be supplied with colors among the other materials, and the application of them is precisely upon the principle of water-color painting.

WEDDING ETIQUETTE:

The etiquette of weddings has changed very little in the last 20 yrs. The groom and the best man are shut up in the vestry until the bridal *cortége* reaches the door of the church; then they come out and stand looking for the bride down the aisle. The organ is playing aloft. Then the ushers, having seated the guests, form themselves into a procession, marching solemnly up the aisle, as they have done for the last 30 yrs. Then the brides-maids come two and two. Perhaps some child bridesmaid precedes the others.

As the *cortége* reaches the lowest altar-steps the ushers break ranks, going right and left; the bridesmaids part and also go to the right and left. The bride comes last, on the arm of her father or the gentleman who gives her away. As she reaches the lower step of the flight which reaches up to the altar the bridegroom advances, takes her by her right hand, and conducts her to the altar, where they both kneel. The clergyman, being in his place, signifies to them when to rise, and then proceeds to make the twain one. The first bridesmaid holds the glove and bouquet, and the best man has the ring; both await the moment when their services shall be required, which is all down in the prayer-book. Formerly brides removed the whole glove; now a finger of one glove is adroitly cut, so that the ring-finger can be exposed; thus the pain and penalty of removing and replacing a long glove may be obviated. Such is a church-wedding, performed a thousand times alike. At the wedding in the church the bridal pair, after receiving the blessing, walk down the aisle, the husband giving his wife his left arm.

In a marriage at home the best man and the bridesmaids can be dispensed with, but they are sometimes retained. The clergy-man enters the parlor and faces the company, the bridal pair follow and face him. A beautiful altar of flowers is generally arranged and a pretty form of flowers covers the group. The bridal pair has a pair of cushions on which to kneel. After the ceremony the clergyman retires and the bridal pair take his place.

If the size of the house will allow, the bridesmaids walk up a long alley through the rooms, which is defined with ribbons. They are followed by the bride, who meets the groom at the extemporized altar, as in a church. This is very pretty. Wedding presents are sent any time within 2 months before the wedding, the earlier the better, as many brides like to arrange their own tables artistically if the presents are shown. A bride writes a personal note thanking every one for his gift. At the proper time the bride retires to change her dress. She puts on her traveling-dress and is met at the foot of the stairs by the groom. The happy pair drives off under a shower of rice, old slippers, and congratulations. It is considered very good luck if the slipper alights on the top of the carriage.

Wedding-cake is no longer sent out. It is neatly packed in boxes, and each guest takes one as he leaves. The best man is the intimate friend, often the brother, of the groom. He accompanies him to the church, follows him to the altar, stands at his right hand, and holds his hat during the marriage ceremony. After this is ended he attends to the clergyman's fee; goes afterward to the reception, where he makes himself useful until the festivity is over.

Of course the bridegroom is allowed to make what presents he pleases to the bride. He is also expected to send something in the shape of a fan, a locket, a ring, or a bouquet to the bridesmaids. He buys the wedding-ring, but is not allowed to furnish cards or carriages. All this is done by the bride's family.

After the marriage invitations are issued the bride does not appear in public nor accept invitations. The bride in America often gives the bridesmaids their dresses, and the groom gives each usher a scarf, a pin, and a pair of gloves. When there are no bridesmaids or ushers, the members of the bride's family precede the bride and her father to the church. The groom takes the bride's mother to her pew in the front row, and then ascends the altar-steps to await his bride. After the father has given him his daughter the relatives ascend and stand about the young couple. When the circle of friends is very extensive, it is customary to send invitations to such as are not expected at the house, to attend the ceremony in the church. This is equivalent to an invitation to the house, and must be treated as such. After a small house-wedding, announcement cards are sent to show that although one's friends were not asked, the friendly feeling remains the same.

If the wedding occurs in the evening, the ushers and groom and best man must be in full evening toilet. If the newly wedded pair commences life in a home of their own, it is customary to issue "at home" cards for some day in the month. Card-leaving by all the guests upon the family of the bride or on the lady at whose house she is married is a rigorous formality, and should be done on the day of the wedding, or at least within 10 days after.

A widow in being married again must not wear veil or orange-blossoms, nor does she have bridesmaids. She is prettier in a bonnet and high dress; let these by as gay as she pleases. If she has a mother living the cards should be sent in her name, and that of her deceased husband, as Mrs. Eastlake becomes Gertrude Severn Eastlake on her cards for her second marriage.

Invitations to a wedding should be engraved in script on a piece of note paper. Cards should accompany them, indicating the invitation to the house.

The best form is the simplest:

Mr. and Mrs. Severn request the pleasure of your company at the marriage of their daughter Gertrude to

Mr. Edward Mortimer,

On Thursday, April 11, at 12 o'clock.

Grace Church

The order of the marriage service is fixed by the laws of the church where it takes place. The best man should go about an hour before to see if the sexton has had the awning, the carpets, etc., arranged properly. The white ribbons must carefully guard that part of the church which is reserved for invited guests. The ushers must also be early, to escort ladies to the proper seats reserved for them. If a lady is accompanied by a gentleman, he follows her to a seat. The ushers should know all the relationships, so that they can place the nearer and remoter kinsfolk of the bridal party in the proper places.

WEEDS, TO KILL:

If one will, when the dew is on, sprinkle a little fine salt on the leaves of any plant he wishes to kill, he will be both surprised and pleased at the result. Beginning some years ago with a few quarts annually, we now use some thousand pounds of salt each year in killing weeds, while no injury to the land or the crops is perceptible.

WELL-BRED GIRL, THE—WHAT SHE DOES NOT DO:

There are some things that a well-bred young lady never does.

- She never accepts a valuable present from a gentleman acquaintance unless engaged to him.
- She never turns around to look after any one unless engaged to him.
- She does not permit gentlemen to join her on the street unless they are very intimate acquaintances.

- She does not wear her monogram about her person or stick it over her letters and envelopes.
- She never snubs other young ladies, even if they happen to be less popular or well-favored than herself.
- She never laughs or talks loudly at public places.
- She never wears clothing so singular or striking as to attract particular attention in public.
- She never speaks slightingly of her mother, and says she "doesn't care whether her behavior meets with maternal approbation or not."

WELLS, TO REMOVE FOUL AIR FROM:

An authority gives an account of an extemporized apparatus for removing carbonic acid gas from wells. It is simply an opened-out umbrella let down and rapidly hauled up a number of times in succession. The effect was to remove the gas in a few minutes from a well so foul as to instantly extinguish a candle previous to the use of the umbrella. Whenever there is an escape of gas in an apartment the adoption of this plan will be found useful.

WELL-WATER, TO PURIFY:

Many people in the country who are compelled to drink well-water are boiling all that is used in the family. The question is frequently asked, how long should it be boiled. The best chemists say that half an hour's boiling is considered sufficient to destroy disease germs, if any exist in the water.

WEN(1), WAYS TO REMOVE:

(1) Wens have been removed by painting them with collodion(2). The pressure that this exerts on the tumor lessons its blood supply, and gradually diminution takes place.

(2) Take yelks of eggs, beat up and add as much fine salt as will dissolve, and apply a plaster to the wen every 10 hours. It cures without pain or any inconvenience.

(3) Dissolve copperas(3) in water to make it very strong; now take a pin, needle, or sharp knife, and prick or cut the wen in about a dozen places, just sufficient to cause it to bleed; then wet it well with the copperas water once daily.

WHITEWASHING AND PAINTING:

Cracks in Plastering: In some cases the plasterer has used too little real plaster

(1) A benign skin tumor or sebaceous cyst.
(2) Made by dissolving gun-cotton or pyroxylin in a mixture of ether and alcohol.
(3) Ferrous sulphate.

and too much lime. Pure plaster of Paris will never crack, but as it sets too quickly for the convenience of the operator a little lime is mixed with it. If you try to plaster with lime alone it will crack all over in drying, and come off in patches. Use as little lime as possible, either in the sand used for brick-laying or in the plaster used for coating the walls.

Brilliant Zinc Whitewash: The Manufacturer and Builder says: "Mix oxide of zinc with common sizing, and apply it with a whitewash brush to the ceiling. After this apply in the same manner a wash of the chloride of zinc, which will combine with the oxide to form a smooth cement with a shining face."

Making Paper Stick to Whitewashed Walls: Make a sizing of common glue and water of the consistency of linseed oil, and apply with whitewash or other brush to the wall, taking care to go over every part, and especially top and bottom. Apply the paper in the ordinary way.

Paint for Kitchen Walls: Paint on the walls of a kitchen is much better than kalsomine, whitewash, or paper, since it does not absorb odors or peel off, and can be quickly and perfectly cleaned. Any woman who can whitewash can paint her own kitchen. The wall needs first to be washed with soap-suds, then covered with a coat of dissolved glue, and then with paint. A broad, flat brush does the work quickly.

Whitewash: Slake the lime with hot water, and to 1/2 pail of whitewash sift through a cornmeal sieve a quart of wood ashes. The finished work will be whiter and better for this addition.

(1) To 5 gallons of whitewash made of well-burned white lime, add 1/4 lb. of whiting or burned alum pulverized, 1/2 lb. of loaf-sugar, 1 1/2 quarts of rice-flour made into a thin and well-cooked paste, and 1/2 lb. of glue dissolved in water. Scrape off old whitewash and apply warm. This is the nature of kalsomine, and gives brilliant and lasting effects.

(2) Slake 1/2 bushel of nice lime with boiling water, covering it to keep in the steam. Strain through a fine sieve, add a peck of salt dissolved in warm water, 3 lbs. of rice-flour made into a thin paste, 1/2 lb. of Spanish whiting, 1 lb. of clean glue dissolved in warm water. Add 5 gallons of warm water to the mixture, and after stirring well let it stand a few days, being covered to keep out dust. It should be put on hot, and for this a portable furnace may be used. A pint will cover a square yard. Any coloring substance may be used except green as the lime destroys the color and the green makes the wash peel off. This last recipe makes the White House whitewash, which is good for fences and out-buildings.

WHOOPING-COUGH, TWO VIEWS OF GIVING MEDICINE:

(1) Dr. Arnold, of Maryland, discussed recently at a meeting of the Medical Association the question of whooping-cough to the following strain: "I am more and more impressed with the little reliability of therapeutic remedies to this disease. We have so many medicines presented for our acceptance; some based upon certain pathological theories, some upon no theory at all, and others based on delusion. In my own family this disease prevailed; I did nothing for it, and it got well in 6 weeks. If I had used medicines I would have thought that I had cured it. We know nothing of its cause; there is great diversity in regard to its pathology, and no unanimity of treatment. Many popular remedies are in use, but in bad cases no remedy seems to be of any great benefit."

(2) Dissolve a scruple of salt of tartar in 1/4 pint of water; add to it 10 grains of cochineal(1); sweeten it with sugar. Give to an infant a fourth part of a table-spoonful 4 times a day; 2 yrs. old, 1/2 spoonful; from 4 yrs., a table-spoonful. Great care is required in the administration of medicines to infants. We can assure paternal inquirers that the foregoing may be depended upon.

WINDOW GARDENING:

A very common error in window gardening is that of attempting too much. Too many plants are crowded into the little space at command, so that it is impossible to give each the air and light it should have. Again, plants of too diverse characters are brought together. It is no uncommon thing to see tropical plants and plants from the temperate zone, if not even Alpine plants, all crowded into the same window and subject to the same temperature and treatment. Better far to have one healthy, well-grown plant, that will yield its flower in perfection, than a dozen sickly, feeble, wretched plants that have no beauty either of leaf or blossom.

Economical devices in the way of window gardening are often very effective. I once saw a window arranged very prettily with a common soap-box and a few plants. The box was fastened by two sticks, reaching from the floor to the box. In the box, which was about two thirds full of earth, were planted geraniums, heliotrope, and the white begonia, sometimes called wax plant. The geraniums, which were of the scarlet variety, were placed in the center of the box, with the begonias round them, then came the heliotrope, in full bloom, and sending the fragrance of its flower all over the room. Around the front of the box moneywort and variegated air-plants were growing almost to the floor, and completely hiding the box.

A bay-window may be decorated in a cheap manner by standing 2 terra-cotta drain pipes on opposite sides of the window, and against the

(1) A red dye made from the female bodies of the cochineal insect.

wall. A small square of oil-cloth will prevent their soiling the carpet. Now, in the one on the sunniest side put a pot containing a barclyana and a scarlet geranium; on the other side put a pot of German ivy with a plant of lantana. Over the top of your pots plant a Kenilworth ivy seed.

Train your vines on wires or strings so as to form an arch, and you will soon have as pretty an ornament to your room as you would wish for. If you have a flat window, where there is very little sun, you may make it beautiful by arranging a box in the manner above described, and filling it with fuchsias. They should be kept warm and moist. Ferns make a beautiful ornament to a room, and can be kept in the shade. A fern basket must always be moist.

Cultivation of Window-Plants: Those who keep plants during the winter will find their success to depend upon supplying them with the needed water, heat, and air, and in preserving them from insects and dusts; matters easily regulated in a greenhouse, but more difficult with plants in window culture. Watering requires judgement. To saturate the earth in a pot by daily soaking is a slow but sure way of killing a plant. The roots need air, which they cannot get if they are surrounded by mud. It is better to allow the plant to flag a little than to over-water it. Carefully watch the plants, and only give water when they show that they need it. Hanging-baskets are best watered by plunging them in a pail or tub of water until the ball of earth is well soaked. Allow the excess to drip, and when this ceases return the basket to its place.

Heat for House-plants: Living-rooms are often kept too hot for plants, as well as for the inmates. The nearer the temperature can be kept at 70 degrees, with a fall of 10 or 15 degrees during the night, the better for both. Cold nights in some localities may injure plants at the windows. Remove them, when severe cold is expected, to the middle of the room, and if necessary cover them with a sheet or with newspapers.

Give fresh air whenever the outside temperature will allow, if for only a few minutes at a time, avoiding a cold draft directly upon the plants. Dust is a great obstacle to successful window gardening. Ivies and all other smooth-leaved plants may be kept clean by washing the leaves with a sponge or soft cloth. Plants with downy leaves should be set in a bathtub or sink, and freely showered by water from a pot with a fine hose, held high above them. When the room is swept the plants should be covered with a thin cloth, or with newspapers, kept from resting on them; these are to remain over them until the dust settles.

Insects: Those who carefully watch their plants can observe the first appearance of insects, and will rarely need any thing more than the thumb and finger, or a brush, to remove them. Where plant lice are numerous, showering with tobacco-water and afterward with clear water will kill them. Scale insects and mealy bugs are easily removed by hand, using a small pointed stick. Chrysanthemums that have bloomed in pots should have the stems cut off as soon as they are out of the flower, and the pots containing the roots removed to the cellar, where they should be looked to and not ever allowed to get so dry as to kill the roots.

WINDOWS, CLEANING:

In cleaning windows the first step is to give them a thorough brushing that will dislodge the dust from sashes, ledges, and chinks. A small whisk-broom is the best for this office, and it should also be used on the outside and inside blinds. Whatever is left on the former will be beaten off on the panes by the next rain, spotting and streaking them, while the dust from the inner shutters can hardly fail to settle on the glass. The brushing having been vigorously done, wipe off the windows with a dry cloth, rubbing them well. Wash the sills and wood-work with a cloth dipped in warm water, and bring a fresh supply before beginning to wash the glass.

Never use soap on windows under penalty of making them cloudy. A little borax, pearline, or household ammonia may be added to the warm water. An excellent substitute for cloths in window-washing is chamois-skin. The glass should be first wiped clean with a dry cloth. The chamois-skin must then be dipped in water, wrung out, and passed rapidly over the glass. A second wetting of the chamois follows; it is squeezed very dry, and again rubbed over the pane. This will dry almost immediately. Both water and chamois-skin must be clean, and the former should be renewed as it becomes clouded. A soft cloth moistened in alcohol and rubbed on the glass adds luster to it. Rubbing with plate powder may perhaps produce a brilliant effect, but it entails extra work in the wiping off of the white dust that will fall from the cloth on the wood-work and carpet.

WOOD-WORK, TO CLEANSE:

Save the tea-leaves for a few days, then steep in a tin pail or pan for half an hour, strain through a sieve, and use the tea to wash all varnished paint. It requires very little "elbow polish," as the tea acts as a strong detergent, cleansing the paint from all impurities and making the varnish equal to new. It cleans window-sashes and oil-cloths; indeed, any varnished surface is improved by its application. It washes window-panes and mirrors much better than water, and is excellent for cleaning black walnut picture and looking-glass frames. It will not do to wash unvarnished paint with it. Whiting is unequaled for cleaning white paint. Take a small quantity on a damp flannel, rub lightly over the surface, and you will be surprised at its effects.

WRINKLES:

The skin has a natural tendency to form wrinkles, even in youth, this tendency naturally increasing with age. Every influence which distends the skin for any time must lead to wrinkles and as a weak or imperfect circulation of the blood will make certain parts of the body swell, it is of the greatest importance to keep the blood pure, and thus prevent bloating, which is sure to be followed by wrinkles. Ladies should take regular exercise in the open air, and keep early hours, deliberately setting their face against excesses in diet, if they wish to keep them free from wrinkles, for when they once come they are most difficult to rid one's self of.

WRITING, FADED, TO RESTORE:

Sometimes a physician's prescription may become faded by water and other fluids, and it may be a matter of life and death to have it renewed or made legible. You can restore faded writing by damping a piece of soft white paper; lay it on the faded writing, press it down closely; put a tablespoonful of spirits of hartshorn in a tin vessel with a candle or lamp under it; hold the soft damp paper over it, so as to receive the fumes of the hartshorn; if the writing is not exhibited on the soft paper plain enough, dampen it again and repeat the whole process until its is plain enough.

WRITING FOR THE PRESS:

It would be a great favor to editors and printers should those who write for the press observe the following rules:

(1) Write with black ink, on white paper, wide ruled.

(2) Make the page small, one fourth that of a foolscap(1) sheet.

(3) Leave the second page of each leaf blank.

(4) Give to the written page an ample margin all round.

(5) Number the pages in the order of their succession.

(6) Write in a plain, bold hand, with less respect to beauty.

(7) Use no abbreviations which are not to appear in print.

(8) Punctuate the manuscript as it should be printed.

(9) For italics underscore 1 line; for small capitals, 2; capitals, 3.

(10) Never interline without the caret to show its place.

(11) Take special pains with every letter in proper names.

(12) Review every work, to be sure that none is illegible.

(13) Put directions to the printer at the head of the first page.

(14) Never write a private letter to the editors on the printer's copy, but always on a separate sheet.

(1) A size of folded writing paper.

YEAST:

(1) Pare and boil 1 dozen mealy potatoes; boil 30 minutes; when boiling put in another kettle 1 handful of loose hops or 2 table-spoonfuls of pressed hops, and 3 quarts of cold water; cover and let boil; when the potatoes are cooked drain off all the water and mash very fine; strain the boiling hop-water into the mashed potatoes; stir well and add 1/2 cup of sugar, 1/4 cup of salt, and 1 pint of flour; when the salt, sugar, and flour are mixed, stir well and strain through a colander; let it stand until blood-warm; stir in 1 cup or cake of yeast; set to rise in a temperature of 75 degrees; keep in a stone jar or pot with tight cover, which should be firmly fastened.

(2) Take 12 common sized potatoes, boil soft and mash hot; pour over 1 pint boiling water; add 1 pint cold water; strain through a colander; add 1 tea-cup sugar, 1 table-spoonful salt; when cold add 1 tea-cup baker's yeast; set in a warm place; allow it to rise light several times and beat down; place in a glass jar, cover tightly and set in a cool place. Half a tea-cupful of this is sufficient for 2 ordinary-sized loaves of bread.

SWELLED BREAST:

"When the breasts are found to be hard and swollen they should be gently bathed with warm hog's lard, and a piece of folded linen saturated with it laid over them."

INDEX

B

C

F

G

H

N

O

S

T

V

W